Vaccines, Vaccination and the Immune Response

Vaccines, Vaccination and the Immune Response

Gordon Ada, D.Sc.
Alistair Ramsay, Ph.D.

Division of Immunology and Cell Biology
John Curtin School of Medical Research
Australian National University
Canberra City
AUSTRALIA

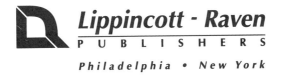

Lippincott - Raven
P U B L I S H E R S
Philadelphia • New York

Acquisitions Editor: Ruth W. Weinberg
Developmental Editor: Renee A. Gagliardi
Senior Production Editor: Molly E. Dickmeyer

Library of Congress Cataloging-in-Publication Data

Ada, G. L., 1922–
    Vaccines, vaccination and the immune response / Gordon L. Ada,
Alistair J. Ramsay.
        p.   cm.
    Includes bibliographical references and index.
    ISBN 0-397-58761-9
    1. Vaccines. 2. Vaccination. 3. Immune response—Regulation.
I. Ramsay, Alistair J. II. Title.
    [DNLM: 1. Vaccines. 2. Immune System—immunology.
3. Communicable Diseases—immunology. 4. Immunization—methods.
QW 805 A191v 1996]
QR189.A33   1996
615′.372—dc20
DNLM/DLC
for Library of Congress   96-31613
                                                                    CIP

Care has been taken to confirm the accuracy of the information presented and to describe generally accepted practices. However, the authors, editors, and publisher are not responsible for errors or omissions or for any consequences from application of the information in this book and make no warranty, express or implied, with respect to the contents of the publication.

The authors, editors, and publisher have exerted every effort to ensure that drug selection and dosage set forth in this text are in accordance with current recommendations and practice at the time of publication. However, in view of ongoing research, changes in government regulations, and the constant flow of information relating to drug therapy and drug reactions, the reader is urged to check the package insert for each drug for any change in indications and dosage and for added warnings and precautions. This is particularly important when the recommended agent is a new or infrequently employed drug.

Some drugs and medical devices presented in this publication have Food and Drug Administration (FDA) clearance for limited use in restricted research settings. It is the responsibility of the health care provider to ascertain the FDA status of each drug or device planned for use in their clinical practice.

9   8   7   6   5   4   3   2   1

The Task Force for Child Survival and Development has nominated 1996 "The Year of the Vaccine." It has been 200 years since Edward Jenner inoculated James Phipps with cowpox and showed that he could then resist a challenge with the smallpox virus. Louis Pasteur died in 1895, and there were many celebrations in 1995 to honor his great contributions to vaccinology and to immunology.

We would like this book to indicate our appreciation of the contributions of these two great scientists. Their pioneering work set the stage for the subsequent research and development efforts that led to the eradication of smallpox (declared in 1980), the elimination of wild poliovirus from the Americas by 1991, and more recently, the elimination of indigenous measles from Finland and the Caribbean Islands.

Preface

About 15 years ago, there was concern that little progress was being made in the development and production of new vaccines. The number of large pharmaceutical firms in the United States producing vaccines was decreasing. The higher safety standards required by the regulatory authorities, the risks of litigation if a new product caused significant side effects, the costs and time involved in bringing a product to market, and the rather poor prospects of a substantial financial return reduced the attractiveness of this area. For example, the opportunity to produce a live attenuated, cold-adapted influenza virus vaccine arose in the late 1960s, but despite all the clinical trials held, it is not yet licensed in the United States, although a similar product has been available in the former Soviet Union for some years. The blood-derived hepatitis B virus vaccine took about 15 years to bring to market.

It therefore comes as something of a surprise to read an article (H. Wigzell, 1995, *The Immunologist*, 3:234) reporting that, according to a survey carried out by the World Health Organization (WHO), about 300 candidate vaccines, mainly against infectious diseases, are at relatively advanced stages of development. Although most of the current vaccines were developed to protect against acute infections, many of the diseases for which vaccines are urgently needed are chronic, persisting infections, caused by agents such as the human immunodeficiency virus (HIV) and plasmodia. What could be the reasons for such a resurgence of interest and activity?

Although many of the new viral candidate vaccines in late-stage clinical trials are still live attenuated preparations, the success of the transfected yeast-derived hepatitis B viral vaccine has provided a great stimulus. Theoretically, the new technologies—peptide synthesis, recombinant DNA technology, and genetic (DNA) preparations—make it possible to develop a vaccine to control almost any infectious disease, and they offer bright prospects for immunotherapy for some noncommunicable diseases such as cancer. However, the experiences with HIV and malaria over the past 10 to 15 years show that advances in knowledge in some other areas are also important. We believe that one of these areas is the recent expansion in our understanding of the immune responses to infections and ways to manipulate those responses.

It is a curious fact that, although the efficacy of a vaccine depends to a large extent on the nature and size of the immune response that it induces, immunologists have not been involved in vaccine design or development until quite recently. Louis Pasteur is rightly described as the "Father of Immunology," and much of his work was directed to the development of a number of vaccines. He coined the terms *vaccine* and *vaccination* in honor of Edward Jenner. In the following one and a half centuries, many of those who made important advances in vaccine development could also be called immunologists because of their contributions. But when the "Second Golden Age of Immunology" began in the middle of the 20th century with the enunciation of the clonal selection theory and the elucidation of the role of T cells, most of the new disciples were much more interested in the study of fundamental aspects of the science. To work directly with viruses or bacteria, instead of dinitrophenyl and keyhole limpet hemocyanin, was sometimes regarded as an unnecessary complication. When Gordon Ada transferred to the John Curtin School in Canberra from the Walter and Eliza Hall Institute in Melbourne in the late 1960s, there was the opportunity to bring virologic and immunologic expertise into a single department. Fortunately, this led to the discovery of major histocompatibility complex restriction in the department a few years later, which went some way to justifying what appeared to be an unusual move at that time. A long association with the WHO began at about the same time, first with the International Agency for Research on Cancer in Lyon, then in Geneva with the Tropical Diseases Programme, the Programme for Vaccine Development, the Vaccine Section of the Human Reproduction Programme, and finally the Global Programme on Acquired Immunodeficiency Syndrome (AIDS). Work then progressed through the Center for AIDS Research at Johns Hopkins in Baltimore and an association with the National Institute of Allergy and Infectious Diseases Division of AIDS.

During the early part of this 20-year voyage, it became clear that virologists, microbiologists, and molecular biologists frequently could be closely involved with vaccinology (a term coined by the late Jonas Salk), but immunologists were involved less frequently. However, with this experience and after writing a number of articles on vaccines, it became increasingly obvious that the development of effective vaccines to control infections by agents such as plasmodia and HIV would be hampered unless the roles of different immune responses to combat infections were better understood and ways to manipulate responses in a desired direction became available. A treatise longer than the average article would provide the opportunity to bring together information about vaccines with a description of the relevant immunologic knowledge about how infectious agents could evade or outwit immune responses and how the immune system might be manipulated to counteract these tricks. It seemed an appropriate time to write this book because the great increase in knowledge in the latter area seems also to offer the prospect of prophylaxis or therapy for tumors, autoimmune disease, and the control of fertility.

We now know that there is a much closer association between components of the innate and adaptive immune responses than was originally realized, and recent advances are making use of this better understanding. Although we have a good appreciation of systemic immunity, most infections occur by other routes, and a better understanding of regional and especially mucosal immunity is needed.

Alistair Ramsay came from Otago University to the John Curtin School in 1988 to develop longstanding interests in viral immunology and in the regulation of mucosal immunity. Vaccine-induced responses in mucosae are notoriously short-lived, but current approaches, including the use of a wide range of antigen delivery systems and adjuvants, particularly cytokines, have been directed toward increasing their longevity. Practical applications of this technology are being explored through membership of the Australian National Centre for HIV Virology and of the Vertebrate Control Centre, which aims to control feral pests through immunocontraception.

This book is organized in six sections. The first gives a brief historical introduction followed by a presentation of current vaccines, vaccines in late-stage clinical trials, future needs, and national and international programs concerned with vaccine development. Section 2 describes features of innate and adaptive immune systems that we consider especially relevant to combating infections. Inevitably, this is a rather short account of a field that is expanding rapidly, with new journals appearing at frequent intervals. Section 3 reports on the way the study of infectious diseases has led to an increased understanding of the immunologic battle between the body and the invader, illustrated to a remarkable extent by findings from the study of HIV, one of the few positive aspects of the HIV pandemic. With the strong move in many situations to reduce vaccine preparations to their simplest components, the ability to selectively enhance immune responses becomes critically important. Section 4 deals with immunopotentiation and methods for the selective induction of different immune responses, such as type 1 or type 2 T-cell responses. Section 5 describes the many new approaches to vaccine development, from oligopeptide preparations to chimeric live vectors, naked DNA, and the possibility of producing some preparations in plants. The final section deals with three situations—tumors, autoimmune diseases, and fertility control—for which new approaches to immunization against self or self-like antigens have gained a new lease on life. Because there is often considerable overlap among sections, the information is presented in a way that we hope facilitates cross-referencing by the reader.

We express our appreciation to colleagues who reviewed various parts of the manuscript: Anand Gautam, Phil Hodgkin, Ian McKenzie, Arno Mullbacher, Bob Seamark, and Dave Willenborg. We would like to express appreciation to Ruth Weinberg for her patience when we fell behind schedule and her help during the production phase. We would also like to thank Renee Gagliardi, Ann Morris and Donna King for their help during production.

Gordon Ada, D.Sc.
Alistair Ramsay, Ph.D.

Contents

Vaccines, Vaccination and the Immune Response

SECTION 1

Past Achievements and Future Needs

CHAPTER 1.1. HISTORICAL BACKGROUND

The discipline of immunology grew out of the observation in ancient times that those who survived a disease seldom suffered a second, similar sickness. Repeated exposure to a disease such as smallpox, which leaves characteristic pocks after the first attack, strengthened this belief. It must have been observed that some persons suffered milder infections than others and that this difference appeared to be related to the site of the disease symptoms, such as early pustules on the arm arising from a skin scratch. This idea led to the practice of deliberate induction of disease by transmission of material from smallpox pus or scabs—the procedure of variolation as it came to be called. The history of smallpox and the final eradication of the causative agent by vaccination illustrates many of the important aspects of vaccine development.

1.1.1. The Story of Smallpox and Its Eradication

The procedure of variolation originated in India and China, probably independently because different routes of administration were used (ie, cutaneous and nasal, respectively).[1] The practice spread westward and not only saved lives but was "commercially important," as Voltaire recorded in 1733. To avoid disruption in the trade of young, beautiful maidens from Circasia to the seraglios of the Turkish Sultan and the Persian Sophy when epidemics of smallpox erupted, the Circassians inoculated their female children with "a pustule taken from the most regular and at the same time, the most favorable sort of smallpox that could be procured." The practice was adopted in the 18th century in many countries, including America.

By modern standards, variolation was a desperate undertaking, because the case fatality rate was 0.5% to 2%, but this compared with 20% to 30% after natural smallpox infection. During the 17th and 18th centuries, 10% of all deaths in London were caused by smallpox, called "the most terrible of ministers of death." The benefit to risk ratio for inoculation was substantial. Benjamin Franklin[1] stated in his autobiography, "In 1736, I lost one of my sons (Francis Folger), a fine boy of four years old by the smallpox. I long regretted bitterly and still regret that I had not given it to him by inoculation. This I mention for the sake of parents, who omit the operation on the supposition that they should never forgive themselves if a child died under it: my example shows the regret may be the same either way, and that therefore the safer should be chosen."

It was observed during the second half of the 18th century in several European countries that milkmaids were rarely pockmarked, and it was believed by many country people that they were protected from smallpox because of an infection acquired from cows. As early as 1774, a farmer called Benjamin Betsy, who considered himself immune to smallpox for this reason, inoculated his wife and children with material from pocks on cows. The family remained free from smallpox infection for about 15 years. However, Jenner is given the major credit, because he performed the critical experiment showing that young James Phipps, whom he had earlier inoculated with cowpox, remained free from disease after deliberate inoculation with smallpox. There was no doubt that infection with cowpox produced a much less severe disease than variolation, and "vaccination" with cowpox rapidly replaced the former practice and hastened the time when many countries would ban variolation.

Vaccination had its critics and opponents, and important changes in the methods of preparation, storage, transport, and administration of the product (finally made routinely in calves) were necessary before it showed its full potential. A major advance was made in the mid-19th century with the introduction of glycerin to preserve the calf lymph and to kill contaminating bacteria. During this half century, the concepts of passaging material to make it less harmful (virulent) and the avoidance of person-to-person vaccination became widely appreciated by interested scientists.

Jenner himself predicted the elimination of smallpox by vaccination. The protection afforded by vaccination, even more so when repeated vaccination was introduced, was so dramatic that it was made legally compulsory in Bavaria as early as 1807, and other countries followed suit. Endemic smallpox was progressively eliminated in industrialized countries.

In 1958, the Soviet Union (USSR) proposed to the 11th World Health Assembly that smallpox should be eradicated globally, and this proposal was approved the following year. Steady progress in eliminating endemic disease by vaccination resulted in increasing numbers of countries becoming free of the disease, but the voluntary nature of this approach had little impact in many developing countries, where the disease remained unchecked. This in part resulted from the less than enthusiastic support of many senior persons, within and outside of the World Health Organization (WHO), together with the burgeoning evidence that a malaria eradication program, begun some years earlier, had run into severe difficulties. In 1966, there were 10 to 15 million cases of smallpox and 2 million deaths from the disease in 31 endemic countries. That year, the 19th World Health Assembly, notwithstanding many private doubts, allocated special funds for the mounting of an intensified campaign to eradicate smallpox. A special program was established in 1967, and a period of 10 years was allocated to achieve a task that had never been set or achieved previously in the history of mankind. The goal was achieved in just over 10 years when the last case of endemic smallpox was located and treated. Three years later, after an intensive, worldwide surveillance scheme had been mounted, the eradication of smallpox was formally announced. The campaign was estimated to have cost $300 million; no figure can accurately portray the savings in human pain and misery. By contrast, the cost of putting a man on the moon was estimated as $24,000 million. Both were fantastic human achievements.

The success of the eradication campaign had a remarkable impact on international and national health programs, because it greatly strengthened the perception of vaccination as potentially a highly effective public health measure. It led to two important later decisions by World Health Assemblies based on the use of two existing successful vaccines, tetanus toxoid and live, attenuated polio virus (see Chapter 1.4). Its impact on national programs was equally great (see Chapter 1.3).

1.1.2. The Pasteurian Era

The second great thrust toward developing immunization as a valid public health procedure for controlling infectious diseases was initiated by Louis Pasteur. The second half of the 19th century saw the acceptance of the concept that infectious disease was caused by germs, and specific agents were identified in many cases. As an example of chance favoring the prepared mind, Pasteur found that a culture of chicken cholera bacillus (now called *Pasteurella multocida*) left exposed to air for some weeks (by accident) failed to produce disease when inoculated into chickens, but these chickens were protected against a later challenge with the virulent organisms (ie, immunity). Although the approach differed, Pasteur saw some similarity between Jenner's use of an organism pathogenic for another host and his own method of "attenuation" of virulence. He proposed that the procedure of inoculation of attenuated microbes be called *vaccination* and that the product used be called a *vaccine*. Both of these approaches are still used to prepare some modern viral vaccines.

Although Koch[2] had isolated in 1876 the anthrax organism and grown it in culture and Davaine[3] had postulated it to be the cause of anthrax, Pasteur had the foresight to wonder and then investigate whether this organism, in a weakened state, could also be used to immunize animals. In a dramatic demonstration at Poilly-le-Fort in 1881, he showed that animals (ie, sheep, cows, and a goat) immunized with his vaccine could survive lethal challenges with the virulent organism, although all of the control (ie, unimmunized) animals died.[4]

In his experiments with rabies, Pasteur adopted a different approach. Aware that the organism resided in the brains and spinal cords of diseased animals, he stored the agent for long periods or passaged it in the brains of other animals, such as rabbits. Administration of the attenuated preparation to humans (instead of animals) raised a storm of protest and temporarily estranged Pasteur from many of his friends, despite the fact that this approach clearly saved many people from fatal disease.

Pasteur can be described as the first great experimental immunologist, although his work and writings suggest that he was more interested in the application of the growing knowledge of microbes to practical use than to elucidating principles and developing concepts.

1.1.3. A Golden Age of Vaccine Development

The demonstration in 1886 by Salmon and Smith[5] that heat-killed cultures of chicken cholera bacilli could protect pigeons from disease showed for the first time that acquisition of immunity did not depend on the interaction of a live microbe with the host. However, some organisms such as diphtheria, although they could be grown in culture, gave poor protection. In 1888, Roux and Yersin[6] showed that immunization with a bacterium-free filtrate of a diphtheria culture would induce a protective response. Von Behring and Kitasato[7] showed that such immunization resulted in the formation of antibodies (initially called antitoxins) that "neutralized" the activity of the bacterial toxin or antigen produced by the bacteria. The discovery of antibodies led to two important findings.

The first finding was that sera from immunized animals could produce rapid cures in infected children, particularly if administered in the early stages of the disease. Repeated transfusions of allogeneic sera led to serum sickness due to the generation of antibodies to the foreign protein and the formation of antigen-antibody complexes. This limited the usefulness of the technique but it is still practised in certain situations by using convalescent (ie, homologous) sera.

The second finding was that the toxicity of bacterial toxins could be modified if they were mixed with an appropriate amount of antibody and the floccule was carefully washed and injected. This approach was replaced by a chemical procedure, treatment with formalin, which detoxified the toxin, converting it to a toxoid.

The close of the 19th century and the early 20th century saw the development of inactivated bacterial vaccines against typhoid fever, plague, and cholera that were composed of the killed or inactivated infectious agent.[8] Although there were attempts to make vaccines composed of live (ie, infectious) bacteria during this period, they were generally unacceptable because of their reactogenicity and the unwillingness of the medical communities and public to accept live bacterial vaccines for human use. (There are strenuous efforts now being directed to developing live bacterial vaccines to control typhus and cholera, because the vaccines containing killed organisms are not highly effective.) This was a highly fertile period, and the basic approaches to vaccine design for the next 70 years, such as live, attenuated organisms, inactivated organisms, and subunit vaccines, were developed during this period. The use of the embryonated chick embryo and the later use of the culture of mammalian cells in vitro for the growth of viruses enabled many additional viral vaccines to be developed.

1.1.4. Development of the Science of Immunology

The late 19th century saw the elucidation of the two major arms of the immune response: the humoral response involving the reaction between antigen and antibodies and the cellular response in which certain cells were directly implicated in immunologic reactions. In the mid-1880s, Eli Metchnikoff[9] studied the way certain cells engulfed and (attempted) to destroy foreign particles, and he called such cells *phagocytes*. In these early days, the reaction between antigen and antibody was seen by many to be more amenable to quantitative analysis.

It soon became apparent that a great variety of substances could act as antigens and induce the formation of antibodies. Antibodies could cause the agglutination of particles such as bacteria or red blood cells or cause a precipitin reaction in a test tube when the antigen bound to the antibody in a certain ratio. Such reactions allowed the standardization of the reagents, such as the quantitation of diphtheria antibodies by Paul Ehrlich.[10] Ehrlich is also remembered for his *side-chain theory of antibody formation* in which he postulated that the white blood cell's surface bore receptors with side chains to which foreign substances (ie, antigens) became chemically linked. This stimulated the cell to produce more receptors, and the excess was secreted into the blood as antibodies. More than 50 years later, Niels Jerne, David Talmage, and Macfarlane Burnet were to return to a concept like this in their formulation of ideas that led to the enunciation of the *clonal selection theory* by Burnet in 1957.[11]

Ehrlich was shown to be wrong in his idea of a chemical linkage between antigen and antibody; the reaction was shown to be reversible, more like the reaction between an acid and base. Marrack[12] later showed that each component might be multivalent such that, at the equilibrium point between both reagents, a "lattice" was formed that resulted in precipitation of the complex.

The question of antibody specificity was examined by studying the properties of modified antigens. Pick and Obermayer showed in 1906 that attaching chemical groups such as nitrate or iodine to a protein changed its antigenic specificity. Landsteiner greatly extended this approach.[13] He coupled low-molecular-weight chemical compounds, some completely synthetic, to proteins and showed that the antigenic specificity was changed. When injected alone, such chemicals did not elicit antibody formation; they needed to be attached to a larger protein, later called a *carrier*. The small chemicals were called *haptens*, and this led later to the concept of hapten-carrier molecules in which the hapten was recognized with great specificity by B cells. So exquisite was this specificity that it was proposed that it could only be achieved by the antigen acting as a template for antibody formation. The *template theory* held sway in immunologic circles until the *selective theory* became generally accepted in the middle to late 1960s. The hapten-carrier concept was most instrumental at about the same time in determining the different roles of B cells and T cells in antibody formation.

The English scientist, A. Glenny, is credited with discovering with his colleagues the principle of primary and secondary antibody responses to antigens.[14] They noticed the differences in response rates to diphtheria toxin in nonimmune animals compared with previously immunized animals. As is discussed in Section 2.2.6, this was a crucial finding on which the scientific basis of vaccination rests. Glenny and colleagues also showed that the injection of soluble antigen preparations into a host resulted in rather brief antibody responses and that this was related to the rapid disappearance of the antigen from the injection site. These researchers were able to show persistence of antigen at the injection site if it (eg, a toxoid) was precipitated with alum before injection. Remarkably, more than 50 years later, alum is the only adjuvant preparation in general use for human vaccines. They also pioneered the work showing that bacterial toxins could be detoxified to form toxoids. The contributions of Glenny and his colleagues to several of the critical aspects of vaccine development were indeed remarkable.

Immune responses were also found to be associated with tissue inflammation in various ways. After the initial demonstration of the phenomenon of systemic anaphylactic shock to toxic substances, it soon became clear that this was a general reaction, obeying what had become "the laws" of immune specificity. Conditions such as asthma and hay fever were clearly in this category and were called *allergies*. The ability to transfer such reactions by serum, particularly subcutaneously, led to the study of immediate hypersensitivity reactions due to reaginic antibodies.

Reactions that took many hours to develop were called *delayed-type hypersensitivity* (DTH) reactions and could only be transferred by cells. Landsteiner and Chase in 1942[15] demonstrated that tuberculin sensitivity could be passively transferred by lymphoid cells from highly sensitized donors but not by their serum. In 1968, Miller and Mitchell[16] demonstrated T-cell help for the production of antibodies by B cells. It became clear that many cell types, but especially T cells, secreted soluble factors (ie, lymphokines or, more generally, cytokines), which in the case of T cells mediated DTH and helper functions.[17]

A new phenomenon then appeared: a class of T lymphocytes derived from sensitized lymphoid tissues could lyse allogeneic cells, as measured by the release of radioactivity from the target cells labeled with the isotope ^{51}Cr.[18] It was found that these two classes of T lymphocytes, helper T cells and cytotoxic T cells, could be distinguished by cell-surface differentiation markers, the former by the CD4 and the latter by the CD8 molecules. Of major importance was elucidation of their mechanisms of recognition and modes of action, the phenomenon of major histocompatibility complex (MHC) restriction discovered by Zinkernagel and Doherty in 1974.[19] This was followed by a remarkable paper in which the role of MHC antigens was for the first time stated to be the mechanism for signaling changes in self to the host,[20] a statement of great importance in understanding the functions of the immune system and the development of vaccines. The events leading up to this work and subsequent studies are reviewed elsewhere.[21]

CD8-positive (CD8 +) cytotoxic T lymphocytes (CTLs) recognized and lysed infected cells expressing class I MHC antigens, and CD4-positive (CD4 +) T lymphocytes, which mediated T-cell help and DTH reactions, recognized cells expressing class II MHC antigens.[22] A history of immunologic discoveries that are relevant to vaccine development is published elsewhere.[23]

The early findings gave rise to the terms *humoral immunity*, mediated by soluble antibodies, and *cell-mediated immunity* (CMI), mediated by different cell types. The recognition that CMI responses were more important than humoral immunity in the recovery from intracellular infections came initially from "natural experiments." Agammaglobulinemic children recover normally from many childhood diseases, particularly intracellular and especially viral infections, but children with thymic dysplasia do not. It became accepted over time that a major role for antibodies was to prevent infections and that the control and clearance of intracellular infections was mainly mediated by T lymphocytes. The terms humoral and cell-mediated immunity are still used widely as a matter of convenience, but they have been supplemented over time by terms that describe the activities of particular cell types (ie, B and T lymphocytes and their subsets) and their products (ie, antibodies and cytokines).

Ehrlich had originally tested the reaction of the body to its own constituents and, because these reactions were negative, he had proposed that, for unknown reasons, the body was unable to mount such a response—hence, his famous dictum, *horror autoxicus*. Despite several studies, such as Metchnikoff's demonstration of antibody formation against self cells such as spermatozoa, it was widely believed these reactions were not typical, and in the formulation of the *clonal selection theory* in 1957, Burnet[11] proposed that the formation of clones of cells against self antigens was forbidden, without specifying any mechanism. Within a few years, however, several studies showed that a substantial proportion of healthy individuals contained antibodies to a variety of self antigens.[24] Many years later, transfer of effector T cells rather than specific antibody was shown to induce several autoimmune diseases (see Section 6.2).

1.1.5. The Hazards of Vaccination: Early Experiences

The history of vaccination has its darker side. It was inevitable that, in the process of vaccine development and without the benefit of prior experience, mistakes would be made and errors would occur. There have been many episodes of substantial morbidity and mortality after vaccination. Most of these events might have been avoided; some could not have been foreseen. The list of infections includes polio, rabies, bacille Calmette-Guérin (BCG), diphtheria, smallpox, yellow fever, and respiratory syncytial virus (RSV, reviewed elsewhere[25]). Several are cited here as examples.

A catastrophe occurred in the city of Lubeck in the early days of BCG administration. Owing to a mix-up in the use of material from different incubators, a batch of vaccine became contaminated with virulent organisms, and 72 of 251 infants immunized with the preparation died.[26] Other than that early episode, this vaccine has had a good safety record, in part because of the availability of drugs for administration to affected recipients. Children immunized with BCG and already or becoming infected with human immunodeficiency virus (HIV) and displaying the symptoms of acquired immunodeficiency syndrome (AIDS) develop a generalized BCG infection.[27]

During the development of a killed poliovirus vaccine in the United States, formalin was used to inactivate the virus. The procedure was checked for safety in animal model systems, and in a very large-scale trial (nearly 2 million children), the vaccine was found to be safe. However, after the vaccine became commercially available and more widely used, cases of paralytic disease in some recipients were reported. It was suspected that some vaccine batches contained residual live virus, and infectious virus was isolated from the suspected batches from a single manufacturer. The problem, traced to incomplete inactivation of viral aggregates by formalin, was solved by the introduction of a filtration step, with subsequent testing for infectivity. Subsequent vaccinations proved to be safe.[28]

The third example is the use of a vaccine composed of inactivated RSV. Shortly after this virus was first grown in tissue culture in the early 1960s, an inactivated viral vaccine was prepared. It induced high antibody and CMI responses in the recipient children with few adverse effects. On subsequent exposure to wild-type RSV, the vaccine not only failed to confer protection, but some vaccinees unexpectedly developed severe respiratory disease.[29] Subsequent investigation showed that the inactivation procedure affected the biologic properties of an important protective antigen.[30] It is also possible that, in the absence of a protective antibody response, the vaccinees who had been sensitized to a DTH response suffered from an enhanced DTH response when infected by the wild-type virus.[31]

1.1.6. Development of Regulations for Testing Vaccines

The occurrence of vaccine-related tragedies has a single advantage in that subsequent investigations reveal the reasons and establish mechanisms to prevent a recurrence. This is the history in many industrialized countries, such as the United States.[32] These events led to the elaboration of a system of discussion, review, and recommendations about biologics, including vaccines, in a country that is held in high regard by health authorities in many other countries. The various additions and modifications that have been carried out since the early 1900s led in 1982 to the existing Division of Biological Standards within the National Institutes of Health being transferred to the Food and Drug Administration and redesignated as The Office of Biologics Research and Review. It was joined with the Office of Drugs Research Review to form the Center for Drugs and Biologics.

The importance of international agreement on standards for biologics was early recognized, and the Health Commission of the League of Nations established a Permanent Commission on Biological Standardization for this purpose. The WHO, which was established in 1948, assumed the tasks of the disbanded League of Nations and greatly expanded such activities. It became a source of advice on many aspects of health for the member states (now more than 190). No less than eight WHO programs are involved with different aspects of vaccine development and testing (see Chapter 1.3).

1.1.7. Definition of Terms and Vaccine Assessment

Immunization describes the process of administering antigen to a live host with the purpose of inducing an immune response for academic or public health purposes. *Vaccination* is used mainly for the latter reason, but the terms are partly interchangeable. The WHO formed the Expanded Programme of Immunization

(EPI) as well as the Programme for Vaccine Development. Vaccination is one form of immune intervention of which there are many; it is defined as a process of antigen administration once or a few times before the host expects to be confronted by a challenge. In the case of infectious diseases, this challenge is infection by the wild-type agent; in the case of a fertility control vaccine, the threat is the possibility of the initiation of pregnancy. In the case of cancer, it may someday be possible to prevent the development of or to cure the lesion.

Vaccines were developed as prophylactic measures to prevent disease caused by infectious agents, and provided their use caused only very low levels of morbidity and especially mortality, their effectiveness and acceptance was based on these criteria. When methods for the quantitative estimation of specific antibody were developed, the practice of estimating seroconversion (ie, the level of serum anti-body after compared with before vaccination) came into general but not universal use. With experience of a particular disease, this could be used to predict the efficacy of a vaccine. In the case of inactivated poliovirus vaccine, serum antiviral immunoglobulin G (IgG) levels of 1:8 and 1:128 were considered necessary for resistance to pharyngeal or intestinal infection, respectively.[33] In many situations, such as influenza infections, most adult hosts have preexisting antibody from earlier exposure to the virus, and in the absence of a natural challenge, the success of the vaccination is judged by the increase in the level of specific antibody.

In some cases, a correlation may not be found between protection and serum antibody levels. Recognition came much later that CMI responses might be important in protection from disease and that these might not parallel the antibody response. An additional criterion was to see whether the immune response in vaccinated hosts after challenge had the characteristics of a secondary response (ie, a more rapid and larger immune response).

Based on the experiences accumulated over many years, regulatory authorities have established rigorous criteria for the assessment of a vaccine's safety and efficacy. The regulations for biologics usually cover four major phases in product development: developmental, investigational (ie, clinical studies), licensing (ie, registration), and post-licensing surveillance.

Before clinical investigations, evidence must be provided of the standards used in the production of the biologic, its final purity, and its safety and potency. Extensive animal tests are required for toxicity and sometimes for teratogenicity. Often, trials in subhuman primates are necessary to assess further the safety, potency, and efficacy of a preparation. The primate species used varies according to its susceptibility, the biologic relevance of the response being measured, or the relevance of the pattern of disease seen in the model to the human case. For some agents, such as hepatitis B virus (HBV) and HIV, the chimpanzee has been used as the only or main relevant model. In the case of HIV, the model does not develop the disease pattern seen in human patients. Similarly, no primate model closely mimics the disease characteristics seen with infection of humans by the agents of malaria or schistosomiasis. Chimpanzees are an endangered species, they are very expensive to maintain, and the rate of breeding in appropriate facilities is insufficient to meet the demand. A call has been made to restrict the use of these primates for this purpose.[34]

Clinical trials usually occur in three stages. In a phase I trial, the product is administered to a small number of normal volunteers. Tests are performed to assess the safety (ie, freedom from adverse reactions), the potency (ie, generation of adequate levels of the desired immune responses), and the effect on appropriate metabolic and pharmacologic activities when this is deemed necessary. It is becoming accepted practice that for vaccines made in a developed country that may be used subsequently in developing countries, at least phase I trials should be carried out in developed countries. One additional advantage of this arrangement is that, for some tropical diseases, volunteers in tropical countries may be already immune and may not give a primary immune response. For example, phase I trials of a leprosy vaccine conducted under the auspices of the WHO were carried out using volunteers in Scandinavia and North America.

After a successful phase I trial, phase II trials are conducted to further assess the previously described aspects but particularly the efficacy of the product in generating high levels of the immune responses that should afford protection against disease or the equivalent after exposure to the live agent. The agent is administered to the vaccinated volunteers (eg, mosquitos infected with sporozoites in the case of malaria or vibrios in the case of cholera); in cases such as HBV or HIV, members of a high-risk group might be included. The trials may sometimes be combined. In two trials of a malaria vaccine,[35,36] 3 of the 6 volunteers in the phase I trial who developed high antibody titers were exposed to infected mosquitos. In each case, one person was completely protected. Planning for a full phase II trial should include agreed values for the level of efficacy and degrees of confidence needed for adequate analysis of the results, because this determines the number of participants required for the trial.

Phase III trials are carried out "in the field." One or more communities are selected for which detailed epidemiologic data and adequate health services are available (eg, knowledge of the risk of contracting the disease naturally, the disease burden, whether the infrastructure for delivery of the vaccine and the assessment of efficacy is in place). Such a trial may involve very large numbers of people.

Post-licensing surveillance is highly desirable and required in many cases. The efficacy of the vaccine to protect against disease and to ameliorate existing disease (as is the case with leprosy) may be assessed. Well-established formulas are available to measure these parameters and criteria such as cost-benefit ratios or cost-effectiveness. Adverse reactions should also be documented. In a country such as the United States, these come from a variety of sources—the manufacturer, physicians, health workers, consumers, and government agencies such as the Centers for Disease Control and Prevention (CDC). Such assessment can establish the ultimate safety and efficacy of the product.

It should be stressed that most of the requirements mentioned have been instituted in the last 20 years, and it is mainly during that time that adverse reactions that occur at a very low frequency have been analyzed. The procedures described for bringing a vaccine to the market should detect and be able to attribute to the vaccine the more frequent side effects of, for example, 1 in 10,000 or fewer vaccinations. But serious and chronic side effects may occur infrequently, and their detection in significant numbers may require the administration of millions of vaccine doses. Large populations must be studied to identify the occurrence and to quantitate the incidence of side effects, apart from establishing their vaccine relatedness. Several examples are discussed in Section 1.2.6. Rare adverse reactions are feared by the regulatory authorities, the vaccine manufacturers, and the public alike. But they act as a catalyst in the drive to develop safer vaccines.

1.1.8. Categories of Countries

In the following chapters, the terms *developed* (or industrialized), *developing*, and *least developed countries* are used. The distinctions are based on socio-economic considerations, of which health is one aspect, by the United Nations and its agencies. Countries form an economic spectrum, and even within a country, there may be great variation. One important component influencing vaccine production and usage is the differences in funds available for total health services. In many developed countries, the figure is more than $1000 per person per year. In least developed and developing countries, it is of the order of $2 and $10 per person per year, respectively.[37] In the WHO/EPI, which is mainly funded from sources within developed countries, a vaccine costing more than $1 per dose could be incorporated into the program only under special circumstances. In the development of vaccines for worldwide application, this figure should be kept in mind. The cost of a vaccine is much less if it is made in developing countries and very large orders are placed. Many of the vaccines used in the WHO/EPI are obtained on this basis.

CHAPTER 1.2. TRADITIONAL-TYPE HUMAN VACCINES AND VACCINATION PRACTICES

Great improvements in personal and community health practices, such as the provision of safe drinking water and sanitation facilities, were major factors in the lessening of the disease burden in communities in industrialized countries after about 1850.[38] Vaccination against the common infectious agents, as it was progressively implemented during the 20th century, has also been important, especially in the case of the highly contagious infections. There are more than 50 vaccines in general use in the medical and veterinary sectors,[39] and the use of medical vaccines in developed countries has reduced many major human diseases to minor public health problems.

This chapter reviews some of the properties of viral and bacterial vaccines that are in general use (ie, have been licensed for human use by the regulatory authorities) or are in trials (ie, phase I and II trials have been carried out, and phase III trials are planned or in progress). In the latter case, the efficacy or safety of the vaccine has not been evaluated to the extent that the vaccine is registered for general use.

This chapter discusses only vaccines that have been developed using traditional approaches, those that do not use peptide synthesis, derivation of monoclonal antibodies, or direct manipulation with subsequent expression of DNA/cDNA. These latter approaches are the subject of Section 5 of this book.

Some idea of the range of microorganisms that may cause disease in humans is given by the list of viruses, bacteria, parasites, and fungi in Table 1.2.1. Those for which vaccines are available or are targeted for vaccine development are presented in this section.

TABLE 1.2.1. *Infectious agents*

Infectious agents	Diseases
Viruses	
Adenovirus	Respiratory disease
Coronavirus	Respiratory and enteric disease
Cytomegalovirus	Mononucleosis
Dengue virus	Dengue fever, shock syndrome
Epstein-Barr virus	Mononucleosis, Burkitt's lymphoma
Hepatitis, A, B, and C virus	Liver disease
Herpes simplex virus type 1	Encephalitis, stomatitis
Herpes simplex virus type 2	Genital lesions
Human herpesvirus-6	Unknown, possibly Kaposi's sarcoma
Human immunodeficiency virus types 1 and 2	Acquired immunodeficiency syndrome (AIDS)
Human T-cell lymphotropic virus type I	T-cell leukemia
Influenza A, B, and C	Respiratory disease
Japanese encephalitis virus	Pneumonia, encephalopathy
Measles virus	Subacute sclerosing panencephalitis
Mumps virus	Meningitis, encephalitis
Papillomavirus	Warts, cervical carcinoma
Parvovirus	Respiratory disease, anemia
Poliovirus	Paralysis
Polyomavirus JC	Multifocal leukoencephalopathy
Polyomavirus BK	Hemorrhagic cystitis
Rabies virus	Nerve dysfunction
Respiratory syncytial virus	Respiratory disease
Rhinovirus	Common cold
Rotavirus	Diarrhea
Rubella virus	Fetal malformations
Vaccinia virus	Generalized infection
Yellow fever virus	Jaundice, renal and hepatic failure
Varicella zoster virus	Chickenpox
Bacteria	
Bacillus anthracis	Anthrax
Bordetella pertussis	Whooping cough
Borrelia burgdorferi	Lyme disease
Campylobacter jejuni	Gastroenteritis
Chlamydia trachomatis	Pelvic inflammatory disease, blindness
Clostridium botulinum	Botulism
Corynebacterium diphtheriae	Diphtheria
Escherichia coli	Diarrhea, urinary tract infections
Haemophilus influenzae	Pneumonia
Helicobacter pylori	Gastritis, duodenal ulcer
Legionella pneumophila	Legionnaires' disease

(continued)

TABLE 1.2.1. *Continued*

Infectious agents	Diseases
Listeria monocytogenes	Meningitis, sepsis
Mycobacterium leprae	Leprosy
Mycobacterium tuberculosis	Tuberculosis
Neisseria gonorrhoeae	Gonorrhea
Neisseria meningitidis	Sepsis, meningitis
Pseudomonas aeruginosa	Nosocomial infections
Rickettsia	Rocky Mountain spotted fever
Salmonella	Typhoid fever, gastroenteritis
Shigella	Dysentery
Staphylococcus aureus	Impetigo, toxic shock syndrome
Streptococcus pneumoniae	Pneumonia, otitis media
Streptococcus pyogenes	Rheumatic fever, pharyngitis
Treponema pallidum	Syphilis
Vibrio cholerae	Cholera
Yersinia pestis	Bubonic plague
Parasites	
African trypanosomes	Trypanosomiasis
Entamoeba histolytica	Amebic dysentery
Giardia lamblia	Diarrheal disease
Leishmania	Lesions of the spleen, tropical sores
Plasmodium	Malaria
Microfilariae	Filariasis
Schistosomes	Schistosomiasis
Toxoplasma gondii	Toxoplasmosis
Trichomonas vaginalis	Vaginitis
Trypanosoma cruzi	Chagas disease
Fungi	
Candida albicans	Mucosal infections
Histoplasma	Lung, lymph node infections
Pneumocystis carinii	Pneumonia in AIDS
Aspergillus fumigatis	Aspergillosis

1.2.1. General Properties of Viruses

Viruses are the simplest of all biologic structures that are able to replicate and produce their own kind.[40] They are metabolically inert and replicate only within cells by making use of the cell's synthetic machinery. They share common features such as the presence of only one class of nucleic acid (RNA or DNA) and of a few to many different proteins. They show great variation in other properties such as size and complexity, with the largest viruses, the pox viruses, being very much larger than the smallest, which are not much bigger than large proteins.

The virion, which is the mature virus particle, has a core of one or several molecules of nucleic acid that may be associated with one or more proteins, sometimes called nucleoproteins. The nucleic acids must be protected from nucleases, and this is a function of the capsid (coat) proteins (capsomers). For reasons of genetic economy, particularly with the smaller viruses, capsomers are composed of repeating units of one or a small number of proteins that pack together symmetrically. With some of the larger and more complex viruses, the capsid is contained within a lipid envelope. This envelope may be "reinforced" on the inside by a matrix protein. Other proteins, peplomers, protrude from the external face; they have hydrophobic (transmembrane) segments that are embedded in the lipid envelope. Peplomers occur in many viruses as repeating units, such as trimers or quadrimers.

Examination of the capsomers or peplomers in the case of enveloped viruses can be useful for identification, and these proteins usually are the target (protective) antigens for viral infectivity-neutralizing antibodies. Their presence in packed symmetric arrays has profound implications for vaccine development. In many instances, many of the epitopes recognized by neutralizing antibodies are found to be discontinuous sequences of amino acids, generated by the folding of closely proximal polypeptide chains from a single or adjacent molecules. Particularly in the case of virions that are formed by budding from the plasma cell membrane, the peplomers are glycosylated to various degrees.

The virion may not only contain proteins that are structurally important, but contain other polypeptides that have enzymatic activity, such as transcription of viral RNA (by the reverse transcriptases of retroviruses), polymerases involved in nucleic acid replication, proteases for the cleavage of precursor protein molecules, and integrases for integration of cDNA into the host cell genome. Some viruses also have regulatory proteins that control these different activities.

1.2.2. Licensed Viral Vaccines for Human Use

Table 1.2.2 lists the commonly used viral vaccines made by traditional procedures. Three general approaches have been used with different degrees of success: attenuation (ie, reduction in viral virulence, which is the ability to cause disease), inactivation with the loss of infectivity, and subunit vaccines in which one or a few of the viral antigens, freed from other viral components, are used.

1.2.2.1. Attenuated Live Viral Vaccines

Most of the vaccines listed in the Table 1.2.2 are attenuated preparations. Four general approaches have been or are being used. The commonest is to prepare host range mutants by prolonged passage of the virulent human pathogen in different hosts or in cell culture (or both), and most included in Table 1.2.2 are in this category. This has largely been achieved on an empiric basis, with continued passage until sufficient attenuation, as shown by a variety of tests but particularly loss of reactogenicity, is achieved without a great loss of immunogenicity.

The development of the 17D yellow fever vaccine illustrates the magnitude of the task that may be involved.[41] The virus, isolated from a patient in 1927, was passaged in sequence as follows: 53 passages in rhesus monkeys and intermittently in *Aedes aegypti* mosquitos; 18 times in whole mouse embryonic tissue cultures; 58 times in whole minced chicken embryo culture; and 160 times in tissue culture using

TABLE 1.2.2. *Traditional viral vaccines for human use*

Agent or vaccine	Source of vaccine (century)	Type of vaccine	Route of administration
Vaccinia	Calf skin (18–20th)	Live, attenuated	ID
Rabies	Sheep brain (19th)	Inactivated	IM
	Duck eggs (20th)	Inactivated	IM
	Tissue culture (20th)	Inactivated	SC
Yellow fever	Mouse brain (20th)	Live, attenuated	SC
	Tissue culture (20th)*	Live, attenuated	SC
Influenza	Chick eggs (20th)	Inactivated	IM
	Chick eggs (20th)	Subunit	IM
	Nonhuman hosts†	Live, attenuated	IN
Polio			
Oral (OPV)	Tissue culture	Live, attenuated	Oral
Inactivated (IPV)	Tissue culture	Inactivated	SC
Measles‡	Tissue culture	Live, attenuated	SC
Mumps‡	Tissue culture	Live, attenuated	SC
Rubella‡	Tissue culture	Live, partly attenuated	Oral
Japanese encephalitis	Mouse brain	Inactivated	SC
Hepatitis B (HBV)	Infected, human plasma	Subunit	IM
	Yeast	Subunit	IM
Varicella zoster	Tissue culture	Live, attenuated	SC
Adenovirus§	Tissue culture	Live, partly attenuated	Oral

IM, intramuscular; ID, intradermal; IN, intranasal; SC, subcutaneous.
*Recommended by the World Health Organization.
†Used in the former USSR.
‡In some countries, used as a trivalent vaccine (MMR).
§For armed forces recruits.

cells from embryo chickens from which the brain and spinal cord had been removed before mincing. Testing at different stages showed that the virus became progressively less neurotropic.

The basis of such attenuation is slowly becoming understood, and polio can be cited as an example. The Sabin polio vaccine, which is used very widely in developed and in developing countries as part of the WHO/EPI, contains three attenuated, antigenically distinct strains of virus, called types 1, 2, and 3 (described elsewhere[28,42]). The aim was to derive virus preparations that had lost their neurotropism in monkeys, and this was achieved by multiple passage of wild-type viruses in nonhuman primates and in tissue culture. The vaccine has been successful in reducing endemic poliomyelitis in many countries.

Reversion to virulence occurs in recipients of types 2 and particularly type 3 in vaccinees, and at a frequency of about 1 to 2×10^6 administrations, a vaccinee and contacts come down with poliomyelitis. The aim has been to determine the basis of this reversion by nucleic acid base sequence analysis. Compared with the wild-type virus, type 1 virus has 57 separate base substitutions, of which 21 code for amino acid changes that are scattered throughout the genome. In practice, this type rarely reverts to virulence, in contrast to type 3. By comparing three different type 3 preparations of virus, it was found that attenuation resulted in at most 10 point mutations, of which three were shown to be amino acid substitutions.[43] The neurovirulent revertant virus was found to differ from the vaccine strain by point mutations at seven positions, of which two may be important in attenuation.[44] The only observed backmutation occurred in a noncoding region, position 472, and there is evidence to suggest that a change at this residue correlates with neurovirulence.[45] These investigations stimulated experiments to construct hybrid viruses that could overcome these reversions, but these hybrids have not progressed to acceptance.

The second approach, the "Jennerian method," is to use as a human vaccine a virus that is pathogenic for another host. The example in Table 1.2.2 is vaccinia. In veterinary medicine, the use of turkey herpesvirus to control Marek's disease in chickens has been successful.

A novel approach can be taken with viruses, such as the orthomyxoviruses, that have a segmented genome. This has been done initially to provide virus that grows well in the chick embryo and to provide a vaccine strain with peplomers, hemagglutinin and neuraminidase, containing the most suitable antigenic specificities. Live, attenuated viruses prepared using this approach and in trials are described later in this section.

The adenovirus vaccine, like the attenuated, live polio vaccine, is given orally. Although the preparation is widely thought to contain unattenuated viral subtypes, this is claimed not to be the case because, although there are no attenuation markers available, genetic analyses show differences between the DNA of the vaccine and the original isolates.[46]

The attenuated virus vaccines that are widely used give long-lasting immunity and generally have good safety records (see Section 1.2.6).

1.2.2.2. Inactivated Viral Vaccines

Inactivated preparations are used as the basis of vaccines for polio, influenza, rabies, and Japanese encephalitis viruses. The inactivating agents used include formaldehyde, the ethylenimines, and β-propiolactone. The extent to which the nucleic acid or protein is affected by these procedures is not always clear; the advantage of the latter reagent is that the excess is rapidly converted in the body to a natural component. Inactivated preparations usually are safer and more heat stable than many live viral vaccines, such as polio and measles vaccines, and this is an important consideration in tropical countries. However, they may be considerably more expensive than live viral vaccines, because a much greater antigenic mass is required, and several injections are frequently required over time to generate lasting immunity. Both of these difficulties are being overcome with viruses that are grown in cell culture. Modern methods of production, such as growth in mammalian cells attached to beads, yield higher titers of virus, and the delivery aspect may be helped by advances in this area (see Section 4).

The contrasts between live and inactivated viral vaccines is well illustrated by the two polio vaccines. Both have their strong advocates. Research to develop each was commissioned at the same time in the United States, but a killed viral vaccine—the Salk vaccine—was developed first and enthusiastically used in the United States and some other, mainly European, countries. It was highly successful and was responsible for the virtual elimination of that disease in the United States and its eradication in Sweden. The attenuated, live viral vaccine—the Sabin vaccine—was first tested and adopted in the USSR and eastern European countries and proved so successful that, over the years, it supplanted the use of the killed vaccine in most countries. The major advantages were oral administration, low cost (because of the small antigenic mass required), no need for adjuvant, effective local immunity (ie, IgA and IgG production), and the expected generation of more comprehensive CMI responses and long-lasting immunity. The main disadvantages (which favor the use of IPV) were heat lability, occasional interference in function because of other infections, and the reversion to virulence, which has already been discussed. The oral poliovirus vaccine (OPV) is used in the WHO/EPI (see Table 1.2.2).

The development of rabies viral vaccines illustrates the importance of effective removal of contaminating substances, particularly when a relatively large antigenic mass is administered. The pasteurian rabies vaccine was grown in brain tissue, and there are still vaccine facilities using this technology in some developing countries that have not been updated since their establishment many years ago. Contamination with myelinated tissue caused neurologic complications. Myelin protein–free vaccines from neonatal mouse brains were introduced in 1956[47] and were used in the USSR and in South America. A duck egg–grown vaccine was made about the same time but proved to be less immunogenic. The vaccine currently used in many countries is prepared from virus grown in human diploid cells,[48] and it is highly immunogenic but relatively expensive.

Experience with the suckling mouse brain–derived rabies vaccine was useful in the later development of a vaccine to control Japanese encephalitis, which occurs in Japan and neighboring countries. This virus is considered by some to be a greater threat to public health than dengue virus infections.

In the western world, inactivated whole virus vaccines to combat influenza are widely used, but in the USSR and in China, live virus vaccines derived by attenuation in nonhuman hosts have been more frequently used. Antigenic drift and shift are major features of the influenza A viruses. Drift occurs because of the accumulation of single-point mutations, particularly in the hemagglutinin (HA) and neuraminidase (NA) peplomers, and shift is caused by the exchange of genes between viruses due to the presence of a segmented genome. The immune response to influenza virus is described in Section 3.2.3.2, where the difficulty of dealing with antigenic variation is considered in more detail.

The decision to develop an influenza virus vaccine was influenced by the memory of the great pandemic that occurred after the First World War and that was estimated to have led to the death of about 18 million people worldwide. The fear of a similar pandemic after the end of the Second World War led to experiments in the United States and Australia to develop a vaccine. The development of an inactivated virus vaccine rather than an attenuated live virus vaccine won the day. Current influenza

virus vaccines are constructed with a standard set of genes coding for internal proteins together with genes for the HA and NA from recent virus isolates. The hope is
that strains causing new epidemics in the oncoming season will be antigenically not
very dissimilar to the HA and NA of the vaccine donor strains. The vaccines are
considered to be about 70% effective during periods of antigenic drift.[49] Annual
revaccination of elderly persons has been recommended in the United States for
many years; a randomized, controlled trial carried out in the Netherlands[50,51] has
indicated that influenza vaccination may halve the incidence of serologic and clinical influenza among the elderly. A safe and effective inactivated hepatitis A viral
vaccine is licensed in several European countries. The virus is grown in tissue
culture and treated with formalin.

1.2.2.3. Subunit Viral Vaccines

Enveloped viruses such as influenza can be disrupted with lipid solvents or detergents. Such preparations may be used as "split" vaccines, but it is more common to
isolate the surface antigens and present them as a subunit vaccine. Such vaccines
have the advantage of less reactogenicity than whole viral vaccines, but they are
poor at inducing some CMI responses.

The isolation from the plasma of infected persons, and subsequent purification
and sterilization of the surface antigen (HBsAg) of HBV to form a safe vaccine is a
landmark in the history of vaccination achievements. A series of three or four injections over some months with adjuvant induces an antibody response in more than
80% of immunocompetent recipients. Revaccination may be necessary after 5 to 10
years.[52] A preparation of HBsAg made in transfected yeast subsequently became
available, and its use as a vaccine is described in Section 5.

These achievements, especially in the case of the hepatitis B vaccine, have been a
major reason for the widely held expectation that vaccination to control a number of
diseases may be achievable with other subunit preparations or with synthetic peptide
preparations (see Section 5).

1.2.2.4. Candidate Viral Vaccines in Advanced Clinical Trials

Table 1.2.2.4 lists viral vaccines that are in advanced clinical trials. The most
striking feature is the extent to which attenuation of viruses remains the most favored way to develop vaccines against what are in most cases acute infections.
There are two examples of viruses, rotavirus and parainfluenza type 3, that are
pathogenic for other hosts and that may be suitable for use as a human vaccine.[53]

Two live, attenuated (reassortant) influenza viruses have undergone extensive
testing.[49] One is a cold-adapted (*ca*) strain, which was derived by continual passage
of virus at decreasing temperatures until a preparation was obtained that grew at
25°C. This strain is temperature sensitive because it does not grow above 37°C, but
unlike other preparations of temperature-sensitive mutants which have proved to be

TABLE 1.2.2.4. *Traditional viral vaccines for human use in late stage trials*

Agent	Source of vaccine	Type
Cytomegalovirus	Cell culture (human)	Live, attenuated; subunit
Influenza virus	Chick embryo	Live, attenuated;* cold-adapted variant
Dengue virus	Cell culture	Live, attenuated
Rotavirus	Cell culture	Live, attenuated NCDV (calf origin) WC3 (bovine origin) RRV (rhesus monkey) Human (?)
Parainfluenza type 3	Cell culture	Live, attenuated
Japanese encephalitis	Cell culture	Live, attenuated
Hepatitis A	Cell culture	Live, attenuated; inactivated

*Reassortant preparations.

unstable, it has proved to be stable. Four of the internal genes of this reassortant have mutations and hence contribute to the genetic stability. A set of six single *ca* gene substitution reassortant viruses was produced from two parents—the influenza A/Ann/Arbor/6/60 (H2N2) parent and the A/Korea/1/82 (H2N2) wild type—to identify the genes that specified the attenuation (*ca*) and temperature-sensitive (*ts*) phenotype. It was found that

A gene for the PA polymerase specified the *ca* phenotype.

A gene for the PB2 polymerase played a major role in specifying the *ts* phenotype.

Genes for a third polymerase protein, PA, and for the matrix protein each contributed to the restriction in viral replication in the upper respiratory tract.

The second reassortant influenza virus in trials was identified because of an observation that most avian influenza viruses recovered from asymptomatically infected water birds were moderately restricted in their replication in the lower respiratory tract of monkeys. An analysis showed that the six genes coding for the "internal" proteins of the virus specified a degree of restriction similar to that of the whole virus. This pattern was also found for reassortant viruses, in which only the two surface glycoproteins were derived from wild-type human strains. Each gene coding for internal proteins was found to contribute to the restriction pattern observed. However, the preparations proved to be unsatisfactory in clinical trials.

The polygenic nature of the mutation pattern augers well for the use of the *ca* mutant as a future human influenza virus vaccine. The data from studies involving more than 500 children,[54] who are the prime target population for vaccination because they are a major factor in the spreading of disease, indicate that the vaccine showed minimal reactogenicity after oral administration, gave superior protection compared with inactivated viral vaccine, induced acceptable antibody levels for 12 to 24 months, and induced IgA and CMI responses. The shed virus was of low titer, and it retained the ca phenotype. Despite these evaluations, this vaccine has not yet been registered for use in the United States, although similar vaccines have been successfully used in the USSR (now Russia) for many years.

Cytomegalovirus, a member of the herpesvirus family, grows only in human cells or persons and may cause disease in the fetus if the mother is infected during the first half of pregnancy. Immunosuppressed patients receiving kidney grafts also have active infections. Vaccines have been developed from virus cultured extensively in human cells,[55] and they induce humoral and cellular responses.[56] When tested in transplant patients, partial protection occurred.

Both inactivated and live, attenuated hepatitis A viral vaccines are being developed. Initially, virus was grown in infected marmoset livers, but the adaptation of the virus to tissue culture made prospects for either type of vaccine more promising. Two attenuated preparations appear to be promising live virus candidates.

Dengue and Japanese encephalitis viruses are members of the flavivirus group, and they cause disease predominantly in countries in southeast Asia, but outbreaks of dengue fever have also been reported in Africa and the Americas. These viruses are vector borne (ie, mosquitos).

Dengue viruses cause fever, and there are four antigenically distinct types (types 1 through 4). Infection with one serotype gives long-lasting homologous immunity but short-lived heterologous immunity. All four types cause dengue hemorrhagic fever (DHF) and dengue shock syndrome. In Thailand, sequential infection with dengue 1, 2, or 4, followed within a few years by dengue 2, seems to be the main cause of DHF, which is an immunopathologically mediated disease. Antibody reacting with the "challenge" dengue virus causes the phenomenon of immune enhancement in which the antibody-virus complex, reacting with Fc receptors on macrophages or monocytes, greatly enhances infection of the cells by the virus. This has dictated the approach taken in the development of vaccines:

1. A vaccine should be polyvalent to protect against all serotypes.
2. Because waning or subneutralizing amounts of antibody favors immune enhancement, the vaccine should give high titers of neutralizing antibody; this should lead to long-lasting and perhaps life-long immunity. This need strengthened the case for a live, attenuated viral vaccine.

Candidate vaccines of types 1, 2, and 4, produced by passaging the viruses in dog kidney cells, have given good immunity. Particularly in the case of dengue 2, the antibody response was monospecific, all vaccinees responded, and levels of neutralizing antibody remained high for at least 3 years.[57] The phenomenon of immune enhancement is discussed at greater length in Section 3.2.3.4.

1.2.3. General Properties of Bacteria

Bacteria (prokaryotes) occupy a position midway between viruses and nucleated cells (eukaryotes).[58] They contain both DNA and RNA, and they can often exist independently of other cells and therefore qualify to be called microorganisms. However, in the protoplast (ie, the interior of the cell), there is no membrane to separate the nuclear material from the cytoplasm, nor is there any evidence of an endoplasmic reticulum or structures corresponding to mitochondria. The lack of an endoplasmic reticulum means that there is no mechanism for the glycosylation of bacterial proteins. The cytoplasm, which contains ribosomes, is contained by the plasma membrane and a cell wall that confers rigidity and shape. The encapsulated bacteria have in addition a layer of polysaccharide next to the cell wall; other types have flagella for motility or have fimbriae or pili, which facilitate adherence to cells.

Two aspects of particular interest are the existence of plasmids and the nature of bacterial antigens. Plasmids are independent replicons that live in bacteria; they are extrachromosomal genetic structures that can replicate autonomously and differ from bacterial phages because they have no extracellular form. They mediate transferable drug resistance, and this property has proved to be extraordinarily useful for manipulating DNA transfer between cells, as is discussed in Section 5.

It has been regarded as axiomatic for many years that, from an immunologist's point of view, the bacterial antigens of most interest are those at the cell surface or secreted from the cell—the extracellular antigens that are toxins or enzymes. Consequently, most attention has been focussed on these two categories. However, all proteins of bacteria that replicate in cells are potential sources of peptides that, when associated with the antigens of the MHC, may be recognized by T cells.

Although simple proteins or saccharides (as part of glycoproteins) are the main antigens of viruses, there is a wide range of bacterial compounds that may be antigens and at least recognized by antibody. These include proteins, complex polysaccharides, oligosaccharides of unusual composition, lipoproteins, lipopolysaccharides (some with unusual fatty acids), glycolipids, glucuronic and other acids, glycans, galactans, and polyamino acids. In addition to random mutations in proteins, this has allowed the mechanisms for antigenic variation to be developed to an extraordinarily high level. Because branched oligosaccharides and polysaccharides favor great antigenic variety, many bacteria exhibit large numbers of different serotypes.

Because they need to exist in many different situations and evade immune responses, some bacteria (ie, encapsulated bacteria) have developed layers of polysaccharide that help to protect against desiccation, phagocytosis, and infection by phages. Lipopolysaccharides are the major antigens of many bacteria, and they induce a variety of biologic effects, some beneficial and some harmful for humans. In view of the requirements for T-cell activation and the "immaturity" of these cells in young children, they are often at greater risk of severe and sometimes lethal infection by many bacteria.

Because of their antigenic complexity, it has taken great effort to establish the important "protective" antigens of many bacteria. In contrast, secreted proteins—mainly toxins—have in a few cases provided the basis for highly effective vaccines.

1.2.4. Licensed Bacterial Vaccines

Table 1.2.4 lists licensed bacterial vaccines made by traditional methods for human use. Like viral vaccines, they fall into three groups: live, attenuated strains; inactivated, whole bacteria; and subunit preparations.

TABLE 1.2.4. *Traditional bacterial vaccines for human use*

Agent	Type	Route of administration	Efficacy
Bacille Calmette-Guérin	Live, attenuated	ID	0–80%
Vibrio cholerae	Inactivated	IM or SC	50–70%
Salmonella typhi	Inactivated	IM	53–88%
	Trypsinized extract	SC	58–68%
	Live, attenuated (Ty21a)	Oral	
Bordetella pertussis	Inactivated	IM	80–90%
	Acellular	IM	
Clostridium tetani (tetanus)	Subunit (toxoid)	IM	>90%
Corynebacterium diphtheriae (diphtheria)	Subunit (toxoid)	IM	>90%
Streptococcus pneumonia (pneumococcus)	Subunit (capsular polysaccharide)	IM or SC	Variable, but up to 70%
Haemophilus influenzae	Subunit (capsular polysaccharide)	IM or SC	40–90% (type b)
	Polys./carrier protein complex	IM or SC	95%
Neisseria meningitidis serotypes A, C	Subunit (capsular polysaccharide)	SC	75–90%
Combination	DTP, DTaP		

ID, intradermal; IM, intramuscular; IN, intranasal; SC, subcutaneous.

1.2.4.1. Attenuated Live Bacterial Vaccines

Unlike the viral vaccines, only one attenuated bacterial vaccine (ie, BCG[59]) has been for many years in common use, forming part of the WHO/EPI schedule. The protection afforded has varied from 80% to almost no protection. A major trial was held in southern India, and the results of a 7.5-year follow-up study were published in 1979, demonstrating little protection by the vaccine. Despite this result, subsequent trials with young children have shown protection to be high, and there appear to be significant differences between the protective responses to the vaccine in adults and older children compared with young children. WHO has recommended that the use of BCG vaccine on a worldwide basis should be continued, especially in infants and children. A positive outcome of the Indian trial was the recognition by WHO that a greater knowledge of the biology of the organism and its protective antigens, particularly for CMI responses, was required. Funds were obtained, initially from the Norwegian government, to initiate a new program on tuberculosis. This later became a component of the WHO Programme of Vaccine Development.

Attenuation of bacterial strains has tended to be more difficult to accomplish than with viruses. When taken together with the advent of antibiotics, which initially seemed to indicate that most bacterial infections could be controlled in this way, the pressure to develop attenuated bacterial vaccines slackened. It became a more urgent research topic after it was demonstrated that antibiotics, although extremely useful, were not the complete answer to bacterial infections, particularly in the least developed countries, sometimes because of cost but more often because of resistance developing to many antibiotics. A live, attenuated *Salmonella typhi* preparation, Ty21a, was licensed for use in the United States.[60] Other mutants are being tested.

1.2.4.2 Inactivated Whole Bacterial Vaccines

Three inactivated whole bacterial vaccines have been in use for long periods: cholera, typhus, and pertussis vaccines. Neither the *Vibrio cholerae* nor the *S. typhi* vaccine has been highly successful, giving only moderate protection for relatively short periods (see Table 1.2.4). One contributing factor to the poor efficacy is that both are intestinal infections, invading at mucosal surfaces, but the vaccines are administered parentally. In contrast, the pertussis vaccine has been quite successful and is given as a trivalent vaccine with diphtheria and tetanus toxoids. However, persisting concern about the reactogenicity of this vaccine has led to the development of subunit (acellular) preparations containing one or more purified bacterial components. Two recently licensed products are recommended for the fourth and fifth doses of vaccine.

1.2.4.3. Subunit Vaccines

1.2.4.3.1. Toxoid-Based Vaccines

Some bacterial infections are noninvasive but are pathogenic because of the secretion of powerful toxins. The ability to detoxify these proteins without loss of immunogenicity was a major achievement. Diphtheria and tetanus are the main examples, and they are regarded as two of the more successful bacterial vaccines. Table 1.2.4.3 reports WHO/EPI data on the immunogenicity of tetanus toxoid and the

TABLE 1.2.4.3. *Tetanus toxoid immunization schedule for women of childbearing age*

Dose	When to give	Expected duration of protection
TT1	At first contact or as early as possible in pregnancy	None
TT2	At least 4 weeks after TT1	1–3 years
TT3	At least 6 months after TT2	5 years
TT4	At least 1 year after TT3 or during subsequent pregnancy	10 years
TT5	At least 1 year after TT4 or during subsequent pregnancy	All childbearing years

From Immunization policy. (1995) Global Programme for vaccines and immunization. World Health Organization Expanded Programme of Immunization, Geneva, 95.3 p. 15.

administration requirements to obtain lasting immunity for women of childbearing age. The two toxoids are administered with pertussis as a trivalent vaccine (DTP). The preparation containing the later acellular derivative is referred to as DTaP.

Both toxoids are used extensively in immunization studies as carriers of haptenic groups for two reasons. Being large proteins, they should contain a number of T-cell epitopes, and because most persons have been vaccinated with one or both toxoids, a secondary T-cell response should be obtained.

1.2.4.3.2. Bacterial Polysaccharide Vaccines

In 1881, Pasteur identified a particular structure—a capsule—associated with a bacterium. The object of this interest is now known as *Streptococcus pneumoniae*, and it is a member of the encapsulated bacterial group that includes pneumococci, streptococci, staphylococci, meningococci, *Haemophilus influenzae*, *Escherichia coli*, *Klebsiella pneumoniae*, and *Bacteroides fragilis*. The polysaccharide coat serves many functions, and it is important for the pathogenicity and immunogenicity of these organisms,[61] enabling them to resist opsonization and ingestion by phagocytic cells and hence clearance from the blood. The capsules may limit the activation of complement, and deposition of C3b on the bacterial surface may be at a site where it is not readily accessible to complement receptors on leukocytes. The classic complement pathway is activated only when antibodies to the specific capsular polysaccharides of the invading bacteria are present.

Beginning in the 1930s, vaccines based on capsular polysaccharides from several strains of pneumococcus were shown to be effective in adults. The current pneumococcal vaccine in the United States, which contains 23 antigenic specificities, was developed following the observation that about 25 of the nearly 100 known serotypes cause about 95% of disease attributable to this organism in that country. It is recommended for those older than 60 years of age. Two other subunit vaccines to control *H. influenzae* type b and *Neisseria meningitidis* are also available and can be effective in all age groups, except children younger than about 2 years of age.

1.2.4.3.3. Conjugates

It was shown as long ago as 1931 that, although pneumococcal polysaccharides were generally poorly immunogenic in rabbits, a conjugate consisting of the carbohydrate coupled to a foreign protein was more immunogenic. This approach has been used to develop several bacterial vaccines. The capsular polysaccharide of *H. influenzae* type b has been conjugated to diphtheria or tetanus toxoid, and these conjugates have exhibited booster effects in experimental animals, as shown by accelerated antibody responses and IgM to IgG switching. Clinical trials that included infants 3 to 14 months of age were promising, and field trials in Finland in which children received the vaccine at 3, 4, 6, and 14 months of age indicated that the rate of short-term protection was about 83%. Two preparations, HBOC, in which a nontoxic mutant of DT, CRM_{197}, is the carrier, and PRP-OMP, in which an outer membrane protein complex of *N. meningitidis* is the carrier, are licensed in the United States for administration to 2-month-old infants. Other preparations containing DT or TT as the carrier are also licensed.

1.2.4.4. Candidate Bacterial Vaccines in Advanced Clinical Trials

Bacterial vaccines in advanced clinical trials are listed in Table 1.2.4.4 and include attenuated strains of *V. cholerae* and *S. typhi* aro A mutant.[60] Two inactivated whole organism preparations have or are undergoing extensive efficacy trials in endemic countries. Inactivated *V. cholerae* plus the toxin B subunit gave encouraging results in Bangladesh.[62]

Mycobacterium leprae can be grown in the armadillo. The bacteria are isolated from the livers and spleens of infected animals, purified, and inactivated. The killed organisms gave strong CMI responses in experimental animals, an encouraging finding. Large-scale phase III trials of BCG with and without the leprosy vaccine are in progress in two tropical countries. After the first 5 years of follow-up of one trial in Venezuela, there is little evidence that BCG plus *M. leprae* offers substantially better protection than does BCG alone.[63] Because of the success of the *H. influenzae* type b/carrier conjugates, other polysaccharide-protein conjugates are under intensive study, and these include pneumococcal- and meningococcal-protein complexes and *E. coli, Pseudomonas aeruginosa, Salmonella typhimurium,* and *K. pneumoniae* conjugates. Serum albumins, toxoids, and bacterial outer membrane antigens are being evaluated as carrier proteins. The use of a homologous bacterial protein as the carrier has the potential advantage that T and B memory cells resulting from vaccination should be stimulated when exposure to the natural infection occurs.

TABLE 1.2.4.4. *Traditional bacterial vaccines for human use in late-stage trials*

Agent	Type	Route of administration
Mycobacterium leprae with/ without BCG	Inactivated*	SC
Salmonella typhi	Aro A mutant	Oral
Vibrio cholerae	Inactivated* plus cholera toxin B subunit	Oral
	Live, attenuated	Oral
Neisseria meningiditis	Subunit†	IM or SC
Protein carrier conjugates	Pneumococcal, meningococcal	

IM, intramuscular; SC, subcutaneous.
*Whole organisms.
†Capsular polysaccharides, serotypes Y, W-135.

1.2.5. Vaccines Against Other Infectious Agents

Because of the great morbidity and mortality associated with some major parasitic infections, especially malaria, there have been intense efforts over the last 20 years to develop vaccines against malaria and, to a lesser extent, against leishmaniasis and schistosomiasis. Many of these have used the newer approaches to vaccination and are discussed in Section 5.

Q fever is a debilitating disease that is particularly prevalent in abattoir workers. It is caused by *Coxiella burnetii* infection. Inactivated whole organisms as a vaccine caused reactions in those previously sensitized by a natural infection. The vaccine is administered to nonsensitized personnel and appears to give complete protection.

Attempts to make a leishmaniasis vaccine based on inactivated whole organisms are in progress. The zoonotic protozoan, *Leishmania chagasi*, is transmitted to humans through dogs. It was reported in late 1994 that 9 of 10 dogs vaccinated with killed promastigotes of *L. braziliensis* plus BCG resisted a lethal challenge of *L. chagasi*, raising the hope that such a vaccine might interrupt transmission to humans from dogs.[64]

1.2.6. Vaccine Safety

A vaccine should be safe, causing no mortality and little morbidity. For vaccines developed by traditional methods, safety and efficacy are often closely interrelated. Vaccines widely used during the smallpox eradication program were found to have a significant level of side effects, as reported in Table 1.2.6.1. These are discussed in Section 5 in connection with the use of vaccinia and other pox viruses as a vector of DNA coding for other antigens.

TABLE 1.2.6.1. *Reported cases (deaths) per million in the United States after smallpox vaccination*

Reported complications	Deaths per million after primary vaccination* (n = 5,959,000)
Encephalopathy	6.5
Encephalitis	2.4
Progressive vaccinia	0.9
Eczema vaccinatum	10.4
Generalized vaccinia	23.4
Accidental infection	25.4
Other complications	11.8
Total	74.7

*There was a much lower frequency of complications after revaccination, and complications occasionally occurred in contacts of vaccinated persons.

Adapted from Lane JM, Ruben L, Neff JM, Miller JD. (1969) Complications of smallpox vaccination, 1968. National surveillance in the United States. N Engl J Med 281: 1201–1205.

imated rates of adverse reactions following diphtheria-tetanus-pertussis
ion compared with complications of natural whooping cough

Adverse reaction	Whooping cough complication rates/100,000 cases	DTP vaccine adverse reaction rates/100,000 immunizations
Permanent brain damage	600–2,000 (0.6–2.0%)	0.2–0.6
Death	100–4,000 (0.1–4.0%)	0.2
Encephalopathy/encephalitis*	90–4,000 (0.09–4.0%)	0.1–3.0
Convulsions	600–8,000 (0.6–8.0%)	0.3–90
Shock		0.5–30

*Including seizures, focal neurologic signs, coma, and Reye syndrome.
From Galaska AM, Lauer BA, Henderson RH, Keja J. (1984) Indications and contraindications for vaccines used in the Expanded Programme of Immunization. Bull World Health Organization 62:357–366.

Table 1.2.6.2 gives data collected by the WHO/EPI, demonstrating the overall safety record of the whole-cell pertussis vaccine. Nevertheless, this vaccine is considered the most reactogenic component of the triple-antigen DTP vaccine. Two of the several categories of reaction recognized—minor local and systemic effects and the protracted bouts of crying with unusual shock-like states—do not have long-term consequences. However, major neurologic reactions may lead to permanent disability. It has been extraordinarily difficult to establish a correlation between such injury and vaccination. The frequency of encephalopathy with residual brain damage 1 year after vaccination is estimated to be about 1 in 300,000 cases, but the correct figure could be 1 in 54,000 to 5,300,000 cases. One study[65] concluded that the pertussis component of DTP may be responsible for rare instances of neurologic damage, but not for all reported cases. These findings were subsequently challenged in an English law court and overturned. Nevertheless, because of the mounting costs of litigation and the inability to obtain commercial insurance, these findings caused two manufacturers to raise the cost of the vaccine in the United States by more than 10-fold. An acellular pertussis vaccine has been in use in Japan for some years, and similar vaccines are now licensed in the United States.

Swine influenza, the serotype that caused the 1918 influenza pandemic, which resulted in about 20 million deaths, was isolated from military recruits at Fort Dix and from a man and a pig from the same farm in Wisconsin in the United States in 1976. A rush program to vaccinate many millions of United States citizens was initiated. The vaccine went through the usual tests before licensing, but in a total of 41.5 million persons who received the vaccine after licensing, about 500 cases of Guillain-Barré syndrome occurred. The chance of detecting and ascribing responsibility for such a reaction in prelicensing trials is negligible. No association of this syndrome with influenza vaccination occurred before or has been seen in later immunization programs, and a definite correlation between the disease and vaccination remains unproved.

Table 1.2.6.3 presents data collected by the WHO/EPI on the estimated rates of serious adverse reactions following measles vaccination compared with the compli-

TABLE 1.2.6.3. *Estimated rates of serious adverse reactions following measles immunization compared with complications of natural measles infection and background rate of illness*

Adverse reaction	Measles complication rates/100,000 cases	Measles vaccine adverse reaction rates/100,000 vaccinees	Background illness rates/100,000 persons
Encephalitis/encephalopathy	50–400 (0.05–0.4%)	0.1	0.1–0.3
Subacute sclerosing panencephalitis	0.5–2.0	0.01–0.1	
Pneumonia	3800–7300 (3.8–7.3%)		
Convulsions	500–1000 (0.5–1.0%)	0.02–190	30
Death	10–10,000 (0.01–10%)	0.01–0.3	

From Galaska AM, Lauer BA, Henderson RH, Keja J. (1984) Indications and contraindications for vaccines used in the Expanded Programme of Immunization. Bull World Health Organization 62:357–366.

cations caused by infection with the natural pathogen.[66] The data indicate that the vaccine is safe and effective. The vaccine is ineffective in the presence of neutralizing antibody, which in endemic countries is present in maternally derived antibodies in young infants up to 9 months of age, when the vaccine is normally administered. In some infants, levels of antibody wane much sooner, and there is a period of a few months when such children are susceptible to infection by the pathogen. This is one reason why 1 to 2 million infants die from measles each year in developing countries. In an attempt to overcome this problem, a high-titer vaccine strain, the Edmonston-Zagreb strain, was developed for administration to 5- to 6-month-old children. Administration of the vaccine to children of this age group in a number of countries induced immune response levels that were similar to those after standard titer vaccines administered at 9 months. The general use of the new vaccines was recommended by WHO in 1989. However, reports began to arrive of mortality, affecting predominantly baby girls, and this resulted in the recall of the vaccine. After long-term follow-up of vaccinated infants, it became clear that the increased mortality rate was confined to populations at the lower end of the socioeconomic scale.[67] Natural measles infection induces a state of immunosuppression. Although the Schwartz vaccine does not induce such a state, the high-titer vaccine may have, opening the way for other infections.

In 1994, the U.S. Institute of Medicine published a report reviewing the evidence bearing on causality and specific adverse health outcomes, mainly within the United States.[68] The possibility of adverse neurologic events after vaccination has fueled much of the concern about vaccine safety. The disorders included demyelinating diseases, such as acute disseminated encephalomyelitis, multiple sclerosis, focal lesions, Guillain-Barré syndrome, and nondemyelinating diseases, such as encephalopathy, subacute sclerosing panencephalitis, residual seizure disorder, sensorineural deafness, and neuropathy. Immunologic reactions to vaccination included anaphylaxis, Arthus reaction, and DTH. Adverse effects after immunization with measles, mumps, polio, and HBV, vaccines; diphtheria and tetanus toxoids; and *H. influenzae* type B (Hib) vaccines were studied. The report contains shorter reports on pertussis and rubella vaccines.

In most cases, the evidence was considered inadequate to accept or reject a causal relation between measles and mumps vaccine and encephalitis or encephalopathy. For example, in uncontrolled studies, the calculated rate of these effects per million doses of vaccines varied from 1 to 11. However, the evidence suggested a causal relation between the trivalent measles-mumps-rubella (MMR) vaccine and thrombocytopenia, but not between the monovalent preparations, and a correlation between MMR and the measles vaccines and anaphylaxis. Because of these effects, there was a causal relation between MMR and death, although the risk was considered to be "extraordinarily low." Natural measles infection induces an immunosuppressive state from which most children recover. This document records only two cases of immunosuppression in immunocompromised children after vaccination with measles vaccine.

The evidence established a causal relation between diphtheria and tetanus toxoids or tetanus toxoid and death from anaphylaxis or Guillain-Barré syndrome. There also seemed to be a causal relation between the unconjugated Hib vaccine (as a first administration) and death from early-onset Hib disease. In both cases, the risk was extraordinarily low.

The evidence was consistent, demonstrating a causal relation between DTP vaccine and acute encephalopathy and shock and "unusual shock-like state" and between MMR containing the RA 27/3 rubella strain vaccine and chronic arthritis. However, the overall impression is that the vaccines studied in this report were particularly safe.

1.2.7. Vaccine Efficacy and Infectious Disease Eradication

Traditionally, vaccine efficacy has been assessed by prevention of disease when the vaccinee is later exposed to the wild-type agent. Perhaps the ultimate test for efficacy is the ability of a vaccine to eradicate an infectious disease. The first success was the eradication of smallpox (see Section 1.1.1), and this was achieved because of a favorable set of factors:

The disease was confined to humans (there was no environmental reservoir).
There was no vector of the agent.
There was no carrier state, and there were no subclinical infections.
There was a very effective, heat-stable, and affordable vaccine, and vaccination required only a single, simple administration.
There was an easy marker (ie, scab) to indicate successful vaccination.

Although this list of advantages may not apply to any other situation, the two most critical points were the availability of a very effective vaccine and restriction of the infection to humans. Two other candidates that fulfilled these requirements were poliomyelitis and measles.

1.2.7.1. Poliomyelitis

In 1985, the Director of the Pan American Health Organization (PAHO) proposed the initiative to eradicate the indigenous transmission of wild-type poliovirus from the Americas by the year 1990.[71] This was extended in 1988 by the World Health Assembly to achieve global eradication by the year 2000. In the Americas, a board representing a consortium of funding agencies coordinated activities, two of which became critical: holding national vaccination days so that whole populations were reached and establishing by mid-1989 nearly 15,000 health facilities throughout the Americas to report regularly on the presence or absence of cases of acute flaccid paralysis. In 1979, there were about 2000 poliomyelitis cases in Brazil alone. Two years later, after the introduction of vaccination days, the incidence had fallen by more than 90%. Near the end of 1994,[70] poliomyelitis was declared eradicated from the Americas, because no case of disease due to indigenous wild-type virus had occurred within the previous 3 years. Earlier in 1994, there was a small outbreak in Canada after the arrival from Europe of members of a religious minority group who had previously refused vaccination and had become infected before leaving Europe.

This success is all the more remarkable because there are several reasons why eradication of poliomyelitis is more difficult than smallpox. Although there is no animal reservoir or vector, the oral vaccine (OPV) is the most heat labile of the EPI vaccines; most infections are subclinical; multiple administrations of the vaccine are required; there is no simple marker of successful vaccination; and cases of polio-myelitis can arise because of reversion to virulence of vaccine strains (see Section 1.2.2.1). Eradication of the disease from some countries in Africa, a continent beset by so many natural and man-made disasters, poses a formidable challenge. One step toward a solution is making the vaccine less heat labile (see Section 1.3.2.3). One milestone of the global program was to eradicate poliomyelitis from the Western Pacific Region, including China and the Philippines, by the end of 1995.

1.2.7.2. Measles

In May 1991, a mass campaign to eliminate measles in one subregion of the Americas was initiated in the English-speaking Caribbean countries. All children between the ages of 1 and 15 years were vaccinated. By early 1994, no laboratory-confirmed indigenous case of measles had been detected. Buoyed by the successes with polio vaccine in the Americas and with measles vaccine in the Caribbean after the introduction of vaccination days, PAHO announced the intention to eradicate measles from the Americas by the year 2000.[71] In nonendemic (ie, many developed) countries, the vaccine is administered, frequently as MMR, at 15 to 18 months of age. In such countries (eg, Australia), localized outbreaks result from inadequate coverage, especially in some ethnic communities and from waning of immunity in some vaccinees, so that a booster vaccination for older children or young teenagers is required.

In the 1970s, measles, mumps, and rubella were rampant in Finland, and in 1982, a national program was initiated in which two doses of a combined live virus vaccine were used. It was reported in 1994[72] that outbreaks of these three diseases had ceased in Finland but that continuing vaccination was needed to protect the population from imported disease.

In the United States,[73] a routine two-dose immunization policy was introduced after the 1990 outbreak, and by 1994, coverage had increased from about 70% to 85%. Surveillance findings and laboratory characterization indicates that the transmission of indigenous strains had been stopped and that the reported cases were from importations.

Because of the high transmissibility of measles, eradication of the disease requires a highly effective vaccine. All the data indicate that the current Schwartz vaccine is effective and safe (see Table 1.2.6.3).

1.2.7.3. Pertussis

Immunization to control whooping cough was begun in England and Wales in the 1950s, and clinical cases of infection and deaths rapidly declined to very low levels as vaccine uptake climbed to more than 80% by the early 1970s. After scares in the media about adverse reactions to the vaccine, vaccine uptake plunged to 30%, and this was followed by a sharp increase in notification of pertussis, particularly in areas where vaccine coverage was low.[74] An intense campaign to boost vaccination coverage resulted in levels reaching more than 90% and very low levels of morbidity by the early 1990s. This is graphically represented in Figure 1.2.7.3.

1.2.7.4. Haemophilus influenzae *Type B*

Laboratory reports of *H. influenzae* infections in England and Wales have fallen dramatically since the introduction of the Hib vaccine in late 1992.[75] This effect has been observed in many industrialized countries, including Australia (Fig. 1.2.7.4).

1.2.7.5. Other Vaccines

Not all vaccines are efficacious. BCG and the early *V. cholerae* vaccines have checkered histories. *Mycobacterium tuberculosis*, because of antibiotic-resistant strains and previously suppressed infections in children with AIDS, has emerged as the biggest killer on a global scale.[76]

The recent outbreaks of cholera in South America and especially in Bangladesh underline the need for improved vaccines. The need for improved vaccines and for

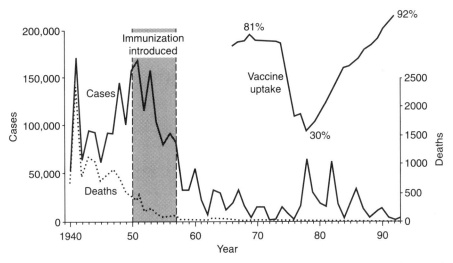

FIG. 1.2.7.3. Whooping cough notifications: cases and deaths in England and Wales from 1940 through 1993. (From Begg N, Cutts FT. [1994] The role of epidemiology in the development of a vaccination programme. In: Cutts FT, Smith PG, eds. Vaccination and world health. John Wiley & Sons, Chichester, pp. 123–137.)

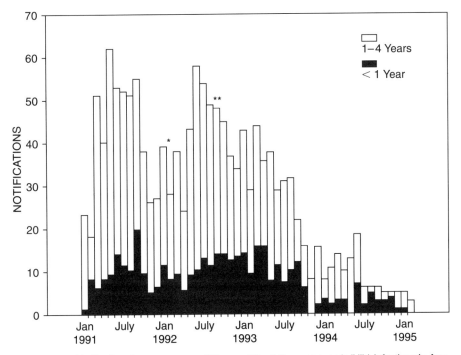

FIG. 1.2.7.4. Notifications by age groups of *Haemophilus influenzae* type b (Hib) infections in Australia from January 1991 to March 1995. The vaccine was introduced during 1992.

vaccines against other diseases is further discussed in Chapter 1.4. The important role of epidemiologic studies in monitoring vaccine efficacy is discussed elsewhere.[74]

1.2.8. Prophylactic Vaccination Versus Immunotherapy

Most vaccines were designed for the prevention of disease on subsequent exposure to the pathogen. Specific infectivity-neutralizing antibody is the first line of defense, reducing the load of challenge infectious agents to the extent that the host's own immune response can control escaped virus without disease occurring. The two situations for which a registered vaccine is knowingly administered to those already exposed to the pathogen are hepatitis B in newborn infants and rabies. In the former case, administration with specific immune serum enhances the level of protection because antibodies in the serum prevent or limit infection until the host has responded to the vaccine.[52]

Rabies infection is characterized by a prodromal phase in which the virus may persist in the body, may replicate in some cells such as muscle, but may take days or weeks to reach the nervous system, which facilitates replication and spread throughout the central nervous system. During this phase, the virus may be neutralized by specific antibody, allowing a window of opportunity to the vaccine to induce a protective immune response even though it has been administered after exposure to the virus.[77]

Potentially, this approach is possible for many slow diseases. Convit and colleagues[78] showed that injection of killed *M. leprae* and BCG into some borderline and polar lepromatous patients caused clinical improvement (positive skin test reactivity), a remarkable result in subjects who previously had been anergic for some years. Similar encouraging results have been obtained with leishmaniasis.[79]

Jonas Salk[80] suggested immunizing asymptomatic HIV-infected persons with the intention[81] of clearing the virus or delaying progress toward AIDS, and others[81,82] soon accepted the challenge. Many groups are now involved in this area. Some early results suggested that immunization stabilized the CD4+ T-cell count, but later the measurement of viral burden in the blood was adopted as possibly a more reliable indicator. However, even this is in doubt following the finding of extensive viral replication in lymphoid tissue,[83-85] resulting in very high levels of virus production up to 10^9 virions per day. Consequently, it may take considerable time to establish how effective immunotherapeutic intervention may be. Possible approaches such intervention may take are discussed in Section 3.

1.2.9. Passively Acquired Immunity

Transfer of immune serum or globulin is regularly used to give short-term protection against infection. There are several major current and potential uses, including protection of travelers on relatively short trips to areas where a particular disease may be endemic (ie, HBV immune serum or globulin is commonly administered for this reason) and protection of neonates or infants born of HBV-infected mothers against HBV infection[52] (ie, administration of immune globulin together with vaccination protects up to 95% of newborns).

Large programs are now underway to protect infants born of HIV-1 infected mothers from infection by passive transfer of pooled high-titer immune globulin to the mother before birth of the child.[86] In many developed countries, about 25% of infants born of infected mothers are infected during delivery; the proportion is higher in some developing countries. The finding that the second-born twin is less likely to be infected than the first-born twin suggests that the amount of virus to which the offspring is exposed is relatively low and is reduced significantly when the first twin is born.

Immune serum or globulin is used to protect immunocompromised patients from severe infections. For example, infection by cytomegalovirus (CMV) is common in patients with AIDS or in those who undergo transplantation. Administration of human IgG with a high anti-CMV titer may prevent about one half of serious CMV-mediated illness, but it does not reduce the incidence of infection.[87] Similarly, administration of large doses of human immune globulin within 4 days after exposure to varicella zoster virus (VZV) prevents or reduces the severity of subsequent disease in immunocompromised patients.[88] In the United States, several commercial preparations of immune globulin are available[89]: CMV, HBV, rabies, tetanus, and VZV.

The potential applications of passive immunization include immunoglobulins for use against Hib, group B streptococcus, *N. meningitidis*, *S. pneumoniae*, and *Bordetella pertussis*. Antiviral candidates are influenza and RSV.[90]

There are two other important developments in this area. CTLs, rather than antibody, are known to be the main mechanism for controlling CMV infections. In a limited but interesting trial,[91] cells were removed from CMV-positive donors of bone marrow cells before the latter were transplanted to patients who had undergone irradiation to dampen their immune systems. The removed cells were stimulated in vitro to generate CTLs to CMV, and after the operation, the effector cells were transfused to the individual patients. No toxicity developed. The CTLs persisted in the recipients, and none developed CMV viremia or pneumonia. In a second case, virus-specific CTLs, obtained by in vitro culture, were adoptively transferred to an HLA-matched sibling with severe chronic, active EBV infection.[92] After each transfer, the patient showed improvement (eg, detection of EBV-specific CTLs, decrease in tumor necrosis factor-α levels) but later died from a bacterial infection.

The disadvantage of using hyperimmune serum or globulin for passive immunization is that only a minor fraction of the product is specific functional antibody. Hybridoma technology has been used to make antigen-specific monoclonal antibodies and to overcome their immunogenicity in humans. Humanization of murine monoclonal antibodies has been carried out by variable domain replacement technology[93] or by complementarity-determining region grafting.[94] These chimeric preparations are being used with some success, but this approach may well be overtaken by the new technology of cloning antibody fragments in phages.[95] The potential and some achievements of this approach are described in Section 5.5.

1.2.10. Maternal Versus Neonatal Immunization

Babies are born into an environment swarming with infectious agents from which they must be protected. Protection is achieved for some months to 1 or 2 years by transfer of maternal antibody through the placenta before birth (IgG) and through colostrum and milk (IgA) after birth. The presence of this antibody can prevent immunization with a live agent, such as measles vaccine (see Section 1.2.6), but it is less likely to interfere with successful immunization with a nonreplicating vaccine (see Section 2.4.4).

Protection of the neonate can be enhanced by immunizing the mother during pregnancy. In the veterinary industry, dam vaccination is used to control infections in the offspring by equine abortion virus, rotavirus infection in cattle, parvovirus infection in swine, and infectious bursal disease in chickens.[96] Maternal vaccination against tetanus is now strongly encouraged in developing countries because of the risk to mother and child of tetanus infection if the umbilical cord is severed under nonsterile conditions. The goal of WHO was to achieve complete protection of pregnant mothers globally by 1995.

Polysaccharide vaccines for Hib, group A and group C meningitidis, and group B streptococcus have been given to pregnant women without adverse effects, and this has resulted in increased amounts of specific antibody in the infants (reviewed elsewhere[97]). Because pneumococci are a leading cause of death in infants and children worldwide, especially in developing countries, one study assessed the effects of maternal immunization with the 23-valent pneumococcal polysaccharide vaccine on antibody levels in the infant.[97] These levels were sufficiently high for the researchers to propose that immunization of pregnant women in this way would be a feasible strategy for developing countries, provided such antibodies did not interfere with subsequent immunization of the infants with the new polysaccharide-protein conjugate vaccines.

Usually, there is concern about immunization of pregnant women with a live agent vaccine, particularly during the first trimester of pregnancy.

CHAPTER 1.3. NATIONAL AND INTERNATIONAL IMMUNIZATION PROGRAMS

1.3.1. International Programs

1.3.1.1. World Health Organization Immunization Programs

Toward the end of the Smallpox Eradication Programme, WHO established EPI in 1974, when only about 5% of children in developing countries were immunized with vaccines against the six common childhood diseases: diphtheria, tetanus, tuberculosis, pertussis, measles, and poliomyelitis. The vaccines were in general use in developed countries. Together with other agencies such as UNICEF, the World

Bank and the United Nations Development Program (UNDP), the EPI has achieved what many initially thought to be an impossible task, to greatly raise the level of childhood immunization globally, which should lead to a great reduction in childhood morbidity and mortality. By 1990, about 80% of children reaching their first birthdays had been fully immunized against these six diseases. It has proved to be more difficult to raise the coverage level to a planned figure of 90%.[98] In the United States, the cost of childhood vaccination is $120 in the public sector clinics and $264 or more in the private sector.[98] The cost of the six basic vaccines for the EPI through UNICEF is less than $1.

The plan is for other vaccines to be progressively added to the basic schedule, with the first one being the hepatitis B vaccine (reviewed elsewhere[98]). For many years, the high cost of this vaccine (about $100 for three doses) in developed countries precluded such a move, but the establishment of vaccine manufacturing plants outside of the major western countries led to supply of the vaccine at a greatly reduced price. For the EPI/UNICEF schedule, the cost of HBV vaccine for three doses is $1.50.[100] The current EPI immunization schedule is given in Table 1.3.1.1.

In the years succeeding 1974, WHO established a number of other special programs that were largely involved with vaccine development to control infectious diseases. The first was the Tropical Disease Research (UNDP/World Bank/WHO Special Programme for Research and Training in Tropical Diseases), which had programs on five parasitic (ie, malaria, leishmaniasis, schistosomiasis, trypanosomiasis, and filariasis) and one bacterial disease (ie, leprosy); Diarrheal Diseases Control, which had a minor component for vaccine development to control enteric infections; Vaccine Development (WHO/UNDP/Programme for Vaccine Development), which initially had committees on acute respiratory viruses, including measles, on dengue and Japanese encephalitis viruses, on encapsulated bacteria, on hepatitis and poliomyelitis viruses, and on tuberculosis. Later, the program assumed responsibility for leprosy and diarrheal diseases. After a few years, a new

TABLE 1.3.1.1. *WHO/EPI recommended schedule for the immunization of infants, mainly in developing countries*

Contact	Age of child	Vaccines
1	At birth	BCG, OPV, and HBV[A]*
2	6 wk	DTP, OPV, and HBV[AB]
3	10 wk	DTP, OPV, and HBV[B]
4	14 wk	DTP and OPV
5	9 mo	Measles and HBV[AB]

BCG, bacille Calmette-Guérin; DTP, diphtheria-tetanus-pertussis; OPV, oral poliovirus vaccine; WHO/EPI, World Health Organization Expanded Programme of Immunization.

*The hepatitis B virus (HBV) vaccine schedule is flexible. Schedule A (HBV[A]) is recommended for populations for whom there is a significant risk of perinatal transmission. Schedule B (HBV[B]) is recommended for populations for whom the risk of perinatal transmission is minimal or immunization at birth is not possible. A third dose of HBV vaccine may be given at 9 months if necessary.

development was initiated, called transdisease vaccinology, which was established to study those aspects that could be relevant to the development of almost any vaccine. Topics included the development of the live vector approach to oral immunization and to immunopotentiators, including controlled release devices. The Global Programme on AIDS was formed and included a section concerned with HIV vaccine development and testing.

The first special program in WHO was on human reproduction (ie, the UNDP/UNFPA/World Bank Special Programme of Research, Development and Research Training in Human Reproduction), initiated in 1971. In 1978, the requirements that a vaccine should meet to control or regulate human fertility were defined, and a committee was established to support research toward the development of vaccines for this purpose.

There has often been close collaboration between these programs and private foundations and governmental agencies. To mention only a few, the Rockefeller Foundation (New York), which initiated the great Neglected Diseases Program (ie, vaccines against parasitic infections), has financially supported some of the previously described programs. The Edna McConnell Clark Foundation (New York) has supported research on vaccines against schistosomiasis and trachoma, and the Population Council (New York) has supported the development of human fertility control vaccines. SAREC, an agency of the Swedish government, supports research on the development and testing of vaccines against HIV and tropical infections.

1.3.1.2. The Children's Vaccine Initiative

A historic event took place in New York in September 1990: holding of a World Summit for Children. Presidents, prime ministers, and other representatives of 159 countries agreed to increase efforts and set specific targets to improve the condition of the world's children in health, education, and children's rights. The targets included[100]

Global eradication of poliomyelitis by the year 2000
Elimination of neonatal tetanus by 1995, and 90% coverage of women of childbearing age
Measles: reduction of deaths by 95% and of cases by 90% by 1995
Maintenance of a high level of global childhood immunization (90%)
Diarrhea: reduction of 50% in children younger than 5 years of age and reduction in the incidence rate by 25%
Acute respiratory infections: reduction by one third of deaths in children younger than 5 years.

In 1991, the Rockefeller Foundation, UNDP, the World Bank, UNICEF, and WHO launched the Children's Vaccine Initiative (CVI). It was a recognition that no single organization has the resources or capability to prevent childhood diseases. The aim is to promote and mobilize resources for the development of single-dose, heat-stable, orally administered vaccines against a wide spectrum of diseases, to be delivered shortly after birth.

The CVI was established in response to the numerous scientific advances in the design and development of vaccines that were being made and to translate those advances into the delivery of new and improved vaccines for the world's children.[101] It is expected to be an initiating, integrating, and propelling force in the development, manufacturing, and use of vaccines. A consultative group was formed to encourage participation by relevant organizations, and it holds annual forums. The operating entities within the CVI are the product development groups of which there are initially two devoted to the development of thermostable oral polio vaccines and to a systematic assessment of microsphere technology for the single-dose delivery of tetanus toxoid. A partner, the Agency for Cooperation in International Health in Japan, is concerned with the development of vaccine production facilities in developing countries such as Brazil, China, and India and with quality control of the products.

1.3.1.3. Reorganization of the World Health Organization's Immunization Programmes

The WHO has responded to these new developments by a major reorganization of its vaccine programs.[102] The Director-General has established the Global Programme on Vaccines and Immunization, which has created three operational components: EPI, Vaccine Supply and Quality (VSQ), and Vaccine Research and Development (VRD). EPI's role is to define global immunization policies and provide technical support to countries through WHO regional offices. VSQ works with countries, vaccine buyers, and vaccine manufacturers to ensure that adequate quantities of safe, fully potent vaccines are available to all national immunization programs at an affordable price. VRD stimulates and supports the research and development activities that may lead to new vaccines and to improved existing vaccines, and it provides the scientific basis for their optimal use.

1.3.2. National Programs

Most countries have programs for the administration of childhood vaccines. Each country has the responsibility of deciding on vaccines to be used in that country and their administration. Sometimes, it is a federal responsibility, and sometimes it is shared between federal and state authorities. In the United States, numerous organizations are involved, including CDC and the National Institutes of Health (NIH), and these have different roles to play. A national vaccine program was established to plan and coordinate relevant activities, but it has been the subject of some criticism.[103] After a measles epidemic in 1989 through 1991, there was a substantial increase in funds to control and finally eliminate vaccine-preventable diseases and to boost the childhood immunization initiative that had been launched in 1988. The

TABLE 1.3.2. *Recommended childhood immunization schedule, United States, January–June, 1996*

Vaccine	Birth	1 mo	2 mo	4 mo	6 mo	12 mo	15 mo	18 mo	4–6 y	11–12 y	14–16 y
							Age*				
Hepatitis B		Hep B-1	Hep B-2			Hep B-3				Hep B	
Diphtheria-tetanus-pertussis			DTP	DTP	DTP		DTaP		DTaP		
Haemophilus influenzae type b			Hib	Hib	Hib		*Hib*				
Poliovirus			OPV	OPV			OPV		OPV		
Measles-mumps-rubella							MMR		MMR or MMR		
Varicella zoster virus							Var			*Var*	

DTP, diphtheria-tetanus-pertussis; DTaP, diphtheria-tetanus–acellular pertussis; Hib, *Haemophilus influenzae* type b; MMR, measles-mumps-rubella; OPV, oral poliovirus vaccine.

*Vaccines are listed under the routinely recommended ages. Bars indicate the range of acceptable ages for vaccination. Italics indicate catch-up vaccination times. Varicella zoster vaccine should be administered to children not previously vaccinated who lack a reliable history of chickenpox infection.

40

schedule approved by the Advisory Committee on Immunization Practices, the American Academy of Pediatrics, and the American Academy of Family Physicians is shown in Table 1.3.2. The goal was to aim for zero indigenous cases of measles, rubella, diphtheria, poliomyelitis, and tetanus in children younger than 15 years and no Hib in children younger than 5 years. Emphasis was to be placed on improving the delivery of services, reducing vaccine costs for children in need, increasing education for parents and providers, and monitoring disease incidence and vaccine coverage.[99]

In the United Kingdom, beginning in the 1950s, immunization levels generally were in the range of 60% to 70%. In the 1980s, the British Health Service introduced a national vaccine registry. The names of all children were entered into a computerized record at birth and their vaccination status regularly updated. By 1988, immunization levels were known nationally from the panels of individual practitioners, and a prosaic approach to increasing the immunization levels was then adopted. Bonuses of increasing monetary values were offered to practitioners as the immunization coverage of children in their panel increased to 70% and then to 90%. All children, regardless of objections and contraindications, were to be counted in the denominator population. The result? The number of physicians achieving bonus targets rose dramatically. The goal of 90% for each of the vaccines was achieved in 1992; it was anticipated that the goal of 95% would be achieved within a few years![104]

CHAPTER 1.4. FUTURE NEEDS AND POSSIBILITIES

1.4.1. The Infectious Disease Burden of Different Populations

Despite the ever-growing list of vaccines available or in late clinical trials, there are still many infectious diseases for which no vaccine is available and that are of great importance in developed and developing countries. One way of assessing the importance of each disease is to consider the number of persons at risk of infection and the morbidity and mortality statistics for that disease.

In 1986, the U.S. Institute of Medicine published data on diseases of importance for the United States[107] and for developing countries[108] with a view to establishing priorities for vaccine development. Although other infections, especially HIV and tuberculosis, have become prominent since then, the basic information made available at that time should still be valid. Readers are referred to the original publications for details.[107,108]

There are great health differences between the first and third worlds. One third of the world's population is exposed to malaria, and at any one time, 200 million persons are affected. In tropical Africa, most children have malaria by 1 year of age, and at least 1 million die each year. At any one time, about 1 billion persons are affected by the six tropical diseases studied in the WHO/TDR programme (ie, malaria, schistosomiasis, filariasis, trypanosomiasis, leishmaniasis, and leprosy), and many have multiple infections. More than 200 million, mainly in southeast Asia, are infected with HBV.

Barry Bloom has outlined some of the statistics of the world's 40 poorest countries[109] and offered a comparison between the first and third worlds. One sentence encapsulates the differences. "This is the Third World in which 75% of the planet's population lives, where 86% of all children are born and 98% of all infant and child deaths occur, and where 10 kids die of vaccine preventable illness every minute."

1.4.2. Emerging and Reemerging Infectious Diseases

Although some statistics remain unchanged, patterns of infectious disease do vary, and some major changes have occurred in the 10 years since the two reports of the U.S. Institute of Medicine were published. The emergence of HIV infection and AIDS in particular has refocused attention on our ability to recognize and control outbreaks of new infectious diseases. A series of scientific meetings have been held since the late 1980s for this purpose. In 1991, a Task Force on Microbiology and Infectious Diseases, appointed by the National Institutes of Allergy and Infectious Diseases, NIH, met to report on five topics, one of which was emerging infectious diseases.[110] In 1992, a meeting was held to discuss emerging viruses,[111] and a comprehensive document on new, emerging, and reemerging infectious diseases was later published.[112]

There appear to be three threatening situations: the emergence of new infectious agents, a newly recognized association between a known agent and a previously unknown disease manifestation, and outbreaks of known, well-defined infectious diseases. Some infectious agents falling into these three categories are presented in Table 1.4.2. There are few truly new agents that were unknown before the latest disease manifestation in humans became apparent. The main ones are HIV, new assortant strains of influenza virus, and *Legionella*. Most agents are listed under the heading of known agents having new associations, epidemics due to a breakdown in vector control, or the emergence of multidrug-resistant strains. There are major outbreaks of classic diseases, such as cholera and tuberculosis. Some of these stress the need for improved or for new vaccines, because this approach in many cases remains the action most likely to be effective. It is also likely that situations such as those previously described will continue to occur, probably at an enhanced rate. The factors involved include increases in urban crowding, in promiscuity, in the penetration by humans into different ecosystems (particularly in tropical countries), in world travel, and in microbial drug resistance.

1.4.3. The Need for Improving Current Vaccines

Although some of the current vaccines are quite effective, there is room for improvement in others for various reasons. Most of the vaccines have been available for many years, and some should be completely replaced because they are of low or

TABLE 1.4.2. *Emerging agents, new associations, and reemerging infectious diseases*

Agent	Disease
Emerging infectious agent	
Human immunodeficiency virus, types 1 and 2	Acquired immunodeficiency syndrome (AIDS)
Influenza viruses	Influenza; new reassortants, mutants
Legionella pneumophilia	Legionnaires' disease; air-conditioning plants
Agents with new disease associations	
Herpesviruses 6 and 7	AIDS
Filoviruses	
Ebola, Marburg, Reston	Transmission to man
Bunyaviruses	
Hanta, Rift Valley Fever	Transmission to man
Arenaviruses	
Lassa fever	Transmission to man
Borrelia burgdorferi	Lyme disease
Helicobacter pylori	Gastric ulcers
Staphylococcus aureus	Toxic shock syndrome
Chlamydia pneumoniae	Pneumonia
Reemerging infectious agents*	
Togaviruses	
Venezuelan encephalitis	Mosquito-borne
Ross River	Mosquito-borne
Flaviviruses	
Dengue	Mosquito-borne
Yellow fever	Mosquito-borne
Japanese encephalitis	Mosquito-borne
Tick-borne encephalitis	Mosquito-borne
Protozoan	
Malaria	Mosquito-borne
New epidemics	
Mycobacteria tuberculosis	AIDS; drug resistance (global)
Vibrio cholerae	Cholera (South America, Bangladesh)
Yersinia pestis	Plague
Escherichia coli, O157:H7	Hemolytic uremic syndrome

*Commonly vector-borne agents, expedited by spraying deficits and drug resistance.

variable efficacy. Others, such as the measles vaccine, are highly effective in many but not all situations. Table 1.4.3 lists some viral and bacterial vaccines that are candidates for replacement, for modification, or for which a supplemental different vaccine would be useful. For some, the cost is a barrier to their wider use; for OPV and measles vaccines, increased heat stability is highly desirable; for others, such as BCG and *V. cholerae* vaccines, preparations of greater efficacy are required.

1.4.4. Infectious Agents Targeted for Vaccine Development

The development of new technologies, particularly those based on recombinant DNA technology, has in theory made possible the development of vaccines to many agents for which vaccine development previously was considered to be difficult or

TABLE 1.4.3. *A need for improvements to current vaccines*

Vaccine	Needs
Viral vaccine	
Vaccinia	Use as a live vector
Rabies	More affordable, as a chimeric virus (?)
Influenza	Attenuated live virus, intranasal inoculation
Poliovirus	More heat stable
Measles	More heat stable, effective in the presence of maternal antibody
Japanese encephalitis	More affordable
Bacterial vaccines	
Mycobacterium tuberculosis	Higher efficacy
Vibrio cholerae	Higher efficacy
Bordetella pertussis	Subunit vaccine, less reactogenic
Additional bacterial capsular antigens/protein conjugates	
Streptococcus pneumoniae	Higher efficacy
Neisseria meningitidis	Higher efficacy

impossible. This has resulted in a reappraisal of the infectious diseases for which no vaccines are currently available. Table 1.4.4 lists some candidates for vaccine development and the different age groups to which they may be administered.[113,114] The major difference from current practices is the large number of vaccines that could be administered to adolescents. Many pathogens cause sexually transmitted diseases, and in view of the changing sexual practices in many societies, the young adolescent seems the obvious target for administration of these vaccines. Not included in Table 1.4.4 are vaccines against diseases that are prevalent in tropical countries. These include the major parasitic infections, especially malaria, leishmaniasis, schistosomiasis, giardia, toxoplasma, and entamoeba, as well as dengue

TABLE 1.4.4. *Some disease agents targeted for vaccine development and for use in infants, adolescents, and adults*

Infants	Adolescents	Adults
Influenza (ca)	HIV 1 and 2	HIV 1 and 2
Parainfluenza	Herpesvirus-2	HTLV
Respiratory syncytial virus	*Chlamydia*	*Helicobacter pylori*
Rotavirus	Gonococcus	Malaria
Hepatitis A virus	Cytomegalovirus	*Staphylococcus*
Dengue virus	*Treponema*	Influenza (ca)
Malaria*	Epstein-Barr virus	Leprosy
	Hepatitis C virus	*Shigella*
	Human papillomavirus	Leishmaniasis
	Borrelia burgdorferi	

ca, cold adapted; HIV, human immunodeficiency virus; HTLV, human T-cell lymphotropic virus.
*In endemic countries.

viruses, Hantaan virus, and the bacterium causing chancroid, *Haemophilus ducreyi*.

It is usually risky to predict the time when vaccines will become available because many factors can influence their development (see Section 5), but of those listed in Table 1.4.4, a few may be licensed within 5 years. The list could include respiratory syncytial, *ca*-influenza, rota, varicella, and dengue viruses. Only time will tell.

SECTION 2

The Mammalian Immune System

CHAPTER 2.1. THE NATURE AND CONTRIBUTION OF INNATE IMMUNITY

The two major types of immune responses are called the specific response and the response due to innate immunity (ie, selective or less-specific responses) of the host. Specific responses are characterized by two main properties, exquisite specificity and memory, which are the exclusive properties of lymphocytes. Innate immunity is important because it is the initial response of the body to an infection, and although components of this response lack the exquisite specificity that can be a feature of the adaptive immune response, at least one component, natural killer (NK) cells, can show a considerable degree of selectivity in distinguishing between infected or malignant cells and normal cells. However, NK cells do not distinguish cells infected by, for example, quite different viruses. Some of the features of this type of response are described in this chapter.

2.1.1. Innate Immunity

Two components contribute to the responses of innate immunity. First, inducible soluble factors, such as the interferons (IFNs), are produced and secreted from a variety of cell types, and they may bind to and affect the activity of other cells. Second, the complement cascade may also be important during the specific response.

One of the earliest manifestations of an infection, particularly an acute infection, may be fever, which is described as the controlled elevation of body temperature above the normal range and is mediated by endogenous cytokines called pyrogens (reviewed elsewhere[115–117]). The body temperature of healthy persons is normally regulated between 36°C and 37.5°C independently of external conditions. The peak temperatures achieved in most fevers rarely exceed 41°C: temperatures above this level are called hyperpyrexia and are caused by other factors. The heat-generating and heat-loss responses take place in the hypothalamus, which contains temperature-sensitive neurons. Heat and cold receptors located in the skin and other parts of the body send impulses to the hypothalamus.

A list of some pyrogens relevant to infectious processes and the cytokines they induce is given in Table 2.1.1.1. The pyrogenic activity of the endotoxins of gram-negative bacteria is caused by the lipid A component, as anti-lipid A antibodies abolish the effect. The pyrogenic exotoxins of *Staphylococcus aureus* and group A

TABLE 2.1.1.1. *Pyrogens involved in the pathogenesis of fever*

Exogenous pyrogens
  Microbial products: lipopolysaccharides such as endotoxins from gram-negative bacteria;
    exotoxins such as those from *Staphylococcus aureus* and group A streptococci
  Host-derived products; antigen-antibody complexes; components of complement; products
    of tissue necrosis

Endogenous pyrogenic cytokines
  Interleukin-1, tumor necrosis factor alpha, interferons, interleukin-6
  Prostaglandins

streptococci trigger pyrogenic cytokine release from macrophages. These exotoxins bind to a segment of certain T-cell receptors (TCRs) present in some persons. Because a high proportion of T cells may be so involved and activated, this binding can cause a massive release of cytokines, which results in fever and shock (ie, toxic shock syndrome). The toxins act as superantigens. Antigen-antibody complexes and the C5a fragment of complement are also pyrogenic.

Some effects of pyrogenic cytokines on different cellular components involved in host defenses are listed in Table 2.1.1.2. Tumor necrosis factor-α (TNFα) and interleukin-1 (IL-1) have a central role. IL-1 is produced by a wide range of cells,

TABLE 2.1.1.2. *Effects of the pyrogenic cytokines, IL-1, TNFα, and IFNγ on cells involved in the early responses to infections*

Natural killer cells
  Enhancement of cytotoxicity (IL-1,* TNFα, IFNγ)
  Induction of IFNγ production (IL-1, TNFα)
Macrophages
  Enhanced chemotaxis (IL-1, TNFα)
  Induction of G-CSF production (IL-1, TNFα)
  Activation of cytotoxic and microbicidal activities (IFNγ)
  Enhanced class I and II MHC expression (IFNγ)
Neutrophils (eg, granulocytes, polymorphonuclear cells)
  Release from marrow storage pool, enhanced endothelial adherence and degranulation
    (IL-1, TNFα)
  Enhanced chemotaxis (TNFα)
  Enhanced oxidative activity (IFNγ)
Eosinophils
  Enhanced endothelial adherence and killing of schistosomes (IL-1, TNFα)
Endothelium
  Secretion of IL-1, expression of adhesion proteins, ICAM-1 and ELAM-1
  Secretion of leukopoietic factors, G-CSF, M-CSF, GM-CSF (IL-1, TNFα)
Fibroblasts, epithelial cells
  Secretion of IFNβ (IL-1?, TNFα?)

CSF, colony-stimulating factor; M, macrophage; G, granulocyte; ELAM, endothelial-leukocyte adhesion molecule; ICAM, intracellular adhesion molecule; IL, interleukin; IFN, interferon; TNF, tumor necrosis factor.
*IL-1 is also involved in the induction of lymphocyte-mediated responses.
Adapted from Root RK. (1996) Host responses to infection: fever, hyperthermia and hypothermia. In: Root RK, Stamm W, Waldvogel F, Corey L, eds. Clinical infectious diseases: a practical approach. Oxford University Press, Oxford.

including macrophages, lymphocytes, and endothelial cells, and it exists in two forms: IL-1α and IL-1β. Although structurally different, both forms of IL-1 bind to similar receptors that are present on many cell types. Injection of TNFα, IL-2, or IL-6 induces fevers similar to those induced by IL-1. The sequence of appearance of these factors in the plasma of humans or rabbits made febrile from lipopolysaccharide injections is TNFα (minutes), IL-1 (within 30 minutes), and IFNγ (after 1 hour). In this case, the IFNγ is secreted from NK cells rather than from lymphocytes.

There seems to be a common mechanism of action by these cytokines: the induction of synthesis and release of prostaglandin, especially PGE_2, probably by endothelial cells in the hypothalamus. PGE_2 can inhibit IL-1 and TNFα production. Substances such as aspirin that inhibit cyclooxygenase prevent the formation of PGE_2.

Because fever in response to infection is such a common phenomenon in vertebrates, it might be expected to be beneficial to the host. Multiplication of some pathogens is inhibited at febrile temperatures. Human neutrophil function and macrophage oxidative metabolism are increased at 40°C but are lost at higher temperatures. The antiviral and antitumor activity of IFNs, IL-1–induced T-cell activation, IL-2 production, and T-cell help for B cells are increased at febrile temperatures. The activity of cytotoxic T lymphocytes (CTLs) is also increased at febrile temperatures.[118,119] Consequently, fever in humans is generally a beneficial response to infection.

2.1.2. Effects of Pyrogenic Cytokines on Cells That Contribute to Innate Immunity

Many cell types respond rapidly to infections, and the nature and effectiveness of this response is the result of the effect of the pyrogenic cytokines. Table 2.1.1.2 summarizes some of the effects induced by these cytokines on six different cell types or groups of cells. Activation of these cells forms the first line of defense of the body, and the activation of some cells is important in the subsequent involvement of the lymphocyte in the adaptive immune response. Neutrophils, mast cells, and eosinophils are important in certain situations.

In humans, a mild influenza infection may be confined to the upper respiratory tract. The ferret demonstrates a similar disease progression, and for this reason, it has been a useful model for studying the early host response at this site. The inflammatory response results in the extrusion of neutrophils onto the mucosal surface, where infection occurs.[120] There is a correlation between the extent of fever and the rate of decline of viral titers, because suppression of fever results in a delayed viral clearance.[121]

Among the most important products of activated cells are the IFNs (Table 2.1.2). IFNα and IFNβ (both are type I) are closely related structurally, but IFNγ (type II, sometimes called immune interferon) is quite different and was initially called an

TABLE 2.1.2. *Properties and activities of the interferons*

Property	IFNα	IFNβ	IFNγ
Nomenclature	Type I, leukocyte	Type I, fibroblast	Type II, immune
Major inducers	Viruses	Viruses, LPS ds-poly RNA	Antigens, mitogens
Cellular source	T, B cells and macrophages	Fibroblasts and epithelial cells	T cells and NK cells
Activities			
Antiviral	+ + +	+ + +	+
Upregulation of MHC antigens	+ (class I)	+ (class I)	+ + + (class I, II)

MHC, major histocompatibility complex; ds, double-stranded; NK, natural killer; LPS, lipopolysaccharides; +, weak; + + +, strong.

IFN because it also had antiviral activity. Studies have subsequently shown that the direct antiviral activities of IFNα and IFNβ are 10 to 100 times greater than that of IFNγ. Conversely, IFNγ is 100 to 10,000 times more active as an immunomodulator than IFNα and IFNβ. The role and importance of IFNγ is discussed in more detail later in this chapter.

Treatment of mice with *Cryptosporidium parvum* before influenza virus infection results in lower lung viral titers and decreased mortality, and this correlates with higher levels of IFNα, IFNβ, NK cells, and activated macrophages in the lung.[122] Mice bearing the *Mx* gene are resistant to influenza virus infection, a finding attributed to an enhanced sensitivity to IFN because the effect is abolished by treatment with anti-IFN antisera.[123]

Most and perhaps all of these cell types secrete various cytokines and bear receptors for other cytokines. From the point of view of immune response induction after immunization, NK cells and macrophages occupy a special position.

2.1.2.1. Neutrophils

Neutrophils (ie, granulocytes or polymorphonuclear cells[124]) are the most abundant white blood cells in the body. Approximately 50% of the cells in the bone marrow are neutrophils and their precursors. Their half-life in the blood is 6 to 10 hours, and about 10 billion are produced daily to maintain the appropriate level in the blood. To expend so much energy on the constant replacement of one cell type can only mean that these cells are crucial for the body's defenses. They are the first line of defense, particularly against bacteria and fungal infections, organisms that can have an extremely rapid replication time. Neutrophils appear within minutes at the site of an injury, followed some hours later by macrophages. Reductions in the number of neutrophils and defects in their function increase the risk of prolonged or recurrent infections with staphylococci, encapsulated bacteria, gram-negative bacilli, and fungi.[125]

2.1.2.2. Natural Killer Cells

NK cells represent a small population of leukocytes and are found in blood and peripheral lymphoid tissues.[126,127] They were initially defined by their ability to kill certain tumor cells and virus-infected cells but not normal cells. They may also contribute to the rejection of allografts, especially in graft-versus-host disease. NK cells do not have the type of receptor found on lymphocytes. In contrast to T cells that recognize peptides associated with major histocompatibility complex (MHC) antigens (see Chapter 2.2), NK cells preferentially lyse target cells that express little or no class I MHC antigens. There appear to be two different families of receptors that can inhibit NK cell activation after MHC recognition (reviewed elsewhere[128]). Two types of other receptor-like molecules have been identified on murine NK cells. Activation of NK1.1 enhances lytic activity, and activation of LY-49 inhibits this activity. NK cells lyse target cells by a mechanism that is similar to that employed by CTLs and that is described in Chapter 2.2. In the absence of lymphocyte-based immunity, as in severe combined immunodeficient (SCID) mice, infectious agents usually are not cleared despite the presence of NK cells.[129]

2.1.2.3. Monocytes and Macrophages

Cells of the monocyte-macrophage lineage occupy a central role in the defense system of the body. Although mouse strains have been developed that do not have functional lymphocytes (eg, SCID mice) or that are deficient in NK cells (eg, NK-deficient C57Bl\6 beige mice), a mouse strain has yet to be developed that does not have functional macrophages. Macrophages are involved from the very beginning of the host response to the very end, when they act as scavengers to clear away cell debris. They can be rapidly activated, they are able to destroy some intracellular microbes, and they function as antigen-presenting cells (APCs).

2.1.3. Interferon Gamma Production and its Role as an Immunomodulator

IFNγ was originally thought to be an exclusive product of T lymphocytes, but the availability of SCID mice changed this view. SCID mice cannot generate rearranged TCRs and immunoglobulin genes and therefore do not have functional T and B cells. It was first found that SCID mice infected with a low (sublethal) dose of *Listeria monocytogenes* resisted the infection and contained activated, class II MHC–positive macrophages. This resistance depended on IFNγ. Mice pretreated with anti-IFNγ before infection failed to develop class II MHC–positive macrophages and died of infection. Spleen cells from SCID mice stimulated in vitro with heat-killed *Listeria* produced IFNγ. This was prevented if the spleen cells were pretreated with anti-asialo GM$_1$ (a surface marker for NK cells) and complement.[130]

Later studies showed that the generation of IFNγ by NK cells depended on macrophages, IL-12 and TNFα. Injection of anti-TNFα antiserum into SCID mice prevented the production of IFNγ and induction of an anti-*Listeria* response. Macrophages from these mice did not have elevated class II MHC expression, and the bacteria were still present in the liver and spleen. In vitro cell depletion studies showed that macrophages were the source of the TNFα. IFNγ production only occurred in the presence of macrophages and bacteria or in the presence of macrophages, soluble bacterial products, and TNFα.

Receptors for IFNγ are ubiquitously expressed on most cells, an indication of the importance of this cytokine. A major function of IFNγ is to increase class I and II MHC antigen expression on most cells, although it inhibits class II expression on B cells.[131] It enhances class I MHC antigen expression by twofold to fourfold, and it induces class I and II MHC expression on cells that normally do not express these antigens. TNFα may synergistically add to this effect.[132]

Cells of the macrophage lineage are a prime target for IFNγ. This cytokine has been shown to promote several actions:

1. Differentiation of immature myeloid precursors into mature monocytes[133]
2. Antigen-presenting capability of macrophages by the upregulation of class II MHC expression and enhancement of the transcription of some auxiliary molecules, such as proteases and peptide transporters that are involved in antigen processing[133]
3. Expression of other cell-surface antigens, such as ICAM, that are involved in macrophage and T-cell interactions[134]
4. Nonspecific cytocidal activity toward many intracellular and extracellular parasites and neoplastic cells by the elaboration of compounds such as reactive oxygen and nitrogen intermediates and TNFα. Mice pretreated with neutralizing anti-IFNγ monoclonal antibodies (MAbs) usually do not resolve low-level microbial infections by organisms such as *Listeria*,[135] *Toxoplasma*,[136] and *Leishmania*.[137]
5. Resistance of macrophages to microbial infection[130]

It appears most likely that the mechanism of intracellular killing of microbes such as some bacteria and parasites, at least in murine macrophages, is by nitric oxide (NO). The enzymatic conversion of L-arginine to L-citrulline generates NO, a reaction catalyzed by nitric oxide synthase (NOS). In mice, intracellular killing of several microbes can be inhibited by treatment with inhibitors of NOS (reviewed elsewhere[133]).

The extent to which these mechanisms are induced by other agents such as viruses is unclear, although the ability of IFNγ to inhibit replication of ectromelia, vaccinia, and herpes simplex viruses in macrophages correlates with the cellular production of NO.[138] Infection of mice by many viruses enhances NK cell activity,[139] and it is to be expected that this would result in IFNγ production. However, some viruses, such as the human immunodeficiency virus (HIV), replicate quite well in macrophages, suggesting that intracellular killing by NO is not a general phenomenon.

Activities of Components of the Complement System

In the absence of antibody, the complement cascade can be activated by a pathway that is initiated by the binding of the third component of complement (C3b) to the surface of an activating particle, such as a bacterium, virus, or parasite. An enveloped virus may be inactivated in this way, and this has been reported for Sindbis virus[140] but not for Ross River Virus (RRV).[141] It is reported that RRV inhibits the cleavage of C3 by the classic or the alternative pathway of activation. This effect may contribute to RRV's success as a human pathogen, because this property could be predicted to retard viral clearance from the blood of infected persons.[141]

Parasites, especially those that live in the blood such as schistosomes and *Trypanosoma brucei*, must develop strategies to resist the action of complement. As many as six mechanisms exist to achieve this purpose (reviewed elsewhere[142]).

Links Between Innate and Adaptive Immunity

The activation and maturation of innate immune responses, culminating in the early production of TNFα and IFNγ, facilitates the effectiveness of the subsequent adaptive responses. During an inflammatory response, T cells leave the circulation and migrate to the sites of an infection. They must first bind to and then pass through the vascular endothelium. A combination of IFNγ and TNFα has been found to enhance the expression of ICAM-1, ELAM-1, and class I MHC antigens on cultured umbilical vein endothelial cells.[143] Enhanced expression of these three proteins was found in skin biopsy specimens of baboons treated with both cytokines.[144]

IFNγ enhances the biosynthesis of some complement proteins in macrophages and increases the expression of complement and high-affinity Fc receptors on monocyte-macrophages,[145,146] promoting subsequent humoral immunity. A transmembrane form of TNFα is present on activated CD4 + T-cell clones and provides a co-stimulatory signal for human B-cell activation.[147] NK cells can donate cytokines that induce B-cell differentiation after exposure to T-cell–independent antigens.[148]

Once activated, fragments of C3, C3dg, and C3d, bind to CD21 on B lymphocytes. CD21 associates with CD19, a B-cell membrane protein that enhances B-cell activation and is required for normal B-cell responses (reviewed elsewhere[149]). Advantage has been taken of these associations by conjugating C3 fragments to an antigen. The result was to greatly increase the immunogenicity of the protein (see Section 4.2.2).

An equally fascinating affiliation is the complementary activities of NK cells and of CTLs. NK cells preferentially lyse cells expressing little or no class I MHC antigens, but the opposite is true for CTLs. This may be of special relevance to the control of tumors and should be considered when designing anti-tumor immunotherapy.

CHAPTER 2.2. THE NATURE OF THE MAMMALIAN ADAPTIVE IMMUNE SYSTEM

Infectious agents can gain entry to their future hosts mainly in three ways: by minor trauma, such as a scratch in the skin (eg, pox viruses) or damage to a mucosal surface (eg, anal sex); by direct access to the circulation, by the bite of a vector such as an infected mosquito, or through an open wound (eg, genital sores); or by infection at a mucosal surface of the respiratory, digestive, or genital tracts. Although the mucosal surface area is far greater than the skin area, with many access routes (and many infectious agents infect by that route), most vaccines are administered parenterally to invoke systemic immune responses. This may change in the future. Chapter 2.3 describes the features of the mucosal immune system that are important for protection from agents infecting by that route.

Most features of the mammalian immune system are common to the systemic and mucosal compartments. There are two parts, the primary and secondary lymphoid organs. The primary lymphoid organs are the bone marrow and the thymus in mammals, but in birds, they are the bone marrow, bursa, and thymus. In these organs, precursor T and B lymphocytes develop and differentiate into mature, immunocompetent cells. In the case of T cells, this includes learning self and nonself discrimination. Most T cells with anti-self specificity are destroyed (a feature of tolerance) in the thymus. In both cases, accomplishing the final goal of immunocompetent cells that respond mainly to foreign antigens to make a protective immune response involves a tremendous amount of cell death. The mature, immunocompetent but antigen-naive cells are seeded from the primary organs to the secondary organs, the spleen and lymph nodes (reviewed elsewhere[150,151]).

Although much of our understanding of the system came about through the use of simple antigens, some semisynthetic or completely synthetic, the use of infectious agents or their products have frequently given a deeper insight into the activity and role of some components.

Recognition of Antigens by B and T Lymphocytes

2.2.1.1. Receptors for Antigens

B cells have two classes of immunoglobulin receptors, IgM and IgD receptors. Both are dimeric molecules with two antigen binding sites, each of which is constructed of the variable (V) segments or domains of two light and two heavy chains. The structure of the dimeric form of IgM is shown in Figure 2.2.1.1.[152] Generally, the affinity of binding of each site of each dimer on antigen-naive cells for the epitopes (ie, antigenic determinants) of antigens is relatively low. If both binding sites are occupied, which may occur if antigens have repeating epitopes, the total avidity of binding is substantially higher. Many infectious agents, particularly viruses, expose at their surfaces such patterns of repeating epitopes. After activation,

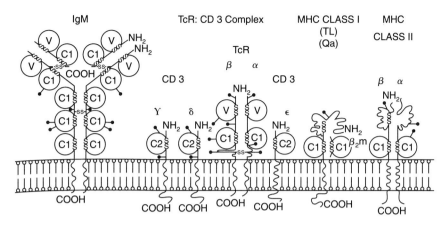

FIG. 2.2.1.1. Some members of the immunoglobulin superfamily. (From Williams AF, Barclay AN. [1988] The immunoglobulin superfamily—domains for cell surface recognition. Ann Rev Immunol 6:381–405.)

B cells may secrete IgM molecules, although in the form of a pentameric molecule (with 10 binding sites) with an attached J chain. In contrast, IgD molecules are not secreted by activated cells. Attempts to define different roles for IgM and IgD receptors have so far been largely unsuccessful. Experiments with knockout mice that do not express IgD receptors showed that, after exposure to antigen, the production of high-affinity Ig was delayed by a few days.[153] After activation and switching of Ig isotypes, memory B cells may express other Ig isotypes—IgG, IgA, or IgE—as receptors for antigen. Their structures are similar to that of the IgM receptor, except that each heavy chain contains only three constant domains.

In contrast, the TCR of most T cells is composed of two short chains, α and β, each composed of only a single variable and constant domain. The variable domains contribute the antigen binding sites. A minor group of T cells has two different chains, called γ and δ. In both cases, the receptors exist as a membrane-bound complex with three chains of a T-cell marker, the CD3 molecule (see Fig. 2.2.1.1).

2.2.1.2. What the Lymphocyte Receptors See

Ig receptors recognize a shape, called an epitope. For proteins and polysaccharides, the basic shape is composed of 5 to 6 amino acids or sugars, yielding a surface area of 250 to 400 A^2. Other adjacent groups may also have a secondary role in the binding such that the total surface area of contact and of interaction may increase substantially.[154] In five cases in which crystals of antigen-antibody complexes have been subject to x-ray analysis, the area of interaction has varied between 700 and 800 A^2, and 15 to 22 amino acid residues of the antigen were identified as being in contact with residues of the antibody.[155] Epitopes may be provided by continuous or discontinuous sequences of amino acids, sugars, or both components of a protein, glycoprotein, or polysaccharide, and some possibilities are illustrated in Figure 2.2.1.2. The antigen is represented by a simple linear polypeptide and shows loop-like structures that are common; there is sometimes crosslinking by disulfide bonds at the base of a loop, which confers greater conformational stability. The area recognized by an antibody or Ig receptor is for convenience designated by a circle. Two examples are given of recognition of continuous linear sequences and of discontinuous sequences.

The conformation of any segment may change according to the amino acid sequence, not only (as would be expected) within an epitope, but also outside the epitope. Two examples of the latter situation are shown with proteins of HIV and of foot and mouth disease virus (FMDV). The antigens gp120 of HIV and VP1 of FMDV contain an important peptide loop crosslinked at the base by a disulfide

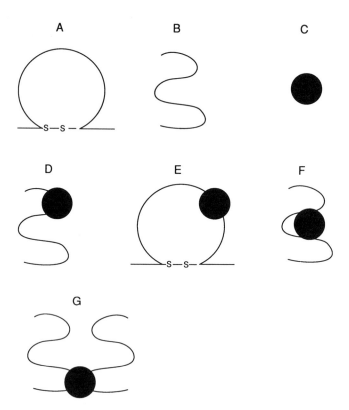

FIG. 2.2.1.2. Examples of continuous (linear) and discontinuous (nonlinear) epitopes (shapes) seen by the antigen-binding sites of antibodies. (**A**) A continuous sequence in the shape of a loop linked by a disulfide bond. (**B**) A linear sequence without a covalent linking bond. (**C**) The epitope seen by the antigen-binding site of the antibody. (**D,E**) Linear sequences are recognized. (**F**) An epitope formed by nonlinear sequences is recognized. (**G**) An epitope can be formed by adjacent sequences of contiguous molecules.

bond. MAbs have been prepared that recognize different epitopes within the loops. However, in each case, a single amino acid change outside the loop interferes with the recognition of the loop by one or more of the MAbs.[156,157] At least experimentally, the Ig receptor on B cells may recognize structures as dissimilar as a small oligopeptide or saccharide and an intact virus particle.

The TCR sees a class I or II MHC molecule that contains a peptide bound in a groove of the MHC molecule that protrudes from the plasma membrane of an APC or a target cell. With class II, the variable regions of the α and β chains contribute to the groove, and the peptide can vary from 12 to 25 amino acids, with a mean length of about 15 amino acids.[158] In the case of class I MHC molecules, there is only a single chain to which another molecule, β_2-microglobulin, binds noncovalently. This attachment is necessary for the subsequent binding of a peptide, which in this case is much more restricted in length (8 to 10 amino acids); the commonest length is a nonamer, a size that allows the peptide to be entirely contained within the groove.[159] In both situations, the peptide and the portion of the MHC molecule forming the groove comprise the epitope recognized by the TCR. In this case, the peptide component is referred to as a *determinant*.

2.2.2. Presentation of Antigen to Lymphocytes

2.2.2.1. Properties of Antigen-Presenting Cells

The efficient presentation of antigen to lymphocytes, especially T cells, requires the APC to have certain characteristics. Table 2.2.2.1 lists the common APCs that interact with and lead to the activation of CD4 + or CD8 + T cells, together with factors that contribute to the interaction.[160] In one case, B cells, which have already seen antigen, are the target cells, and the events that occur here are described in Section 2.2.5.2.

Follicular dendritic cells (FDCs) also act as APCs. Dendritic cells should not be confused with FDCs (see Table 2.2.2.1 and Section 2.2.5.2). Both have extensive cytoplasmic protrusions, called dendrites, providing very large surface areas. Their origin and method of antigen presentation differ. Dendritic cells were originally called "veiled cells" because of the extensive folding of their plasma membrane.

The main APCs, sometimes called professional APCs because of their efficacy, are macrophages, dendritic cells, and B cells. They display two basic properties: expression of class I or II MHC antigens, depending on the cell to be activated, and one or more types of co-stimulator molecules. *Co-stimulation* is a term invented[161] to describe the need for an additional signal and presentation of antigen to a TCR to activate a T cell. Different co-stimulator molecules have been described, but B7, which exists in two forms, B7.1 and 7.2, is the most important. T cells must express a corresponding ligand for interaction, and this is predominantly the CD28 molecule. Expression of these molecules is enhanced by other cytokines, such as IFNγ, and this interaction also leads to cell activation. The cytokine IL-7,[162] which is

TABLE 2.2.2.1. *Properties of antigen-presenting cells involved in activation of CD4+ and CD8+ T cells*

APC	Expression of class II MHC antigens	Expression of class I MHC antigens	Expression of co-stimulator	Modulation by cytokines	Target cells
Macrophages	Constitutive, IFNγ enhances		Present, activation enhances	IFNγ enhances, IL-10 inhibits	CD4 + T-cells
		Present, activation IFNγ enhances	Present, activation enhances?	IFNγ enhances	CD8 + T cells
Dendritic cells*	Constitutive, high		High	GMCSF, IL-1 enhances (in culture)	CD4 + T cells
		High	High	?	CD8 + T cells
B cells	Constitutive, IL4 enhances	Low	Higher after activation	Enhances APC capacity	CD4 + T cells
CD4 + T cells	Constitutive (in humans)	High	Higher after activation	IFNγ enhances	CD4 + T cells
			Higher after activation	IFNγ enhances	CD8 + T cells

APC, antigen-presenting cells; MHC, major histocompatibility complex; IFN, interferon; IL, interleukin; GMSCF, granulocyte-macrophage colony-stimulating factor.

*Including Langerhans cells. Follicular dendritic cells (FDCs) present antigen, in the form of antigen-antibody complexes, to B cells. The complexes are attached by FcR and CR to the outside of the plasma membrane and are involved in the generation and subsequent recruitment of memory B cells to form antibody-secreting cells. FDCs also express class II MHC antigens. Whether the antigen is ever endocytosed, processed, and serves to activate passing T cells is unknown.

Adapted from Unanue ER. (1993) Macrophages, antigen-presenting cells and the phenomena of antigen handling and presentation. In: Paul WE, ed. Fundamental immunology. 3rd ed. Raven Press, New York, pp. 111–144.

important in the induction of CTLs,[163–165] is also a potent inducer of co-stimulator molecules.[166]

In vivo, macrophages develop from a progenitor cell in the bone marrow under the influence of several colony-stimulating factors (CSFs). They leave the blood-stream and settle down and persist for very long periods in sites such as the sinus of lymphoid tissues, where they are exposed to foreign antigens. A major activity of macrophages is scavenging, and they actively phagocytose particulate material such as bacteria (reviewed elsewhere[160]).

The other principal APCs for T cells, dendritic cells, are more mobile. They are present in the blood, and such cells in the afferent lymph are deposited in the T-cell–rich areas of the draining lymph nodes—an effective way to deliver and present foreign antigens, particularly intracellular material, to organized lymphoid tissues. One form of dendritic cell, the Langerhans cell, is found in the epidermis, skin appendages, and squamous mucosal epithelia, such as that in the vagina, cervix, and esophagus. These cells also carry foreign material to the draining lymph nodes. Once located there, they are referred to as "interdigitating cells." Dendritic cells are poorly phagocytic, unlike macrophages.

2.2.2.2. Antigen Processing

Noninfectious preparations often may be internalized by a receptor-mediated process (eg, by Fc or C receptors) into endosomes, which then fuse with lysosomes to form an endolysosome. Proteolysis in the prevailing mild acid conditions generates peptides. Elsewhere, class II MHC molecules as αβ dimers complex with an invariant chain and move to the trans-Golgi network, where they are targeted to the endosome. In this mildly acid environment, they bind the antigenic peptides and discard the invariant chain, and the peptide-MHC complex is transported to the cell surface, where it may be recognized by a CD4+ T cell. This is called the *exogenous antigen pathway* of antigen processing.

An infectious particle, such as a virus, bacterium, or parasite, may infect an APC, productively or abortively. A virus, for example, may enter the cell by receptor-mediated endocytosis (eg, influenza) or by fusion with the plasma membrane (eg, Sendai) and is delivered to an endosome. An enveloped viral particle may fuse with the endosome membrane and, in so doing, liberate the RNA or DNA into the cytoplasm. This opens the way for translation and transcription of the nucleic acid, with the synthesis of new viral protein, some of which is degraded to peptide by enzymes that form part of a large multifunctional protease (ie, proteasome). One possibility is that during synthesis the protein is particularly susceptible to degradation by proteases, such as before the conformationally intact antigen is formed. The peptides are moved into the lumen of the endoplasmic reticulum by a transporter of antigenic peptides (TAP); they combine with class I MHC antigens and are translocated to the cell surface, where the complex may be recognized by a CD8+ T cell.

This is called the *cytosolic or endogenous pathway*. Most or all newly synthesized proteins, including self proteins, contribute peptides through this pathway.[167]

Some exogenous antigens of infectious agents are presented by means of the endogenous pathway (reviewed elsewhere[168]). Some bacteria and parasites infect mainly macrophages and replicate in endosomes. However, *L. monocytogenes* and virulent *Mycobacterium tuberculosis* secrete cytolysins that allow escape of the bacterial proteins from the macrophage endosome into the cytoplasm. Other bacteria, such as *Mycobacterium bovis* and *Salmonella typhimurium*, replicate in the endosome, and the peptides from degraded antigens bind mainly to class II MHC molecules. Using specific transporter systems, some antigenic peptides escape into the cytoplasm and bind to class I MHC molecules. Similarly, some parasites infect cells and replicate in vacuoles or phagolysosomes. A major surface protein of *Toxoplasma gondii* escapes into the cytoplasm after the membranes of the infected cell's vacuoles and those of the parasite fuse. Some antigens of *Leishmania major* also seem to escape from the infected phagolysosome into the cytoplasm.

Processing of antigens by either route results in activation of APCs, which may increase the expression of different components. External stimuli such as IFNγ induce or enhance the expression of co-stimulators and MHC antigens. APCs also may liberate a variety of factors that enhance the activities of other cells (Table 2.2.2.2). As well as secreting a variety of cytokines that promote fever (see Section 2.1), macrophages secrete factors that affect connective tissues, complement proteins, and CSFs; that regulate lymphocyte responses; and some that promote tissue repair.[160]

Because the peptides are bound noncovalently to the MHC antigen, direct exposure of APCs to other appropriate peptides may result in attachment to already exposed but "empty" MHC molecules. This has proved to be a convenient means

---

TABLE 2.2.2.2. *Secretory products of macrophages*

Proteins involved in defense and inflammation
Complement proteins, C2, C3, C4, C5
Lysosyme, fibronectin
Growth and differentiation regulatory factors
G-CSF, M-CSF, GM-CSF
Cytokines that regulate lymphocyte responses
IL-1, 6, 8, 10, 12
IL-1 receptor agonist
Factors that promote tissue repair
Platelet-derived growth factor
Fibroblast growth factor

CSF, colony-stimulating factor; G, granulocyte; IL, interleukin; M, macrophage.
Adapted from Unanue ER. (1993) Macrophages, antigen-presenting cells and the phenomena of antigen handling and presentation. In: Paul WE, ed. Fundamental immunology, 3rd ed. Raven Press, New York, pp. 111–144.

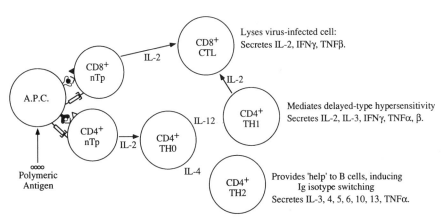

FIG. 2.2.3. Antigen presentation and T-cell activation APC, antigen-presenting cell; ♈ and ♥, class I and II MHC antigens; ○, ●, peptides from degraded antigen bound to MHC molecules; ∨, T-cell receptor; CD4, △, and CD8, ▲, T-cell differentiation antigens; �, co-stimulator molecules on APC; ⨆, ligand on T-cell recognizing co-stimulator molecules; nTp, naive precursor T cells; TH0, early activated CD4 + T cell; Il, interleukin; TH1, TH2, and CTLs, regulatory on effector T cells. (From Nathanson N. [1996] Viral pathogenesis. Lippincott–Raven Publishers, Philadelphia.)

for preparing APCs for stimulation of specific T-cell responses and for making appropriate target cells to be used in CTL assays. There are a number of methods other than the use of infectious preparations for inducing class I MHC expression of peptides of particular antigens, as described in Section 4.2.3.

2.2.3. Activation and Differentiation of T Cells

Figure 2.2.3 illustrates the interaction between the APCs and the naive, immunocompetent T cells and the subsequent replication and differentiation of the T-cell subsets. The TCR (see Section 2.2.2) in association with the CD4 or CD8 molecule recognizes the peptide-MHC complex, and the induced co-stimulator on the APC is recognized by the corresponding ligand on the T cell. This initiates activation of the T cell, which first produces IL-2 and then the IL-2 receptor (IL-2R). This leads to differentiation of the cells to the regulator or effector state.

2.2.3.1. CD4 + T Cells in Mice

It was originally thought that CD4 + T cells formed a single population with two main functions: to help B cells produce antibodies (ie, helper T cells) and to mediate delayed-type hypersensitivity reactions. The ability to clone T cells led to the discovery that these cells could be divided into at least two subclasses, which were called TH1 and TH2.[169] The distinction was based on the pattern of cytokines secreted by the cells and their biologic activity. This categorization has largely stood

TABLE 2.2.3.1. *Characteristics of T-cell subsets*

CD4 + T cells	
TH0	Secretes IL-2, 4, 5, 10 and IFNγ
	Provides help to B cells
TH1	Secretes IL-2, 3; IFNγ; TNFα, β
	Provides help for IgG2a (mice) and IgG1 (humans) production
	Mediates DTH reactions
	Primary cells may but usually do not lyse infected cells
TH2	Secretes IL-3, 4, 5, 6, 10, 13; TNFα
	Provides help for IgG1, IgA, and IgE production
CD8 + T cells	
Primary and cloned cells	Secretes Il-2, IFNγ, TNFβ
	Lyses infected cells shortly after infection
	Usually a poor mediator of DTH reactions
Mature cells cultured with	Fail to produce IL-2 or IFNγ; loses CTL activity
IL-4 or mitogens or	Secretes IL-4, 5, 10
allostimulated	Helps B cells to produce antibody

CTL, cytotoxic T lymphocyte; DTH, delayed-type hypersensitivity reaction; IFN, interferon; Ig, immunoglobulin; IL, interleukin; TNF, tumor necrosis factor.

the test of time, with some modifications.[170] The pattern originally proposed is still largely valid, but a population of cells (TH0) were later discovered that had a composite cytokine profile.[171,172] The cytokine secretion patterns and some activities of CD4 + T-cell subsets, as well as those of CD8 + CTLs, are shown in Table 2.2.3.1. There is some similarity between the profiles of TH1 and CTLs. One suggestion was that TH0 cells might be precursors to TH1 and TH2.[172] One difficulty with this proposal was finding that, at least in vitro, some cytokines are antagonistic. IL-4 and IFNγ are mutually inhibitory, and IL-10 inhibits the production of IFNγ. In situations like this, it is conceivable that the secretion pattern of cloned cells may be different, quantitatively or qualitatively, to that of an uncloned precursor as it exists in the body.

2.2.3.2. Roles of Interleukin-4 and Interleukin-12 in Murine Infections

In many model infections in which TH1 and TH2 cells are found, there are a few examples in which one or the other greatly predominates. *Leishmania* infection in mice has become the classic example. This organism elicits a strong TH1 response in C57 Bl/6 mice that recover from the infection. In contrast, BALB/c mice develop a TH2-type response and develop severe disease.[173,174] IFNγ seemed to be responsible for the protective response as a single injection of an anti-IFNγ MAb converted resistant mice into susceptible mice; in contrast, treatment of susceptible mice with an anti-IL-4 MAb cured the disease.[175,176]

It was later found that the macrophages of mice injected with heat-killed *L. monocytogenes* produced a new cytokine, IL-12, that induced the TH1 response.[177]

Administration of IL-12 cured mice infected with *L. major*.[178] The NK cells of these mice released high concentrations of IFNγ. IL-4 and IL-12 are considered to be critical cytokines that determine the subsequent balance between the CD4 + T-cell subsets, with IL-4 favoring a humoral response and IL-12 initiating cell-mediated immunity.[179] This dichotomy is reflected in Figure 2.2.3. However, it has also been demonstrated[180] that both beneficial or detrimental effects can be seen in mice, depending on the dose of LCMV (a noncytopathic virus) administered. Higher doses favored increased viral replication. The important roles of IL-2 have been reviewed in detail elsewhere.[181]

An alternative approach to selecting a TH1- or TH2-type T-cell response, revived by Peter Bretscher, is to induce states of immune deviation by varying the dose of antigen administered.[182,183] Subcutaneous injection of high doses of *L. major* into susceptible BALB/c mice induced a transient cell-mediated immunity (CMI) response, which decayed as increasing amounts of antibody were produced. In contrast, injection of very low doses of parasites induced only a CMI response; no lesion or a small lesion that resolved with time was seen. Later challenge of these mice with a high dose of parasite showed that they had become resistant. These observations were consistent with the type of cytokine profile seen. It was proposed that this might be a suitable strategy to test with vaccination against tuberculosis and leprosy.

2.2.3.3. CD4 + T-Cell Subsets in Humans

For a time, it seemed uncertain whether TH1 and TH2 T-cell subsets could be demonstrated in human immune responses, but accumulating evidence supports this scenario. For example, the examination of T-cell clones isolated from a donor who was immune to purified protein derivative and to a canine parasite showed a TH1 and TH2 cytokine pattern, respectively.[184] Other examples have been reviewed elsewhere.[185]

There has been consuming interest in the suggestion that a TH1 response is associated with resistance to HIV infection and that the TH2 cytokine pattern is more often related to disease susceptibility.[186,187] This has led to the hypothesis that a switch from TH1 to a TH2 pattern during infection might occur and be relevant to the progression toward acquired immunodeficiency syndrome (AIDS).[186] Despite intense investigation and discussion (reviewed elsewhere[187]), a consensus has not been reached. One of the difficulties in this area is that, other than the pattern of cytokines secreted, the two T-cell subsets cannot be distinguished. It also was rather belatedly realized that the cytokine profiles of CD4 + TH1 and CD8 + CTLs were rather similar and that, in the case of intracellular infections, effects attributed to TH1 T cells might be related to a significant extent to CTLs. To allow for this, there is recognition that the terminology, TH1 and TH2, should be changed to type 1 and type 2 responses, with the former including CD4 + TH1 and CD8 + CTL cells.

2.2.3.4. CD8+ T Cells in Mice

Figure 2.2.3 suggests that CD8+ T cells may arise directly from the naive pre-cursor CD8+ T cell (nTp) or that it requires help from a CD4 TH1 cell. In vitro and in vivo studies support the latter hypothesis,[188] but there is increasing evidence that, at least in some viral infections of CD4+ T-cell knockout mice, quite strong CTL responses occur.[189] It has been shown that an activated CD4+ T-cell and a B-cell mitogenic but not a nonmitogenic influenza virus induce a CD4+T-cell–independent CTL response. The explanation is that only the two former agents stimulated strong co-stimulator activity of the APC[190] and that this was sufficient to promote CD8+T-cell proliferation and differentiation.

CTLs have two major functions: to lyse infected target cells and to secrete cytokines. The original description of MHC restriction of lysis of virus-infected target cells by CTLs[19] led to an avalanche of publications demonstrating the existence of these cells in many infections caused by viruses and by some intracellular bacteria and parasites. It proved difficult to demonstrate, however, that the same mechanism that was so effective in vitro, direct lysis after cell-to cell contact, also occurred in vivo.[191] This was later established.

In one investigation,[192] mice were depleted of CD4+ and CD8+ T cells so they could not make antibody or T-cell responses. Transfer of LCMV-specific CTLs from syngeneic infected mice to the treated mice after the latter had been infected with LCMV (a noncytopathic virus) soon followed by the appearance in the blood of the viral internal nucleoprotein, NP. (The ability of these mice to make anti-LCMV antibody would have blocked detection of the NP.) The NP seemed to have been released as a direct result of the transfer of specific CTLs. The transfer of CD4+ T cells did not result in the production of anti-NP antibody unless CTLs were also transferred.

In vitro, CTLs and NK cells exocytose perforin-containing granules that cause lesions in the membrane of nondividing target cells, resulting in their lysis.[193] It had been shown previously that recovery from an LCMV infection was attributable to CTLs rather than to NK cells. Construction of perforin-negative (ie, knockout) mice offered a direct approach to demonstrating whether lysis of infected cells in vivo was an important mechanism for clearing an intracellular infection by a potent pathogen. Such mice were found to have a greatly impaired ability to clear an LCMV infection,[194] suggesting that other contact-dependent signals or secretion of cytokines such as IFNγ are insufficient in this case. Similarly, the resistance of IFNγ knockout mice to the intracellular *L. monocytogenes* is severely impaired compared with wild-type mice. However, immunization of such mice with an attenuated *L. monocytogenes* strain conferred greatly increased resistance to challenge with a virulent strain, and this appeared to be mediated by CD8+ T cells.[195] This could be explained by the earlier finding that protection against this bacterial infection was achieved by perforin-dependent CD8+ T cells.[196]

This finding may not apply to all infections, because it has been shown that clearance of vaccinia virus, which is not a natural pathogen for mice, can be achieved by IFNγ in the absence of CTLs.[197] In this case, IFNγ may function as an antiviral cytokine and/or stimulate macrophages and NK cells.

It was earlier shown that only clones of CTLs that secreted IFNγ would clear an influenza infection.[198] Furthermore, transfer of virus-specific CTL and administration of anti-IFNγ MAb to vaccinia virus–infected mice ablated the protective effect of the CTL.[199] In these experiments, the IFNγ may have had a direct antiviral effect or upregulated class I MHC antigens on infected cells to make them more susceptible to lysis. On the basis of these few findings, it has been proposed that control of cells infected with noncytopathic viruses, such as LCM, involves cell lysis, whereas control of cells infected with cytopathic viruses is via cytokines such as IFNγ.[200] However, perforin-negative mice (C57Bl/6 background) infected with a dose of ectromelia virus, Moscow strain (a cytopathic virus and a natural mouse pathogen), die of uncontrolled virus replication in the liver and spleen after subcutaneous inoculation of a virus dose that is sublethal for wild-type C57Bl/6 mice (G. Karupiah, personal communication). This admittedly limited series of experiments suggest that lysis of infected cells by CTLs may be critical for protection against infection by a virulent virus, regardless of whether the virus kills the infected cell.

Mice lacking the cellular receptor for IFNγ have been developed and found to have increased susceptibility to *L. monocytogenes* and vaccinia virus infections,[201] even though they had normal CTL and CD4+ T-cell responses. IFNγ may have had direct antiviral effects or upregulated class I MHC antigen expression.

2.2.3.5. Lysis of Target Cells by CD8+ or CD4+ T Cells

In mice, primary CD4+ T cells are generally noncytotoxic; otherwise, MHC restriction would not have been so clear-cut and might not have been discovered. However, there is ample evidence that, once cultured or cloned, these cells can lyse infected target cells.[202–204] However, primary CD4+ T cells in infected B_2-microglobulin–deficient (knockout) mice (but not in the controls) lysed target cells as though in the absence of classic CTLs, CD4+ T cells could develop this activity.[205] A potential hazard of such a response is that activated B cells may be lysed after interaction with the CD4+ T cells occurred and the isotype switch would not occur. One investigation using these mice reported a great decrease in IgG antibody production during a viral infection.[206] Whether the described mechanism is the explanation for this result or antigen-stimulated B cells are protected from lysis by CD4+ T cells is being studied.[207] The relative roles of CD4+ and CD8+ CTLs in mice have been discussed elsewhere.[208]

2.2.3.6. Cytokine Modification of CD8+ T-Cell Activity

In 1992, it was found that the culture of CD8+ T cells with IL-4 profoundly changed the properties of the cells.[209] Using mitogens or allostimulation in the presence of IL-4, the cells switched to IL-4, IL-5, and IL-10 production, and they lost cytotoxic activity and did not secrete IFNγ or IL-2[210] (ie, they had properties like type 2 T cells). Perhaps not surprisingly, further culture with IL-2 or IL-12 produced cells that were able to secrete IFNγ and IL-2 on reactivation.[211]

Do these modified cells occur in vivo? Cloned CD8 + T cells of the T2 type have been developed from the blood of HIV-1–infected people with low CD4 + T-cell counts,[212,213] but in each case, the cloned cells were developed by stimulation with a mitogen. Formally, it remains to be seen whether such cells can be isolated after stimulation with specific antigen.

One of the most fascinating implications of these findings with cytokines, especially IL-4 and IL-12, on the properties of T cells is the likelihood that they provide an explanation for a series of findings that divided the immunologic community for many years—the question of suppressor T cells. Several eminent immunologists demonstrated marked suppressor effects, many attributed to CD8 + T cells. Although these cells expressed a characteristic marker, I_J, analysis of the chromosomal DNA of such cells could not identify sequences coding for this marker on the putative suppressor cells. This lack of a specific coding sequence concerned many other immunologists, and the disagreement remained unresolved for many years. This latest information on the effects of dominant cytokines on subsequent immune responses may contribute to an understanding of the earlier findings (see Section 3.1.4.1).[214,215]

2.2.3.7.   CD8 + T Cells in Human Infections

Six years after the demonstration of MHC restriction of CTL activity in mice, a similar finding, human leukocyte antigen (HLA) restriction, was made in humans by McMichael and colleagues,[216] and this group has remained at the forefront in human studies ever since. Studies with influenza infections in mice showed that the internal NP was a major source of CTL determinants, and this was also found to be so in human influenza studies.[217] It was later found that the HA2 subunit of influenza A H1 and H2 subtype viruses induces a crossreactive (H1/H2) CTL response.[218] Theoretically, CTLs should be formed in all human viral infections, unless the infection induces a suppressor mechanism to prevent their formation.

Another example of CTL formation is found in dengue virus (a flavivirus) infections. In mouse infections, the nonstructural proteins were found to be the major source of CTL determinants.[219] CD8 + T-cell clones have been developed from lymphocytes of a dengue strain 4–infected adult.[220] Three patterns of specificity were found: one specific for dengue 4, one crossreactive for dengue 2 and 4, and one crossreactive for all four dengue strains. All of the clones were HLA-B35 restricted and recognized a nonstructural protein (ie, NS3).

In most such investigations, CTLs are derived by re-stimulation and culture of memory T cells in the peripheral blood. Such cells may persist for many years. For example, vaccinia-specific CTLs could be developed from a person vaccinated 14 years earlier, and the likelihood of reexposure to this virus in the interim is minuscule.[221]

In experimental models, effector CTLs (ie, in vitro stimulation and culture is unnecessary) can usually be isolated from target organs for several days after viral replication has occurred and before the infection is controlled by the CMI response. In human infections, such manipulation is usually not possible, and frequently, only memory CTLs are present in the blood, even with a persistent infection such as with Epstein-Barr virus.[222] However, in many individuals infected with HIV, effector CTLs are present in the blood for some years after infection (reviewed elsewhere[223]). This response may reflect the very high level of viral replication in lymphoid tissues,[83–85] which presumably continually stimulates such a potent CTL response that effector CTLs spill over into the circulation. The immune response to HIV is discussed in greater detail in a later section.

CTL activity has been demonstrated in many model infections by intracellular bacterial or parasitic agents.[168] Reports of this response in the corresponding infections in humans have been appearing for some years, as in patients with tuberculoid leprosy,[224] tuberculosis,[225] and malaria.[226] Mice were protected against a *Plasmodium* infection by CTLs directed to the circumsporozoite protein,[227] and human CTL preparations have since been made that recognize sequences within this protein.[228,229] Among malaria-immune Africans, HLA-B53–restricted CTLs recognize a conserved peptide in another liver-stage–specific antigen.[230]

2.2.4. Activation and Differentiation of B Cells

Antigens that react with B cells are divided into two groups. The first are those that are also processed by APCs and that result in activation of T cells, which then may aid the process of B-cell replication and differentiation. The proliferation and differentiation of B cells by such antigens is called a T-cell–dependent process; the second group contains some antigens, notably oligosaccharides or polysaccharides, that are not processed by APCs. The T cells therefore do not contribute to theactivation of B cells that react with these antigens. This is called a T-cell–independent process.

2.2.4.1. T- and B-Cell Interactions

An individual B cell may recognize an epitope on a monomeric antigen or epitopes on a polymer (Fig. 2.2.4.1). The receptor-antigen complex is endocytosed by the cell, it enters the endosomal-lysosomal pathway, and degradation of the complex proceeds. If other antigens are physically associated with the protein bearing one or more epitopes recognized by the receptor, they may also be endocytosed and processed. It is not necessary for the two (or more) antigens to be covalently linked, as was once thought. It is conceivable that an intact or largely intact virion may be

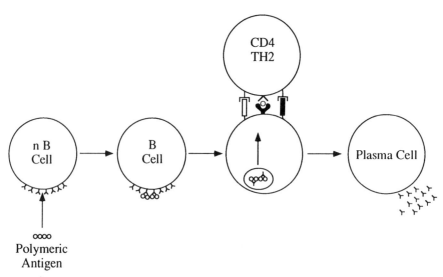

FIG. 2.2.4.1. Antigen presentation and B cell activation. nB cell; immunocompetent, naive B cell; ooooo; polymeric antigen; ⅄, Ig receptor; ⅄, class II MHC receptor; o, peptide from degraded foreign antigen; ⅄, T-cell receptor; ⎜⎜ co-stimulator molecule on the B cell and the corresponding ligand, CD28, on the T cell; ▮, CD40 differentiation antigen on the B cell and the corresponding ligand on the T cell; ⅄ ⅄ ⅄, secreted Ig molecules. (From Nathanson N. [1996] Lippincott–Raven Publishers, Philadelphia.)

taken up by a single cell in this way. The process is highly efficient; the concentrations of endocytosed material in the cell are orders of magnitude higher than the level in the external media. Appropriate peptides may bind to class II MHC molecules, and the complexes are transported to the cell surface.

Two other events are initiated after the interaction of the antigen with the cell receptor (reviewed elsewhere[231]). One is an increase of the level of co-stimulator molecules such as B7.1 and B7.2 on the B-cell surface. The second is a migration of the B cell to a region of the lymphoid tissue, the T-cell–enriched area, where it has the opportunity to meet T cells, especially those already activated by prior interaction with the antigen. The B-cell co-stimulator molecules engage with the CD28 ligand on the T cell. This mutual activation leads to engagement of the CD40 differentiation antigen on the B cell with the corresponding ligand on the activated T cell. The formation of the CD40 ligand and its interaction with CD40 is essential for the subsequent events, beginning with B-cell proliferation. The T cell may secrete IL-4, IL-5 (mice) or IL-2, IL-4, IL-10 (humans), and this leads to differentiation of the B cell that results in the switching to production and secretion of one of the many different isotypes of Ig.[232] Blocking of the interaction of CD40 and its ligand prevents the subsequent events.[233,234] The binding and uptake of a complex of associated antigens should have the advantage that many different MHC-peptide complexes may be expressed at the cell surface and attract the attention of many T cells with different receptor specificities.

The interaction of B cells with a multivalent self antigen leads to deletion of the B cells,[235,236] but the binding of an oligovalent or monovalent self antigen results in a state of anergy or apparent nonresponsiveness.[236,237] The ability of such cells to induce co-stimulator after receptor engagement is reduced,[238] such that a carrier-primed T cell is less efficient at subsequent activation.[236] Anergic B cells can be activated and function if they are exposed to sufficient stimulation by CD40 and lymphokines.[239] However, the life span of B cells, whether stimulated by self or foreign antigens, appears to be short unless they receive T-cell help.[231]

2.2.5. B- and T-Cell Replication and Differentiation in Secondary Lymphoid Tissues

B cells are released from the bone marrow and T cells from the thymus into the periphery as immunocompetent but antigen-naive cells. In the thymus, T cells have already gone through negative selection to remove most self-reacting cells and positive selection to differentiate to immunocompetent cells with the appropriate antigen-receptor repertoire such that mainly exogenous antigens are subsequently recognized (reviewed elsewhere[240,241]). T and B cells have their first contact with antigen in secondary lymphoid tissues, the lymph nodes and spleen. Once exposed to an infectious agent, B cells must be continually mobilized for long-lasting production of specific antibody, in case a second exposure to the same infectious agent occurs at a later date. Because the evidence indicates that antibody-secreting cells usually are short lived, type 2 CD4 + T cells must also be continually available for activation to facilitate antibody production. In contrast, specific effector CTLs need only be present while the infectious agent is present. They are not needed again until reexposure to that agent occurs. Consequently, they persist as memory cells (see Section 2.2.6.). This section briefly describes the elaborate procedure that ensures the first objective of continuing production of antibody after exposure to antigen, a critical requirement if a vaccine is to be effective.

2.2.5.1. Lymphoid Tissue Architecture and Lymphocyte Traffic

Figure 2.2.5.1A illustrates the architecture of a lymph node, and Figure 2.2.5.1B shows the events that occur in the node. A similar series of events occurs in the spleen.[242] In Figure 2.2.5.1A, afferent lymphatic vessels convey the antigen into the cortical and medullary areas. The cortex is rich in B cells, and the paracortex is rich in T cells (ie, the T-zone). Incoming antigen, especially particulate material, may be phagocytosed by macrophages in the medulla, and this, with uptake also by dendritic cells, initiates the immune response.

Circulating lymphocytes, including IgD + , IgM + B cells, T cells, and dendritic cells, enter the paracortex through the high endothelial venules (lymph nodes) or

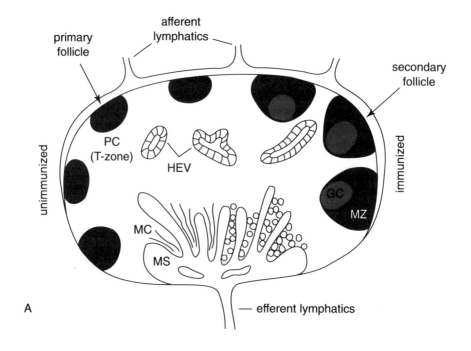

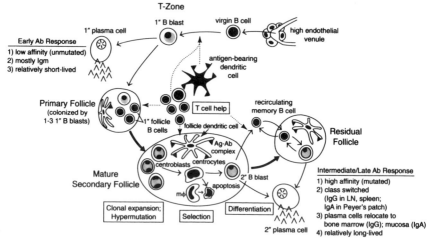

FIG. 2.2.5.1. **(A)** Architecture of a lymph node. Schematic representation of lymph node structure. Afferent (incoming) lymphatic vessels empty into the convex aspect of the lymph node adjacent to the lymph node cortex. The cortex consists of the predominantly B-lineage lymphoid follicles and the predominantly T-lineage paracortex (PC; also called the T-zone). In a resting (unimmunized) lymph node, primary follicles (*left*), composed of resting B cells, are the predominant lymphoid follicle. After immunization, secondary follicles (*right*), composed of activated germinal center (GC) B cells surrounded by resting mantle zone (MZ) B cells, predominate. Within the paracortex are the specialized high endothelial venules (HEV) that function in lymphocyte (particularly virgin lymphocyte) recruitment. The lymph node medulla consists of alternating medullary cords (MC), which in an immunized lymph node are typically filled with plasma cells

70

marginal zone (spleen). Unstimulated lymphocytes may traverse the T-zone and exit through the efferent lymph. After presentation of a T-cell–dependent antigen to B cells, primary blast cells are formed. Some of these cells rapidly differentiate to form relatively short-lived plasma cells, producing mainly low-affinity Ig but also some other antibody isotypes. B cells that respond to a T-independent antigen such as a polysaccharide become IgM-secreting cells. Because of the high avidity of IgM, however, this may be an important early defense mechanism. For example, one or a very few molecules of specific IgM with complement may result in the phagocytosis of certain bacteria.[243]

Some of the antibody formed early during this initial response combines with the antigen. Such complexes together with associated complement components become attached by complement or Fc receptors to the external surface of very specialized cells, the FDCs. The FDCs occur in a diffuse pattern in primary follicles, are non-motile, are generally long lived, and have a very large surface area. With associated antigen, they have been appropriately described as forming a library of past antigenic experiences.[244]

Some activated T cells and a few B-cell blasts may colonize a primary follicle, where under the influence of the FDC-associated antigen, B-cell blasts undergo further clonal expansion to form centrocytes. During this process, the character of the follicle changes to form a germinal center in which the antigen-bearing FDCs move to form a cap while rapid cell replication proceeds beneath it. Antibody isotype switching occurs, and IgG-, IgA-, and other isotype-producing cells are formed. Most importantly, somatic hypermutation of the B-cell receptors takes place at this time, and the centrocytes with mutated receptors move toward the antigen depot. Those with receptors of highest affinity for the antigen are selected by the antigen to further differentiate to become plasma cells or memory B cells. The cells that fail to receive the positive signal from antigen die by apoptosis and are consumed by macrophages. Plasma cells and memory B cells exit the node through the efferent lymphatics. The plasma cells migrate to the bone marrow (IgG) or the Peyer's patches (IgA), and the memory B cells recirculate. When the latter revisit germinal centers retaining specific antigen, they may process some of the antigen

---

(*right*), and medullary sinuses (MS) that coalesce to form the outgoing or efferent lymphatic vessels. (**B**) A model of B-cell maturation in secondary lymphoid tissue. The diagram shows the B-cell response to a new T-dependent antigen to which T-cell help is not limiting. The diagram demonstrates what is thought to occur in lymph node or mucosa-associated secondary lymphoid tissue, although with minor alterations (ie, the entrance of virgin B cells is through HEV rather than by MZ sinuses); it is equally applicable to spleen. The events shown are for the first exposure to a given antigen, although the response to reexposure to the same antigen can be easily extrapolated from this model. Reimmunization would result in massive stimulation of the memory B cells (*lower right quadrant*) and their differentiation into secondary plasma cells. The secondary antibody response is functionally equivalent to the intermediate late phase of the primary response (ie, high affinity or class switched antibody), but because of the preformed memory B-cell population, it is much more rapid. (From Picker LJ, Siegelman MH. [1993] Lymphoid tissues and organs. In: Paul WE, ed. Fundamental immunology, 3rd ed. Raven Press, New York, pp. 145–198.)

"shed" by the FDCs in the form of iccosomes,[245] present it to specific T cells within the germinal center, and differentiate to plasma cells. This continuing cycle of plasma cell and memory B-cell formation, with the latter always available for recruitment to form more plasma cells, ensures a continual production of antibody of high affinity.

B cells that recognize a T-cell–independent antigen may also migrate to follicles. In the case of some antigens, such as an $\alpha(1\text{-}6)$-dextran, this may lead to the formation of germinal centers, where antibody-secreting cells are produced over a considerable period, and a limited amount of somatic hypermutation takes place.[246] Germinal centers can be formed independently of the interaction of T and B cells.

2.2.5.2. Follicular Localization and Persistence of Antigen

The previous brief description is derived from a vast amount of experimental work, and the sequence of events outlined has important implications for vaccine design. B cells and FDCs are interdependent because FDCs do not form in the absence of B cells, as demonstrated in SCID mice.[247,248] One of the most important early demonstrations was that the antigen that localized on the FDCs retained its original conformation.[249] Many of the high-affinity antibodies that, for example, neutralize viral infectivity recognize discontinuous sequences that are often formed by adjacent antigen molecules. If this outline of events is correct, it implies that single molecules of antigen and, during infections in particular, complexes of similar or different antigens from infectious agents may complex with antibody specific for one or more of the antigens in the complex and attach to the FDCs. Infectious HIV virions have been identified on lymph node FDCs in humans during infections.[250] The binding is complement dependent,[250] and it is known that even if HIV immune complexes formed by neutralizing antibody are held there, the HIV remains infectious, despite the presence of an excess of neutralizing antibody.[251] For HIV, this is a superb way for infectious virus to be transported into the lymph node, and the virus then has the opportunity to contact and infect CD4+ T cells which continually pass through the follicle.

The question of the length of time antigen persists in the follicles or germinal centers and whether this is the only mechanism involved in the long-lasting production of antibody is further discussed in Section 3.3.1.1.

2.2.5.3. Principles of Antigen Handling

The described method of antigen handling and presentation gives rise to an important principle demonstrating a dichotomy in the immune system.[252] Antigens for immunization or vaccination that contain (especially) discontinuous B-cell epitopes important for protective humoral immunity should be administered in a form that retains the native conformation. Because most such antigens are at the surface of the agent, they should be resistant to proteases (for the agent to survive in nature). Once inside a cell, the antigens should be readily degraded to peptides (mechanisms reviewed elsewhere[252]). Although it has not been formally shown that resistance of FDC-bound antigen to proteases is important in this respect, such an effect was seen in early experiments using flagella particles from *Salmonella*. These are composed of repeating units of the monomeric protein flagellin, which is easily prepared by exposing flagella to mild acid.[253] The antibody (IgG) response to a single injection of flagella to rats (in the absence of adjuvant) was more prolonged than the response to a similar injection of flagellin. Radiolabeled flagella persisted in the lymph node follicles longer than radiolabeled flagellin, and in vitro, the flagella were much more resistant than flagellin to trypsin, which is not surprising because the former, when attached to the bacterial body, must remain functional in the gut. Some bacterial polysaccharides such as $\alpha(1\text{-}6)$-dextran, which are very resistant to degradation, can persist on FDCs for long periods and induce long-lived production of antibody.[246]

2.2.6. Generation and Persistence of Immunologic Memory

Memory is one of the two major characteristics of the vertebrate immune system, and the feasibility of vaccination or immunization completely depends on the formation and eventual activation of memory T and B cells. Compared to the study of specificity, it has been a difficult area, and our knowledge is still far from complete.

2.2.6.1. Generation of Memory

The precise mechanism of formation of a B memory cell is unknown. The precursor is the rapidly dividing B cell, the centrocyte, within the forming germinal center, which undergoes somatic hypermutation and selection by antigen for further differentiation. But the trigger that decides the fate thereafter is unknown. Three possible models[254] have been proposed: the immediate precursor becomes a memory or a plasma cell by an unequal division; differentiation occurs under the influence of different lymphokines from other cells; or memory and plasma cells originate from different precursors further back in the B-cell lineage (ie, in the bone marrow). Further research may clarify the picture.

Even less is known about the individual steps involved in the generation of memory T cells from naive precursor cells. There is no indication that this occurs in a special site corresponding to the germinal center.

2.2.6.2. Properties of Memory Cells

The most obvious marker of memory B cells is the presence of immunoglobulin isotypes other than IgM and IgD, such as IgG, IgA, or IgE. Evidence is accumulating that precursor B cells express high levels and memory B cells express low levels of an antigen recognized by the MAb JIID.[255] Several findings are consistent with this distinction:

1. In transfer experiments using SCID mice, JIID[hi] cells gave a primary antibody response, but JIID[lo] cells gave a secondary response.[256]
2. Somatic mutations are found only in the IgV regions of JIID[lo] cells.[257]
3. On transfer, only JIID[lo] cells give rise to germinal centers.[258]

It could be expected that memory B cells express enhanced levels of those lymphokine ligands that are important in interaction with activated CD4 + T cells, because memory B cells seem to be more easily stimulated by antigen and by noncognate bystander mechanisms[259] than are primary cells. It also could be expected that memory B cells might present antigen more effectively to T cells than naive cells, but this remains to be demonstrated.

In the case of T cells, the fact that the TCR isotype neither changes nor somatically mutates (although there may be selection based on avidity) adds to the difficulty of distinguishing between activated, effector, and memory T cells. Many markers are said to be expressed at higher levels on memory than on naive T cells,[254] but the one for which there appears to be the strongest evidence is the CD45 molecule. A low-molecular-weight isoform, CD45RO, in humans is claimed to characterize memory cells.[260] CD45R[lo], the low-molecular-weight isoform, cells were more effective in providing help for B cells.[261] Adoptive transfer of CD45R[hi] cells to rats gave rise to CD45R[lo] cells,[262] findings consistent with but not proving the validity of these markers. As is the case for memory B cells, the requirements for stimulation of memory T cells are less stringent than for naive T cells.[263]

Although the activation of primary self-restricted CTLs in vitro requires the conditions provided by special APCs such as dendritic cells or by lymphokines such as IL-7,[209] secondary responses do not.[210] Moreover, the co-stimulatory molecule CD80 or CD86 must be expressed on the APC to interact with CD28 on CTLs for their differentiation from naive splenocytes. Memory CTLs do not require this co-stimulatory interaction.[264]

2.2.6.3. The Life of Memory Cells

There is a general consensus that memory B and T cells persist in the body for long periods. On the basis of the previously described considerations, memory B cells are thought to have a long half-life. There has been some disagreement over the half-life of memory T cells, but some reports[265,266] indicate that it is very long and probably lasts a lifetime in mice. A study of vaccinia virus–specific memory CTLs in adults who had been immunized against smallpox when children and who, it is presumed, had no contact with this virus since that time led to the conclusion that this T-cell immunity can persist for as long as 50 years after immunization against smallpox.[267]

It has been claimed that memory T and B cells only persist in the infected or immunized host if the specific antigen is present.[244,268] Antigen in its correct conformational state persists in the lymphoid tissues, and B memory cells are recruited by contacting the antigen. Whether the memory cells periodically need to contact antigen to survive and whether they can remain as memory cells after such contact remains to be established.

The claim that memory T cells can only persist if antigen persists, particularly in the case of class I MHC–restricted T cells, has since been shown to be wrong. From a practical aspect, there would seem to be little need for antigen persistence for memory T-cell maintenance. Antigen persists for the continual formation and recruitment of B cells to form antibody-secreting cells, because there is a need to have the continual presence of antibody. It allows advantage to be taken of the somatic hypermutation of the B-cell receptor, so that higher-affinity antibody is produced while the amount of persisting antigen on FDCs declines. Moreover, in the absence of infected cells that would continually provide specific nonapeptides, how would the antigen persist? It seems unlikely that it could exist for weeks or months as a peptide-MHC complex at the surface of a previously infected cell. Because only antibody and not effector T cells can prevent a second infection, it is more economical for the host to have a pool of memory CTLs that can be rapidly activated to become effector cells when a second, similar infection occurs. The TCR, unlike the B-cell receptor, does not undergo somatic hypermutation, offering an additional argument against antigen persistence.

Three papers have convincingly demonstrated that the longevity of memory CTLs does not require the persistence of antigen.[269–271] These researchers showed that memory cells could be transferred into noninfected, irradiated recipients or into mice genetically rendered unable to express MHC class I antigens (β_2-microglobulin knockout mice), where they persist for long periods. These cells could subsequently be activated with the typical shortened kinetics and increased potency that are the hallmarks of a memory response.

2.2.6.4. Increase in Antigen-Specific Lymphocytes After Stimulation

After immunization or infection, the number of T and B cells of a given receptor specificity are assumed to increase markedly. A traditional way to assay such increases is, after immunization or infection, to remove the cell population and restimulate with the antigen or infectious agent in vitro for 5 to 6 days under limiting dilution conditions. This approach has regularly shown a substantial increase in specific cell numbers. For example, the precursor frequency of virus-specific precursor CTLs in the lungs of mice before and after infection with influenza virus increased from about 20-fold to more than 100-fold, depending on the virus used in the experiment.[272] In this type of experiment, the assumption is made that cells from the lungs of uninfected mice will respond almost as well as the memory cells from the infected mice. In a similar approach, the increase in the number of anti-influenza antibody-secreting cells (as plaques) was measured, and values corresponding with 100-fold to 1000-fold increases were found.[273] However, in this experiment, no allowance was made for a possible increase in numbers arising from antibody-secreting cells already present in the population before in vitro stimulation was carried out.

More accurate figures are likely to be obtained if assays can be carried out without involving in vitro stimulation. One example of the latter approach was measurement of precursor B-cell frequency in the spleens of mice before and after immunization with phycoerythrin.[274] By 35 days after immunization, the frequency had risen from $5/10^6$ to about $1/10^4$ and remained within the range of 0.5 to $1.5/10^4$ for up to 196 days, which was about a 50-fold increase (A. Mullbacher, personal communication).

Memory in both lymphocyte compartments has two components: a qualitative change in the properties of the cells and an increase in numbers of cells of that specificity. Both factors contribute to the essential role of the immune response—a quicker and more effective response to the challenge infection by a vaccinated or immunized host.

CHAPTER 2.3. THE NATURE OF THE ADAPTIVE IMMUNE SYSTEM: REGIONAL IMMUNITY

The body is separated from the environment by thin layers of cells in two main areas: skin and mucosa. Some microorganisms infect through the skin, by a scratch or by an insect bite. Most microorganisms infect through the mucosa. The difference in area between these two sites is profound. The surface area of mucosa in an adult is equivalent to that of a tennis court, and it is not surprising that most infectious agents infect through this route. Although the immune responses described in the previous section also occur in the skin and mucosa, the responses that occur at these latter sites have additional characteristics.

2.3.1. Epithelial Immunology

The epithelium of the skin has two special immunological characteristics: the presence of a type of dendritic cell, the Langerhans cell (see Section 2.2.2.1), and a class of T cells, called intraepithelial lymphocytes (IEL), which have $\gamma\delta$ receptor chains, in contrast to the $\alpha\beta$ chains of most T cells. IEL are also abundant in mucosal epithelial tissues.

The role of the Langerhans cells is to take up and transport foreign material to the draining lymph nodes, where the immune response is initiated. This has been dramatically demonstrated in experiments in which DNA-coated microscopic gold particles were fired by a "gene gun" into the mouse skin. Histologic examination at different times thereafter showed some of these particles being conveyed by Langerhans cells to the draining lymph nodes (see Section 5.4.9).

In mice, the IELs normally represent a relatively small proportion of the total T-cell compartment. Much needs to be learned about their properties and roles in

TABLE 2.3.1. *Distribution of γδ T cells as a percentage of lymphocytes in each organ or site*

Organ	Humans (%)	Mice (%)
Blood	0.5–16	0.5–2
Thymus		0.5–1.5
Spleen	2–30	0.5–2
Lymph node	5	0.5–3
Intestine	10	50
Skin (epidermis)		+
Other epithelia		+

+, present.
From Haas W, Pereira P, Tonegawa S. (1993) Gamma/delta cells. Ann Rev Immunol 11:637–686.

defense, but because they proliferate in response to viral, bacterial, and parasitic infections, they are likely to play a role in defense against infections (reviewed elsewhere[275,276]). Most develop independently of αβ T cells, and some occur in nu + / nu + mice. They are found particularly in the epithelial spaces of regions such as the skin, gut, lung, genital tract, and tongue. Because they circulate, like αβ T cells, they are present in most tissues. Their distribution in several regions in mice and humans (Table 2.3.1) indicates some substantial differences between these two species.

These cells differ in several additional major respects from αβ T cells. Only a small proportion of mouse γδ T cells recognize class I or II MHC antigens, and they are broadly crossreactive for the products of different alleles. The remainder seem to recognize nonclassic MHC antigens, possibly small molecules such as peptides presented by nonpolymorphic proteins from the TL antigen region. Most lack many of the cell markers that characterize αβ T cells, including the CD3, CD4, and CD8, but on stimulation, all seem to produce a range of cytokines, and they can lyse target cells.

In the presence of APCs, human and mouse γδ T cells mount strong proliferative responses to killed mycobacteria and some to extracts that contain heat shock proteins. Like αβ T cells, γδ T cells also respond to superantigens.

These and other findings suggest that these cells do not normally provide help to B cells. The possible direct role of these cells in several different infections is discussed in Section 3.1.4.2.

2.3.2. Mucosal Immunology

The existence of a mucosal immune system that appeared to function at least partially independently of systemic immunity was first proposed by Besredka in 1919,[277] based on his observations that rabbits were protected from fatal dysentery after oral immunization with killed *Shigella* bacillus, regardless of antibody titers in their sera. It was not until 1963 that this local immune system was characterized in a molecular sense, when Tomasi demonstrated that the fluids that bathe mucosal surfaces contained high levels of a new immunoglobulin isotype, which came to be called IgA and contrasted with the low levels of this isotype found in the serum. Moreover, salivary IgA was shown to contain two additional components, one called the secretory component[278] and the other a J chain that linked two Ig monomers together.[279] Both of these distinguish most IgA in external secretions from IgA in serum.

In adult humans, epithelial tissues comprising an area of over 300 m^2 overlie the mucosae and represent the major portal of entry into the body for most pathogens and allergens. Cooperation between a range of innate and local adaptive immune mechanisms serves to protect these tissues. The migration of specific B and T cells from mucosal inductive sites, such as the gut- and bronchus-associated lymphoid tissues (GALT and BALT), to the various mucosal effector tissues forms the basis of adaptive immunity at the mucosae. Local T cells mediate cytotoxic and helper functions, and vast numbers of B cells, which largely produce IgA antibodies, populate regions adjacent to the exocrine glands. About 10^{10} antibody-producing cells are found in each meter of human bowel, about four times as many as in bone marrow, spleen, and lymph nodes combined. As many as 80% of such cells found in humans and mice are located in the intestinal tissues.[280]

2.3.3. Mucosal Lymphoid Tissues

The cells of the muscosal immune system are found in the mucosa-associated lymphoid tissues (MALT) or in transit between these sites. MALT has three main functions[281]: to protect mucosae against invasion and colonization by pathogenic organisms; to block uptake of undegraded dietary and microbial antigens; and to prevent the development of potentially harmful immune responses if the antigens penetrate the mucosal barrier.

Because mucosae are continually exposed to foreign matter, MALT must regulate appropriate effector mechanisms to optimize responses and avoid local tissue damage. As shown in Figure 2.3.3, MALT consists of anatomically discrete lymphoid compartments, such as the Peyer's patches of the small intestine, other isolated lymphoid follicles and the appendix (all comprising GALT), the components of nasopharyngeal tonsillar tissue (ie, Waldeyer's ring), the BALT, and tissues in the genitourinary tract. It is in these tissues that local immune responses are initiated, and these are mediated by the great number of lymphoid cells migrating to the mucosal parenchyma. The putative link between these tissues is referred to as the "common mucosal immune system," whereby immunocytes sensitized at one site, particularly GALT, may transfer immunity after homing to other mucosal and glandular sites.[282,283] Hopes of widespread exploitation of this system for improved mucosal immunoprophylaxis may be compromised by restrictions on the degree to which migration and subsequent differentiation of immunocytes actually occurs be-

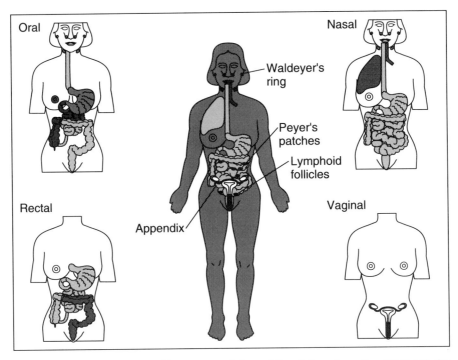

FIG. 2.3.3. Regional spheres of immune reactivity and the sIgA system. Consistent with the concept of a common mucosal system, contingents of IgA-secreting B cells can migrate from the site of initial encounter with antigen to other mucosal tissues. Depending on the site where the encounter with antigen takes place, IgA-committed B cells disseminate preferentially to certain privileged, mainly regional mucosal organs, where they differentiate into IgA-secreting plasmocytes. The route of administration of antigens determines the anatomic distribution of secretory IgA antibody responses. (From Czerkinsky C, Holmgren J. [1995] The mucosal immune system and prospects for anti-infectious and anti-inflammatory vaccines. The Immunologist 3:97–103.)

tween different mucosal tissues. For example, although the adenovirus vaccine is administered orally and protects at a respiratory site, extensive migration of cells between the gastrointestinal and respiratory tracts may not normally occur.

2.3.3.1. Gut-Associated Lymphoid Tissues

The GALT is the most highly characterized of the organized mucosal lymphoid tissues and comprises the small intestinal Peyer's patches and thousands of single lymphoid follicles scattered throughout the gut wall. Peyer's patches possess distinct B-cell, T-cell, and APC populations, particularly in the dome region, and they are covered with a specialized reticular epithelium containing a high proportion of cells adapted for antigen sampling. These microfold or membrane (M) cells possess small microvilli and thin processes extending around lymphocytes. The M cells do not degrade antigen, but rather pass it onto the underlying cells.[284] Lymphoid folli-cles containing germinal centers occur beneath the dome and are thought to be sites of high-level antibody isotype switching and affinity maturation, giving rise to large numbers of cells bearing surface IgA.[285,286] The retention and presentation of antigen on FDCs facilitates this process. The follicles do not, however, give rise to high numbers of antibody-producing cells, unlike systemic lymphoid tissues. Adjacent T-cell zones contain a full complement of T-cell subtypes, although more than one half are CD4+ helper T cells, which appear to regulate IgA responses, while CD8+ T cells are also present in abundance. With the aid of local macrophages and dendritic cells, these cells give rise to specific effector cells. More work is required to delineate the best means of stimulating GALT with different antigens, particularly soluble antigens whose fate is not well known, in order to optimize the production of appropriate effector populations.

2.3.3.2. Other Organized Mucosal Lymphoid Tissues

Local immune responses are also induced in the BALT and the tonsillar tissues of Waldeyer's ring. The nodules of lymphoid tissue comprising BALT are found near the branches of airways or between bronchi and arteries, although the occurrence of these tissues in species other than rabbit and rat is highly variable.[287] BALT consists of lymphoid follicles with structures resembling germinal centers and containing FDCs, and they are covered by epithelia apparently specialized for antigen uptake. These epithelia contain lymphocytes and display membrane processes extending into the lumen, but they are not entirely analogous to those overlying GALT. Most evidence suggests that BALT is not a common feature of healthy human lungs, although it has been described in cases of autoimmune disease and immunodefi-ciency.[288] It is likely therefore that other respiratory tissues function in antigen up-take and processing in humans. There is little evidence for organized lymphoid structures at other mucosal sites, such as the genitourinary tract (see Section 6.2.) and mammary and salivary glands. Nevertheless, immune responses occur in these tissues after the migration of immunocytes from GALT and other inductive sites and, in some cases, as a result of local generation in draining lymph nodes.

2.3.3.3. Mucosal Effector Tissues

After exposure to antigen and stimulation in MALT, specific immunocytes un-dergo a process of migration and populate mucosae, where their effects are medi-ated (Fig. 2.3.3.3). In the best characterized of these processes, antigen-specific T cells and B cells induced in the Peyer's patches migrate through the efferent lym-phatics, thoracic duct, and systemic circulation to effector sites such as the lamina propria of the gut wall and the respiratory and reproductive tracts and glandular tissues. These cells express adhesion molecules that bind to addressins on mucosal and glandular epithelia. For example, the α4β7 integrin expressed by Peyer's patch

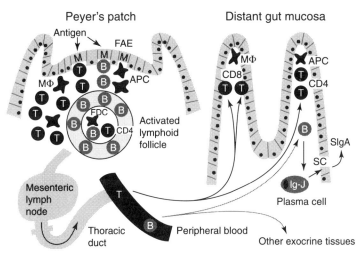

FIG. 2.3.3.3. Scheme for induction of intestinal immune responses and cell traffic in the integrated mucosal immune system. Luminal antigens are mainly transported into the Peyer's patch through M cells (M) of follicle-associated epithelium (FAE) and are presented to T cells (T) by macrophages (MO), other types of antigen-presenting cells (APCs), and probably B cells. Lymphoid follicles become activated and generate high-affinity memory B cells by retaining and presenting antigen to follicular dendritic cells (FDC) under the influence of CD4 + regulatory T cells. Primed T and B cells migrate to the peripheral blood circulation and extravasate mainly into the intestinal lamina propria but also into other exocrine tissues. Intestinal B cells differentiate in the lamina propria under the influence of MO, APCs, and CD4 + T cells into plasma cells. These produce mainly polymeric immunoglobulin (Ig) with J chain (Ig-J; predominantly pIgA) that is transported to the lumen by the epithelial transmembrane secretory component (SC). Most CD8 + T cells migrate into the villus epithelium, perhaps to mediate oral tolerance to food antigens. (From Brandtzaeg P. [1995] Basic mechanisms of mucosal immunity. The Immunologist 3:89–96.)

B and T cells appears to be an important factor for their localization in intestinal lamina propria,[289] but cells expressing $\alpha E\beta 7$ appear to migrate deeper into intestinal epithelium and are retained by binding of this molecule to E-cadherin expressed on epithelial cells.[290] The widespread migration of cells sensitized in GALT forms the basis of the common mucosal immune system and has obvious implications for mucosal immunoprophylaxis.

The gastrointestinal lamina propria is the major mucosal effector tissue of the body and contains an anatomically diffuse cell population comprising about 30% B cells, mostly IgA plasma cells, and about 50% T cells, as well as macrophages, eosinophils, and mucosal mast cells. Most T cells are CD4 + types and regulate antibody production in these tissues. A discrete population, the IELs, is found between intestinal epithelial cells. The IELs comprise NK cells, allospecific CTLs, CTL precursors, and mast cells. Unlike lamina propria T cells, most IELs bear the CD8 marker, and approximately one half are of thymic origin, with the remainder migrating directly to the gut from the bone marrow.[291] Human IEL cells display cytotoxic activity specific for epithelial cells and have been implicated in the development of oral tolerance[292] (see Section 2.3.7). IELs also contain a significant sub-population of cells expressing the γδ TCR. It is possible that these cells play a role in surveillance of mucosal tissues by eliminating infected or damaged epithelial cells. However, their restriction specificity and antigenic repertoire remain to be elucidated.[293]

The lung parenchyma contain significant numbers of interstitial lymphocytes and NK cells, of the order of 10^{10} cells in humans, but the degree to which these cells represent a pool with specific functions separate from circulating systemic cells is unclear.[296] At least in the upper respiratory tract, large numbers of cells secreting IgA antibodies are generated after antigen stimulation of the large mass of organized local lymphoid tissue through the intranasal route. The male and female reproductive tracts contain large numbers of APCs, B cells, and T cells and possess epithelia capable of synthesizing the secretory component.[294] Although some studies have reported the secretion of IgA antibodies in response to locally administered antigens in these tissues, the relative importance of local generation of these responses, as opposed to migration of sensitized cells from tissues such as GALT, remains to be clarified.

2.3.4. Regulation of Mucosal Immune Responses

The induction of mucosal IgA responses strongly depends on help provided by CD4+ T cells generated in MALT,[295] and the co-stimulatory molecules and cytokines that they express may play major roles at different stages in the mucosal immune response (reviewed elsewhere[296]). Antigen activation of B cells in MALT apparently leads to immunoglobulin heavy-chain switching, which results in the expression of surface IgA by IgM-bearing cells. The interaction of the CD28 and CD40 ligand molecules on local T cells with the B7 molecule on APCs and CD40 on B cells, respectively, provides important co-stimulatory signals for this process.[297]

Type 1 and 2 helper cells are found in approximately equal numbers in MALT,[298] but in effector tissues, T-cell cytokine production is strongly biased toward type 2 responses.[298,299] In vitro, IL-4 promotes immunoglobulin heavy-chain switching to IgA in murine B-cell lines,[300] but results from studies of cytokine gene knockout mice showed that the ability of mucosal B cells to undergo switching to IgA production did not depend on the presence of this factor.[301] Transforming growth factor-β (TGFβ) is probably more important as an IgA switch factor in mice[302] and humans.[303] IL-4 is nevertheless important for the development of type 2 T cells and for the normal development of MALT.[301]

After migration from MALT into mucosal effector tissue, primed IgA B cells undergo further differentiation into plasma cells. Local T-cell–derived IL-5, IL-6, and IL-10 are thought to be important mediators in this process and are abundantly produced in these tissues, although mice deficient for IL-5 production displayed no defect in their ability to mount mucosal IgA responses.[304] In contrast, IL-6-deficiency resulted in a marked reduction in numbers of IgA-producing cells at mucosae and deficient responses to conventional B-cell antigens such as soluble proteins and viruses.[305] However, the IgA-producing capacity of B1 cells, which largely bear the CD5 marker and derive from the peritoneal cavity rather than MALT, appears unaffected by the absence of IL-6.[306] Most attention has been given to MALT-derived conventional B cells as the source of secretory antibodies at mucosae, although as many as 50% of IgA + B cells in the gut wall may arise from this self-replenishing peritoneal CD5 + population.[307] These B1 cells appear to differ from conventional bone marrow–derived B cells in their migratory patterns, responsiveness to cytokines, and antigen repertoire,[308] responding well to bacterial surface antigens such as lipopolysaccharides. They deserve greater attention as targets for immunization to achieve improved specific IgA responses.

2.3.5. Production and Function of Secretory Antibodies

The primary function of secretory antibodies, especially secretory IgA, is to cooperate with the many innate immune mechanisms that function at mucosae to prevent microorganisms from invading the body and to neutralize toxins. This process of *immune exclusion* usually does not involve inflammation, which could be disastrous given the volume of such antigenic material to which mucosae are exposed. For this reason, it is important that secretory IgA antibodies do not bind complement.

These antibodies provide an early line of defense for the body and are produced by the vast numbers of activated B cells that migrate to secretory mucosae and exocrine glands and localize beneath the epithelial basement membrane. IgA is produced largely in dimeric form, although some is tetrameric. The units are joined by the J chain.[279] The molecule reaches the lumen by active transport through secretory epithelial cells.[309] Secretory antibodies must function in a highly proteolytic environment and the intrinsic resistance of these molecules is enhanced by their binding of the secretory component.

Secretory IgA antibody is present at the point of initial contact with pathogens, particularly viruses, and the molecules' multivalency makes them effective at neutralizing virus. Nevertheless, the mechanisms of neutralization are not entirely clear; the simple binding of these molecules to viruses so that cellular penetration is prevented is an oversimplification. IgA may also form immune complexes in the mucosal lamina propria,[309] and in vitro studies suggest that it may also bind virus within infected epithelial cells.[310] Influenza virus that has been bound by IgA may still enter receptive cells through their plasma membranes and may reach the nucleus, but viral mRNA is not transcribed from such neutralized virions[311] (see Section 3.1.2).

IgA may also inhibit a broad range of bacteria from infecting mucosal epithelia by carbohydrate-specific interactions that are independent of specific antibody activity. For example, mannose-containing oligosaccharide side chains on the IgA heavy chain are recognized by specific lectins on bacterial fimbriae.[312] Secretory

IgA and serum IgA also are able to potentiate the antibacterial effects of innate factors such as lactoferrin and lactoperoxidase present in secretions.[313] These molecules may also mediate local antibacterial antibody-dependent cell-mediated cytotoxicity (ADCC) by binding Fc receptors on monocytes and CD4 + T cells, particularly against *Salmonella* and *Shigella* species.[314]

2.3.6. Mucosal Effector T Cells and Cell-Mediated Immunity

Mucosal tissues in humans and experimental animals also contain cells expressing cytotoxic activity (ie, CTLs, ADCC, and NK cells). Such cells are present in the lamina propria and among the IEL population.[315] Alloantigen-specific CTL clones derived from IELs in orally immunized mice displayed one of two phenotypes, a classic CD8 + cytolytic T-cell population and an unusual subset that mediated nonspecific lytic activity when activated by IL-2.[316] IELs also contain significant numbers of γδ TCR + cells, whose function remains uncertain but that may play a role in eliminating infected epithelial cells.[293] Classic antigen-specific CTLs were shown to be induced in GALT after oral administration of vaccinia virus,[317] reovirus, or rotavirus.[318] They were detected in draining lymph nodes and, in some cases, in systemic lymphoid tissues such as the spleen. There is an advantage in inducing effective CMI responses in tissues where most infectious agents are first encountered. Another particularly good example of this is the demonstration of specific CTLs in the vaginal mucosa of monkeys infected with simian immunodeficiency virus.[319] More work is needed to optimize the generation and activation of such mucosal T-cell populations by vaccination.

2.3.7. Induction of Tolerance in the Gut-Associated Lymphoid Tissues

Mucosal administration of antigens may, in addition to eliciting local antibody and cell-mediated immune responses, induce a state of systemic tolerance. This phenomenon was first described in 1911 by Wells,[320] who found that guinea pigs fed hen egg proteins did not develop anaphylactic responses to subsequent systemic challenge with the same antigen. Many later studies have shown that ingestion of a range of proteins can lead to poor systemic immune responsiveness to those particular antigens.[321,322] Oral tolerance, as this process has come to be called, may represent a natural mechanism for the avoidance of dangerous inflammatory reactions to ingested proteins. The GALT, where specific mucosal immune responses are generated, is also the site in which the events leading to oral tolerance may be initiated.

The primary mechanisms governing decreased T-cell responsiveness differ according to the amount of antigen that is ingested. They are the clonal anergy of antigen-specific T cells and the generation of cellular suppressive mechanisms. The development of clonal anergy is favored by ingestion of high doses of protein,[323] probably after its entry into the systemic circulation intact or in fragmented form.[292] Active suppression occurs in response to low doses of antigen and is mediated by immunosuppressive cytokines, such as TGFβ, IL-4, and IL-10, produced at systemic sites by T cells generated in GALT.[324] The most commonly demonstrated correlate of oral tolerance to fed antigen is a diminished delayed-type hypersensitivity response. Such responses are normally mediated by TH1-type cells and are inhibited by IL-4 produced by TH2-type cells. GALT appears to favor the development of T cells producing type 2 factors, including IL-4. The GALT may also give rise to a CD4+ T-cell subset that secretes predominantly TGFβ and mediates helper function for mucosal IgA responses but immunosuppression toward systemic type 1 responses.[292] Immunohistochemical studies have shown that IL-4 and TGFβ are upregulated in systemic target tissues of autoimmune disease in animals fed low doses of autoantigens.[292]

The prospects of using mucosally induced tolerance as a means of treating autoimmune diseases are enticing. Some success has been reported using this approach in animal models, such as chronic experimental immune encephalomyelitis, and human trials for the treatment of rheumatoid arthritis, multiple sclerosis, and uveitis are underway.[292] The major problem is to overcome ongoing autoimmune disease. Earlier workers have met with limited success, noting a requirement for large doses of tolerogen and repeated immunization for anything but a short-term immunosuppressive effect.[281]

Czerkinsky and colleagues[325] showed that the development of peripheral tolerance to fed erythrocytes was profoundly enhanced if they were conjugated with recombinant B subunit of cholera toxin (CTB), presumably through improved efficiency of antigen presentation in GALT. This occurred despite the induction of strong mucosal IgA responses to the erythrocytes and CTB in the gut. Prior experience with CTB and the cholera toxin from which it was purified suggested that both preparations could break tolerance to conjugated proteins in addition to their activity as potent mucosal immunogens.[326] It appears, however, that the former property may have been a function of trace amounts of contaminating cholera toxin in the CTB preparation. Experiments with conjugates of a range of particulate and soluble antigens with CTB, including autoantigens, suggest that this molecule dramatically reduces the amount and number of doses of tolerogen required to induce peripheral tolerance and may also act in this way after a systemic immune response has been initiated.[281] A single oral dose of myelin basic protein conjugated to CTB, given before or after disease induction, protected rats against experimental immune encephalomyelitis. This approach offers great promise for the use of oral tolerance induction to treat human autoimmune diseases and other conditions occurring as a result of inappropriate immune responses (see Section 6.2).

CHAPTER 2.4. THE IMMUNE SYSTEM OF THE NEONATE

In 1948, Burnet and Fenner[327] proposed that, up until about the time of birth, exposure of the human fetus to environmental antigens, including infectious agents, would induce a state of tolerance to those antigens, because the immune system of the fetus was unable to mount an effective immune response. The ability to mount an immune response to environmental antigens would be progressively acquired within months after birth. Medawar and colleagues[328] later showed that newborn mice could accept and not reject foreign white blood cells. These two observations led to the award of the Nobel Prize to Burnet and Medawar in 1960. It was fortunate that humans and mice showed rather similar characteristics in this respect and that foreign cells were a form of foreign antigen that could persist and were not a severe challenge to the host.

Three childhood vaccines are commonly administered at or near birth: bacille Calmette-Guérin (BCG) vaccine, oral poliovirus vaccine (OPV), and hepatitis B virus (HBV) vaccine. BCG is known to persist for long periods after vaccination; children immunized at birth who later become infected with HIV may suffer an outbreak of a progressive mycobacterial disease. At least three administrations of OPV and hepatitis B vaccines are given over many months (see Table 1.3.1).

2.4.1. Development of B and T Cells

In humans, B-cell development begins within the fetal liver and the omentum[329] and T-cell development within the thymus at 7 to 8 weeks' gestation.[330] Pre-B cells express μ chains but no light chains in the cytoplasm, but the later expression of the light chain leads to the expression at the cell surface of monomeric IgM molecules, which serve as a functional receptor. By 10 to 12 weeks, the fetal liver contains about equal numbers of pre-B and receptor-bearing B cells, and by 15 weeks, the proportion of B cells in the blood and spleen is similar to that in postnatal life.[331] In the thymus and fetal liver, intracytoplasmic CD3 is found in pre-T cells before the expression first of the β chain and then of the α chain of the TCR. T cells with the CD3-TCR complex occur in the fetal liver at 10 weeks of gestation and occur thereafter with increasing frequency.

2.4.2. Development of Repertoire Expression

Early experiments, particularly those using larger animals such as sheep, seemed to indicate that the fetus might develop the ability to respond to different antigens at different times during fetal development. Findings with inbred mice also suggest an ordered expression of antibody specificities. Antibodies to different antigens, particularly carbohydrate antigens, are frequently dominated by a few clonotypes in late fetal or very early postnatal life[332,333] and occur at a predictable time. The fact that some of these clonotypes are not expressed in adult life suggests that these patterns of expression at different stages are not an artifact. In mice and humans, the early expressed clonotypes tend to secrete polyreactive antibodies;[333] many of the producer B cells express the CD5 marker and produce autoreactive antibodies. In mice, this period of restricted diversity lasts for about 3 weeks, beginning about 1 week before birth. Histologic evidence suggests that the newborn mouse is equivalent in this respect to the 12-week human fetus.[329] This early restricted variable heavy chain use may indicate that fewer epitopes on different antigens may be recognized.

2.4.3. Maturation of the Human Immune Response

By 16 weeks' gestation, fetal B cells may express the IgM, IgD, IgA, and IgG receptors, which are present in "adult" numbers in the blood.[334] Individual cells, however, may express IgM and IgD, as well as another isotype, such as IgG or IgA.[335] To judge from adults with certain B-cell deficiencies, this property is characteristic of immature phenotypes.

Neonatal T cells exhibit poor helper function because of a deficiency in their production of IL-2 and of IL-4 or IL-6. The T cells produce sufficient cytokine to induce B-cell proliferation but not enough to drive efficient terminal differentiation. Supplementation of the cultures with these cytokines results in increased performance of the B cells.[336] It seems that neonatal B cells require higher levels of these cytokines than adult B cells. Compared with adults, only a small proportion of the neonatal T cells express the CD45RO (ie, memory) phenotype; the remainder with the CD45RA phenotype suppress the activity of the former.[337] It would be useful to know the nature of the antigens recognized by the CD45RO cells.

Less is known about the properties of the neonatal APCs. It would be of interest to see the effect of immunizing neonates with an antigen together with selected cytokines and measure any difference in the immune response. The findings from such experiments may be relevant to the goals of the Children's Vaccine Initiative.

2.4.4. Maternal Immunization to Prevent Infectious Disease in the Neonate

Immunization during pregnancy is thought to be desirable if the infection to be avoided is dangerous for the mother and the offspring (see Section 1.2.10). There is an international program to immunize pregnant women in developing countries against tetanus because of the danger of infection to mother and child if the delivery occurs under unhygienic conditions.

Transplacental passage of maternal IgG, the only Ig isotype transferred, begins during the first trimester and increases until delivery.[338] The IgG binds to Fc receptors on the trophoblast cells in the placenta; endocytosis and active transport follow. IgG1 and IgG4 are most effectively transferred and reach maternal blood levels by about 35 weeks' gestation.[339] The half-life of the acquired IgG is thought to be 3 to 4 weeks.[340] It follows that, to be effective, vaccines for maternal immunization should induce predominantly IgG responses. Highly effective vaccines should produce in the female responses lasting many years (like a natural infection) so that antibody transfer could provide protection during successive pregnancies. Although there is concern about vaccinating during pregnancy with live attenuated vaccines and the practice is often discouraged, it is much safer than infection with the wild-type agent.[90]

Breast milk of immunized mothers may also contribute to their infants' protection. Pregnant women immunized with the *Haemophilus influenzae* type B (Hib) polysaccharide vaccine have elevated levels of antibody in the breast milk.[341] In experimental animals, antigen-activated lymphocytes home to and are retained in mammary glands.[342] An increase in antibody levels in the breast milk was seen with lactating Pakistani women immunized after delivery with cholera and polio vaccines.[343] Such women may have been exposed to the wild-type infection at a mucosal surface before immunization.

2.4.5. Effect of Passive Antibody on the Neonate's Immune Response

Maternally derived antibody may protect the infant against a specific infectious disease but prevent immunization against that infection if the vaccine used is a live attenuated preparation. The classic case is measles in developing countries (see Section 1.2.6). This inhibition is less likely if the vaccine is a noninfectious preparation. Vaccination with tetanus toxoid,[344] with serogroup A and C meningococcal polysaccharide,[345] or with Hib polysaccharide[346] during pregnancy did not affect the response of the infant to the same vaccines if immunization was carried out 6 to 18 months after birth, although there are examples of transient immunosuppression.[90] There are some reports[327,347] that neonates may become immunized after maternal vaccination (eg, tetanus toxoid), as shown by the presence of IgM and T-cell proliferative responses at birth and in later childhood. The precise mechanism involved is not clear, but some evidence suggests that the formation of maternal anti-idiotype antibodies after immunization can alter the establishment of antibody repertoires in the offspring. Cells in the cord blood of neonates of mothers with parasitic infections showed specific T-cell responses to idiotypes expressed on antibodies specific for the particular parasites.[348] These cases suggest that the transferred antibodies induced in the neonate anti-idiotypic T cells that were specific for the idiotypes on the maternal antibody, although anti-idiotypic reactions to maternal antibody have been demonstrated only rarely in human neonates.[349]

Anti-HBV Ig given at birth temporarily protects the neonate against infection until the vaccine, given at the same time, becomes effective. The net result is an apparently improved efficacy of the vaccine (see Section 1.2.9). A similar finding has been reported for tetanus toxoid.[341] It could be expected that, at the correct concentration, passive antibody might enhance an immune response to an antigen by favoring uptake of the antigen-antibody complex into APCs and by rapidly targeting some antigen to FDCs in lymphoid follicles (see Section 2.2.5.2).

SECTION 3

Immune Processes and Their Evasion by Infectious Agents

CHAPTER 3.1. IMMUNE RESPONSES IN THE PREVENTION, CONTROL, AND CLEARANCE OF INFECTION

3.1.1. Sequence of Responses to Infections

It is convenient to divide the infectious process in a host into several stages: infection of susceptible cells, replication of the agent, partial limitation of replication by the early-induced innate responses (see Section 2.1), induction of cell-mediated immune responses, and induction and maturation of the humoral immune response. Usually, IgM is the first immunoglobulin isotype to be produced, followed by IgG, IgA, or IgE.

There can be very great variation in the times for appearance of these responses. In a model system with an acute but sublethal infection, such as influenza virus in the mouse lung after intranasal inoculation, responses such as α and β interferons (IFNα and IFNβ) and increased natural killer (NK) cell activity are detectable within 24 hours of the infection. Helper T cell activity may be detected within 24 to 36 hours and cytotoxic T lymphocyte (CTL) activity within 4 to 5 days. Depending on the size of the original inoculum, peak infectious virus levels are reached by days 3 to 6, after which levels fall, and infectious virus cannot be recovered from the lung after 9 to 12 days. Effector CTL activity reaches a peak 2 to 3 days after maximum viral levels and then decreases, finally disappearing 2 to 3 days after infectious virus can no longer be recovered. Specific IgM-secreting cells are first seen 5 to 6 days after infection is initiated, and IgA- and IgG-secreting cells are found 3 to 4 days later. Peak levels of these cells do not occur until about 2 months, and levels then slowly fall, but there are always some IgG-secreting cells present until at least 18 months later.[350]

Some of these responses are represented in Figure 3.1.1*A*. Memory CTLs are found by day 14 and persist for many months. Maximum levels of memory antibody-secreting cell production are seen about 2 months after infection is initiated (Fig. 3.1.1*B*). Based on the finding that infection of mice with a recombinant vaccinia virus containing the gene for IL-4 was shown to greatly reduce the later production of effector CTLs,[351] it is tempting to speculate that IL-12 may be expressed very early in the infection and that this is followed at days 6 to 7 by IL-4 production dominating, which prevails for some time (Fig. 3.1.1*C*). The net effect of this primary response is that, at almost any future time, this mouse has high levels of specific antibody and of memory CTLs. The human response to influenza has not been followed to the same extent, but the infection is acute, and recovery occurs within a few days to a week.

The human response to human immunodeficiency virus (HIV) infection is very drawn-out. It has been proposed[352] that, after infection at a mucosal surface, virus-infected cells reach draining lymph nodes and initiate cycles of replication that result in viremia, occurring some weeks after the infection began. A temporal association between the substantial decline (but not disappearance) of bloodborne virus and the presence of CTLs has been shown,[353,354] and antibody is detected at later

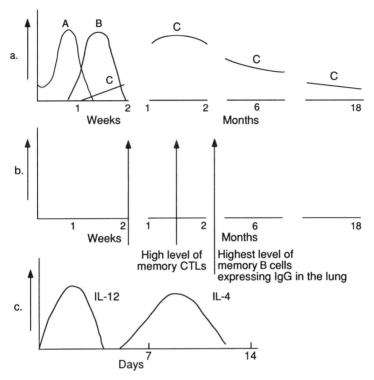

FIG. 3.1.1. Time sequence of the infectious process (ie, influenza virus) and subsequent specific immune responses (ie, cytotoxic T lymphocytes [CTLs] antibody) in the mouse lung after
intranasal infection. (**A**) Ordinate, increase in infectivity or effector cell numbers; abscissa, time
(weeks, months) after initiation of infection. Curve A, titer of infectious virus; curve B, appearance and disappearance of specific CTL activity; curve C, appearance and continuing presence
of specific antibody-secreting cells, mainly IgG, but initially also IgM and IgA. (**B**) High levels of
memory CTLs (by limit dilution analyses) are found at 2 and 6 weeks. Memory B cells reached
their highest levels in the lung at about 2 months but remained at high levels in the spleen for up
to 18 months. (**C**) Postulated levels of interleukin-12 and interleukin-4 in the infected mouse lung
and draining lymph node after infection. (From Ada GL, Jones PD. [1986] The immune response
to influenza infection. Curr Top Microbiol Immunol 128:1–54.)

times. In some individuals, neutralizing antibody is not detected for many months
after the infection was initiated. The temporal sequence of the different responses in
these two infections is similar.

3.1.2. Prevention of Infection

3.1.2.1. Neutralization of Intracellular Agents by Specific Antibody

The amount of an infectious agent that reaches susceptible cells may be limited in
several ways. Cilia in the lung air passages may sweep some organisms into the

trachea, and they are then swallowed. Complement may directly lyse some enveloped viruses (see Section 2.1.4). Bacteria on the skin may be killed by acid components of the skin and sebaceous secretions. However, the only mechanism that has the potential for completely preventing infection is specific antibody, which may be present after a previous infection. The formation of substantial titers of neutralizing antibodies has been the principal aim of most vaccine developers. Although the titers reached in vaccinated individuals are rarely sufficiently high to completely prevent infection—the induction of so-called sterilizing immunity—the antibody should limit the infectious dose to such an extent that a resulting infection is subclinical (ie, disease is prevented). Not unexpectedly, many infectious agents have devised ways of subverting antibody-mediated prevention of infection (see Chapter 3.2).

Infection usually results in the production of specific antibody that may be directed against different epitopes of all components of the agent. This antibody has several roles. First, it may prevent infection (ie, neutralize the infectivity of intracellular and extracellular infectious agents). Second, in the case of an intracellular infection, it may recognize antigens on the surface of infected cells, and this may lead to complement-mediated lysis (see Section 3.1.4). Third, non-neutralizing antibody may combine with the infectious progeny of infected cells; these complexes infect or enhance infection of other cells possessing Fc or C receptors, such as macrophages (eg, flaviviruses) or transport the agent to the surface of follicular dendritic cells in lymphoid follicles, where the virus may contact other susceptible cells (eg, HIV). Fourth, antibody may help in the disposal of debris from infected cells. Antibody serving the first three functions, and particularly the first, is usually only a small fraction of the total antibody produced. Typically, only one or a few antigens of an infectious agent are important in these respects, because only a few of the potential epitopes on a single antigen may be the target of neutralizing antibody.

3.1.2.2. In Vitro Neutralization of Infectivity

In vitro neutralization of infectivity is performed mainly with cells in culture, but occasionally the technique is applied to embryonated eggs or the equivalent. It measures the ability of an antibody preparation to prevent infection of the cells. Usually, the antibody is mixed with the agent for a defined period, such as 30 minutes at 37°C, before the mixture is added to the cellular substrate and incubated, often for hours or days (and sometimes even longer), depending on the agent and the ability of the cells to support replication. Because the neutralization titer is viewed as a surrogate marker of the ability of the antibody to prevent infection in vivo, the nature of the assay is important. The most accurate and sensitive assay is one based on determination of the decrease in the actual number of cells infected, such as by counting plaques (ie, infected cells). Decreases of 10-fold to 100-fold and sometimes 1000-fold may be measured with considerable accuracy. With many situations, plaque assays are not possible, and estimates of a decrease in the production of a viral or bacterial antigen or enzyme (eg, the reverse transcriptase of HIV-1) are made. Frequently, reductions of only up to 10-fold can be calculated (with variable degrees of accuracy) in such situations, and the end result may be less reliable and meaningful.

Neutralizing epitopes for a number of viruses and bacteria (and the occasional parasite) have been described, and several are cited to establish principles. Antibodies binding to five sites of the hemagglutinin (HA) of influenza virus neutralize infectivity (reviewed elsewhere[350]). The sites were identified by analysis of sequence changes in mutants derived under immune selection in the presence of neutralizing monoclonal antibodies (MAbs); analysis of the three-dimensional structure of HA molecules; and comparison of sequences from related epidemic and mutant strains. The sequences at these sites are mainly nonlinear and discontinuous. Panels of MAbs specific for four of the sites were exposed to denatured HA, monomeric HA, and trimeric HA (the form in the virion). None bound to denatured HA, and MAbs bound preferentially to the trimer compared with the monomer in three of the four sites.[355]

A similar situation is found with many RNA viruses, because they frequently have a mosaic consisting of repeats of antigens at their surface,[356,357] but there are exceptions. Poliovirus,[358] the foot and mouth disease agent,[359] and HIV-1 viruses have in addition linear peptide loops. The principal neutralizing domain of HIV-1 is a linear, disulfide-bonded loop of up to 33 residues.[360]

Epitopes in bacterial proteins are often linear sequences. Antibodies directed against the major outer membrane protein of *Chlamydia trachomatis* neutralize infectivity.[361] This protein has hydrophobic sequences held in the bacterial membrane, and these are interspersed with hydrophilic sequences exposed to the exterior. Four regions of these latter sequences possess different amino acid sequences that vary for each serovar, and these segments are interspersed with five constant regions.[362] Vaccine studies in monkeys and humans have shown that protection by antibody is serovar restricted,[363] indicating that the variable sequences provide the epitopes recognized by neutralizing antibody.

How do antibodies prevent infection? Neutralizing antibodies change the isoelectric point of polioviruses.[364,365] A high-resolution study of influenza virus neuraminidase/Fab crystals showed a conformational change in the neuraminidase.[366] This type of change resulting from interaction with antibody may be a common occurrence. The major cellular receptor for HIV-1 is the CD4 molecule. The binding site on the viral envelope protein, gp120, is discontinuous, and antibodies to this region neutralize more broadly than those to the V3 loop. After CD4/gp120 binding occurs, fusion of viral and host cell membranes occurs, allowing virus entry.[367] However, it has proved to be difficult to raise high titer antibodies to this region of gp120.

Substantial differences in the mechanism of monomeric (IgG, IgA) compared with oligomeric (IgM, secretory IgA) forms of antibody in neutralizing influenza virus infectivity have been described.[368–370] The oligomeric forms reduced the attachment of the virus to the cell so that the virus was not internalized. In contrast, virus complexed with neutralizing monomeric Ig was internalized. In the case of IgG, the block in replication seemed to be at the viral transcriptase level. This implies that a conformational effect of antibody on the HA affected another antigen in the virion.

The generation of different Ig isotypes may also be important. IgG_2 antibody is critically important for immunity to *Staphylococcus* mastitis in ruminants. This isotype mediates protection by opsonizing staphylococci for phagocytosis by neutrophils, and this is the major mechanism for controlling bacterial infections in the mammary gland. Although live *Staphylococcus aureus* vaccines stimulated good IgG_2 responses, inactivated bacterial vaccines administered with Freund's adjuvant did not. The use of a different adjuvant, dextran sulfate, induced the formation of IgG_2 responses.[371]

Most bacteria that colonize the exterior of the body are harmless, living on the nutrients present, as in the gut. Some, however, secrete powerful toxins, such as the *Corynebacterium* and cholera organisms, which target intracellular components. Staphylococci and group A streptococci secrete toxins that act as superantigens by binding to those T-cell receptors of class II T cells expressing the V_b gene, and this results in a massive secretion of ILs. Other toxins may bind to receptors on susceptible cells. In each case, antibody prevents this interaction. Some bacteria have specialized mechanisms such as proteases that facilitate penetration of the epithelial cells into the deeper tissue. Antibody to the components of the bacteria that bind to the cell, such as the pili, can prevent this penetration. If penetration does occur, the organism may meet mast cells sensitized with specific IgE. Interaction with these cells causes degranulation, initiating an acute inflammatory reaction that may result in the destruction of the invader.

These examples illustrate the diversity of ways in which antibody can prevent infection. Such knowledge can be useful in designing vaccines.

3.1.3. Limitation of Replication

During the early period after initiation of infection and before effector lymphocytes are formed, various components of the innate immune system may contribute to limiting the replication of an infectious agent (see Section 2.1). In humans, a mild influenza virus infection may be confined to the upper respiratory tract. In a similar infection in the ferret, the inflammatory response consists mainly of polymorphonuclear neutrophils that are extruded onto the mucosal surface at the site of infection.[120] There is a correlation between the rate of decline of nasal virus titers and the extent of the fever, because suppression of the fever results in delayed viral clearance.[121] Pretreatment of mice with *Cryptosporidium parvum* results in lower lung viral titers and mortality rates, and this correlates with increased levels of IFNα and IFNβ, increased NK cell activity, and activated macrophages recovered from the infected lungs.[122] Mice bearing the *Mx* gene are resistant to influenza virus infection, and this is attributed to an enhanced sensitivity to IFNs, because the effect is abolished by pretreatment with anti-IFN antibody.[123]

The difference in the response between susceptible and resistant strains of mice to cytomegalovirus (CMV) infection is seen within 2 to 3 days of infection and is in part a function of NK cells, because NK-deficient C57Bl/6 beige mice are more susceptible to this virus than their heterozygous litter mates.[372] Treatment of mice with anti-asialo GM$_1$ antibody, which depletes NK cells, enhances the growth of CMV, vaccinia virus, and mouse hepatitis virus but not that of lymphocytic choriomeningitis virus (LCMV).[373]

Theoretically, in previously immunized or infected individuals, antibody-dependent cellular cytotoxicity (ADCC) that has been demonstrated in vitro would be expected to contribute to the control of intracellular infections in vivo. This activity has been reported for a number of viral infections. In the case of HIV-infected persons, NK and monocytes have been shown to act as ADCC effector cells and to be directed to the gp120. In contrast, complement-mediated antibody-dependent cytotoxicity has not been observed in HIV-infected individuals (reviewed elsewhere[374]). It is difficult to assess the extent to which such reactions contribute to restricting or clearing infections.

In the case of some extracellular bacteria such as infections by pneumococcus, deposition of some components of complement, particularly C3, can lead to liberation of proinflammatory peptides that attract macrophages and granulocytes that help to limit the spread of the infection (discussed elsewhere[375]).

3.1.4. Control and Clearance of Infections

3.1.4.1. Extracellular Infectious Agents

Many bacteria and some parasites live and replicate outside the host cells. In such situations, specific antibody of the appropriate isotype in conjunction with phagocytosis by cells with the appropriate Fc receptor provides the major mechanism for limiting replication and controlling infection.

In the case of parasites, macrophages, neutrophils, mast cells, basophils, and eosinophils have all been implicated as effector cells in ADCC reactions, at least in vitro. Eosinophils in particular have been thought to play an important role in the host defense against helminths such as schistosomes (*Schistosoma mansoni*[376]) and *Trichinella*.[377] However, studies in IL-5 deficient mice which do not show eosinophilia, indicate that these cells do not play a critical role in the control of the helminth, *Mesocestoides corti*.[304] IgG and IgE may be important, and some studies show a strong correlation in humans between resistance to these parasites and the presence of specific IgE.[378,379] In attempts to define the role of different cytokines and hence the roles of T1 and T2 lymphocytes in helminth infections, experiments using mice have provided a spectrum of findings, which have raised some doubt about the relevance of the murine model for this infection (reviewed elsewhere[380]).

The contribution of the adaptive immune response to the control of extracellular bacteria is twofold. First, the presence of specific antibody arms effector cells so they can kill the bacteria by ADCC mechanisms. Second, if effector T1 and T2 cells

TABLE 3.1.4.1. *Properties and functions of components of immune responses to the control of extracellular infectious agents*

Type of response	Components			Importance at different stages of the infectious process		
	Complement	Cell type	Cytokines	Prevent	Limit	Control or clear
Innate immunity	+	M'phages*	IL-1, TNFα	−	+	+
Adaptive immunity						
CD4+ T2/antibody	+	T and B cells, APCs	IL-3,4,5,6†	+ + +	+ + +	+ + +
CD4+ T1	−	T cells, APCs	IL-2, TNFα,β, IFNγ†	−	+	+ +

APCs, antigen-presenting cells; IFN, interferon; IL, interleukin; M'phages, macrophages; TNF, tumor necrosis factor.
*Other cell types are listed in Table 2.1.2, and additional properties are listed in Table 2.2.2.1.
†For a more complete list, see Table 2.2.3.
+ + + Very important
+ + Important
+ Contributes
− No role

are formed during the adaptive immune response, these secrete cytokines such as IFNγ and tumor necrosis factors (TNFα, TNFβ), which further activate phagocytic cells and contribute to the destruction of the bacteria. This synergy between components of the innate and adaptive immune systems is illustrated in Table 3.1.4.1.[381]

3.1.4.2. Intracellular Infectious Agents

3.1.4.2.1. Innate Immunity

It is likely that the mechanisms of components of the innate immune system contribute to recovery from some infections, but there is no evidence that they are responsible for clearing any infection. For example, despite the high level of NK cell and macrophage activity in nu−/nu− mice, infectious influenza virus persists in foci in the lungs.[350] The synergy between components of the innate and adaptive immune systems in the case of intracellular infections is illustrated in Table 3.1.4.2.1.

3.1.4.2.2. Role of Antibody

Once inside a cell, an infectious agent is usually inaccessible to antibody, although there are some exceptions. Patients with lepromatous leprosy have very high titers of specific antibody, but to no avail. Because agammaglobulinemic patients recover from many viral infections, antibody may not be essential for recovery from such infections. However, antibody can be beneficial, because it may modify the disease due to influenza virus infection[382] and Junin virus in humans,[383] and animal studies point to the same conclusion. Passive transfer of immune serum to mice early after infection reduces lung viral titers.[384] In infected nude mice, passive anti-

TABLE 3.1.4.2.1. *Properties and functions of components of immune responses to the control of intracellular infectious agents*

Type of response	Components			Importance at different stages of the infectious process			
	Complement	Cell type	Cytokines	Prevent	Limit	Control	Clear
Innate immunity	+	M'phages	IL-1, TNFα	−	+ +	+	−
Adaptive immunity							
CD4 + T2/ antibody	+	T and B cells, APCs	IL-3,4,5,6*	+ + +	+ + +	+ +	+
CD4 + T1	−	T cells, APCs	IL-2, TNFαβ, IFNγ	−	+	+ +	+ +
CD8 + CTLs	−	T cells, APCs	IL-2, TNFαβ, IFNγ	−	−	+ + +	+ + +
γδ T cells	−	T cells, APCs	IL-2, TNFαβ, IFNγ	−	?	+ + ?	+ ?

APCs, antigen-presenting cells; CTLs, cytotoxic T lymphocytes; IFN, interferon; IL, interleukin; M'phages, macrophages; TNF, tumor necrosis factor.
*For a more complete list, see Table 2.2.3.
+ + + Very important
+ + Important
+ Contributes
− No role

body prevents virus dissemination, but the effect is transient, because virus shedding reappears as the antibody titer wanes.[385] Infected mice in which the antibody response is suppressed by anti-IgM antibody from birth recover from the infection.[386] However, it has been shown that severe combined immunodeficient (SCID) mice infected with influenza virus and later given specific antibody cleared the virus. The virus was egg-grown, and the dose used was apparently quite small, because control mice took as long as 3 weeks to die.[387]

There are two other examples of antibody clearing a viral infection. Some MAbs to the fusion protein of respiratory syncytial virus (RSV) were found to protect against infection and to clear an established RSV infection. At 6 days after infection (the time of maximum lung viral titers), these MAbs were able to clear the infection within 6 hours of administration.[388] Of the different parameters measured, the only biologic property that correlated with this activity was prevention of syncytia formation by the virus. It seemed likely that these antibodies were endocytosed into the infected cell and could prevent viral formation. In the second example, MAbs or hyperimmune serum specific for Sindbis virus were able to clear this virus from infected neurons in SCID mice, even when administered some days after the original infection.[389] This finding is of interest because neurons are one of the few cell types in the body that do not express (or express at very low levels) class I major histocompatibility complex (MHC) molecules. It was thought that CTLs might not be able to clear such infections,[390] but this is not universally the case, as described subsequently (3.1.4.2.3).

In the face of such findings, it becomes a challenge for vaccine developers to see whether, in appropriate cases, the generation of high antibody titers would have a major role in controlling and clearing an infection in addition to preventing the infection.

3.1.4.2.3. Role of Effector CD8+ T Lymphocytes

There are three general arguments supporting an important role for CTLs. One is the clearing of many viral and some bacterial and parasitic infections. A list of some murine viral infections for which viral levels were greatly reduced by the transfer of CTLs is provided in Table 3.1.4.2.3A.[391-398] Although some of these refer to clearance of virus from individual organs, others refer to experiments in which mice were protected from an otherwise lethal dose of virus. Impaired antigen presentation resulting in defective CTL formation can affect susceptibility to neurologic damage by some viruses.[399-400] Persistent viral infections may occur when the generation of CTLs is subverted (see Chapter 3.2).

The second argument is based on the fact that, with few exceptions, all cells in the body express class I MHC antigens; the exceptions are red blood cells, gametes, cells of the trophoblast, and neurons. Plasmodia have employed the fact that red blood cells do not express MHC antigens by using them as hosts. However, the fact that a cell type does not express class I MHC antigens does not necessarily protect those cells, if infected, from CTL activity. CTLs specific for LCMV on transfer to the brains of mice infected with LCMV cleared the infection from infected neurons.[390] In this case, the adjacent glial cells were infected and were probably the direct target of the CTLs so that secretion of cytokines such as IFNγ may have cleared the virus from the neurons—a bystander effect.

The third argument is that virus-infected cells become susceptible to CTL lysis shortly after infection and long before viral progeny is produced.[401,402] This provides a considerable period for effector cells to find infected host cells and prevent an additional cycle of infection in other host cells. As was colorfully expressed,[403] CD8+ CTLs are auditors that unceasingly monitor molecular events at cell surfaces: "without this constant vigilance, the body, like a company, would be out of business very quickly."

In theory, it might be expected that CTLs would be formed and would contribute to at least the control of an intracellular infection and sometimes to the clearance of

TABLE 3.1.4.2.3A. *Clearance or control of virus in animal models after transfer of virus-specific CD8+ cytotoxic T cells*

Virus	References
Poxvirus (vaccinia)	391, 395
Arenavirus (lymphocytic choriomeningitis)	392
Orthomyxovirus (influenza A)	393, 397
Alphaherpes (herpes)	394
Paramyxovirus (Sendai)	395, 396
Pneumovirus (respiratory syncytial)	397
Betaherpesvirus (murine cytomegalo)	398

Adapted from Ada GL. (1994) Vaccines and the immune response. In: Webster RG, Granoff A, eds. Encyclopedia of Virology. Academic Press, New York, pp. 1503–1507.

the infection. Judging from the studies of animal and human infections (see Section 2.2.3.7), it is expected that this frequently turns out to be the case.

HIV infections in humans continue to provide new insights into the control or loss of control of a viral infection. An association exists between the decrease in viremia and detection of CTL activity among white blood cells.[353,354] Many infected individuals thereafter have active CTLs among their white blood cells for several years. It is as though there is such a tremendous production of cells, virus, and infected cells[83–85] that the corresponding large production of CTLs in the lymph nodes results in a constant spillover into the blood (see Section 2.2.3.7). Although CTL activity finally decreases and disappears as disease becomes more apparent, an association between CTL activity and a slower progression to disease has been observed.[404]

A decade ago, CD8+ effector T cells isolated from HIV-1–infected persons were shown to inhibit HIV replication in tissue culture, and this activity was due to soluble factors and was not human leukocyte antigen (HLA) restricted. A similar effect was subsequently seen with CD8 T cells from simian immunodeficiency virus (SIV)–infected monkeys (reviewed elsewhere[223]). Two groups have identified such factors having this effect. IL-16 was found to have this effect, but relatively high concentrations were required.[405] Three other factors were found to be active at lower concentrations, RANTES, MIP1a, and MIP1b.[406] The extent to which these factors may be useful therapeutically is unknown.

Four groups of observations suggest that a CTL response may be critical in certain circumstances. There are a few well-documented examples of seronegative, virus-negative individuals whose CTLs recognize HIV-1 determinants. The first group includes infants born to HIV-1–infected mothers.[407,408] The second comprises individuals who are in heterosexual contact with HIV-infected patients. Among six seronegative contacts, there was an unusually high frequency of HIV nef-specific CTLs. Nef is one of the earliest expressed viral proteins in the infected cell.[409] A third group includes female prostitutes in two African countries who were almost certainly exposed to HIV-infected partners.[410] Although host factors may also be involved in these situations, the virus to which these individuals were first exposed may have been defective in some respect. Seven of 20 health care workers exposed accidentally once to HIV were found to possess CTLs to the env antigen; all 20 controls were env-CTL negative.[411] This latter finding has special significance for future vaccine strategies and is discussed in more detail in Section 4.2.3.

CTL activity (see Section 2.2.3.7) has been reported in murine and in human infections with some bacteria (eg, listeriosis, tuberculosis, leprosy) and some parasites (eg, *Plasmodium falciparum* [malaria], *Trypanosoma cruzi*). Two examples indicate the progress being made in understanding the role of CD8+ T cells in two of these diseases.

Leprosy patients show a spectrum of disease patterns; those with the tuberculoid form demonstrate strong cell-mediated immune (CMI) responses, and those with the severe disease, lepromatous leprosy, have high antibody titers and weak CMI responses (ie, resistance to the infection correlates with strong CMI responses). Messenger RNA profiles from cells in human lesions from the resistant and susceptible forms were found to code for IL-2 and IFNγ and for IL-4, -5 and -10, respectively.[412] Clones of CD8 + T cells from resistant forms secreted IFNγ, and those from individuals with widespread infection secreted IL-4,[413] supporting the earlier demonstration of suppressor CD8 + T cells in lepromatous leprosy skin lesions.[414]

The second example is the presence of CTLs in *Plasmodium*-infected individuals. It was shown some years ago that mice[415] and human volunteers[416] immunized with irradiated plasmodia sporozoites were protected from challenge with the live sporozoites. In mice, in vivo depletion of CD8 + T cells eliminated this protection, and adoptive transfer of antigen-specific CTL clones protected. The major antigen is the circumsporozoite protein (CSP), and there has been much interest in defining possible CTL determinants in this protein and seeing whether CTLs directed to these or other sporozoite determinants could be detected in the peripheral blood lymphocytes of malaria-infected individuals in endemic regions. Experiments with mice[417] and humans seemed to indicate that only one determinant in the CSP was recognized, and this was in the variable region.[418] A search for CTLs in infected individuals was initially unsuccessful,[419] but later efforts demonstrated the presence of CTLs, although at low levels.[420-422] The low levels may reflect the low antigenic stimulus induced by relatively few sporozoites. The encouraging finding was that responses to several determinants were found, some of which were in conserved regions.[422] The determinants between them could bind to different HLA molecules that were present in up to 75% of the population.[423]

Two overlapping CTL determinants, one of which is conserved, have also been found in the sporozoite surface protein 2 of *P. falciparum*.[424] Both are HLA-B8 restricted. The challenge is whether vaccination procedures can be devised that prime strongly for responses to all of these determinants, including the less dominant ones. Despite the central role played by CTLs in this infection, CD4 + T cells also have an important if poorly defined role in protection against sporozoite infection.[425]

T. cruzi infects a wide variety of cells in susceptible and resistant strains of mice. Immunization with an avirulent strain protects against infection with a virulent strain. Depletion of CD8 + T cells increases the susceptibility of the mice to infection and reverses vaccine-induced immunity.[426]

There has been great interest in the possibility of predicting the presence of CTL determinants in proteins. Two approaches were used to detect and assay peptide determinants from known proteins. One was the isolation and characterization of peptides from peptide–class I MHC complexes from the surface of virus-infected cells,[427] and the other used peptides to sensitize MHC-compatible target cells to lysis by CTLs.[428] From a knowledge of the crystal structure of the MHC-peptide complex, it became clear that certain residues at a given peptide position could be detrimental for binding. This led to the realization that binding peptides had a motif specific for MHC molecules of different allelic specificities and that there were usually two anchor positions that were critical for peptide binding. It became possible to screen proteins of known amino acid sequence for such peptides, and such lists are growing in length almost daily (see Table 3.1.4.2.3A).[429]

Pure peptide binding motifs can be misleading in the search for natural ligands for several reasons, such as protease specificity during antigen processing and the specificity of peptide transporters. If the list of peptides obtained is to be used as the basis for construction of peptide-based vaccines, there may be an additional restriction. Even though a given peptide will bind firmly to an MHC molecule of a given specificity, not all hosts with an MHC haplotype, which contain that allelic specificity but differs in the rest of the haplotype, will respond to that peptide in vivo. This is because of cross tolerance with different self peptides, a phenomenon that is discussed in more detail in Chapter 3.3.

Table 3.1.4.2.3B gives some indication of the advances made within 7 to 8 years toward documenting ligands (ie, naturally occurring determinants isolated from infected cells) and peptide determinants (ie, peptide sequences from isolated antigens that sensitize target cells for lysis by CTLs) from a variety of infectious agents. The reader is referred to the original publication[429] for details. Proteins from more than 20 viruses have been studied in this way, but few have been from bacteria and parasites. Most were identified using known motifs from proteins of known amino acid sequence.

Influenza A virus and HIV have been examined in this respect in considerable detail. As early as 1992, 66 determinants from the three major proteins of HIV-1 (env, gag, pol) identified from one motif and restricted by HLA-A2 had been described.[430] Such information is useful for the design of vaccines, but it has also been used[410] to establish whether HIV-exposed but uninfected Gambian women had HIV-1–specific CTLs. Four HIV-1 and HIV-2 crossreactive peptides were used to

TABLE 3.1.4.2.3B. *Identified peptide ligands* and peptide determinants† that react with class I major histocompatibility complex antigens and come from proteins of various infectious agents*

Class of infectious agent	Infectious agent and protein source of peptides
Viruses	Adeno (5EIA); EBV (LMP2, EBNA); Human CMV (gpB); HCV (core); Hepatitis B (sAg, cAg, nucleocapsid); HIV-1 (gp120, gp41, gag, nef, RT); HPV 16 (E7); HSV-1 (CP27, gpB); HTLV-1 (tax); Influenza B (NP); Influenza A (HA, **MP**, MP, **NP**, NP, NS1, BP1); LCMV (gp, NP); Measles (HA, NP); Murine CMV (**pp89**); Rabies (NS); Rota (VP 3,6,7); RSV (M2); Sendai (NP); SV40 (T); VSV (**NP**)
Bacteria	*Listeria monocytogenes* (**gp60**), listeriolysin
Parasites	*Plasmodium falciparum, P. berghei, P. yoeli* (CSP)

Adeno, adenovirus; EBV, Epstein-Barr virus; CMV, cytomegalovirus; HCV, hepatitis C virus; HIV, human immunodeficiency virus; HSV, herpes simplex virus; HTLV, human T-cell lymphotropic virus; LCMV, lymphocytic choriomeningitis virus; RSV, respiratory syncytial virus; VSV, vesicular stomatitis virus; Rota, rotavirus; Sv, sarcoma virus.

*Peptides isolated from the class I MHC/peptide complexes on infected cells. Peptides in bold type were identified as ligands.

†Peptides of known sequence derived from antigens which bind to class I MHC and to target cells which are then recognized by specific CTLs.

Data from Rammensee HG, Friede T, Stevanovic S. (1995) MHC ligands and peptides motifs. Immunogenetics 41:178–228.

elicit HIV-specific CTLs from three of six of these female prostitutes with HLA-B35, the most common Gambian class I HLA molecule. Other determinants have since been identified to which two of the other three prostitutes have responded (A. McMichael, personal communication). The intriguing question was whether such a finding might indicate protective immunity to HIV infection (see Section 3.4.2).

3.1.4.2.4. Role of Effector CD4+ T Lymphocytes

Type 2 T cells are important for antibody production in all infectious situations. The role of type 1 T cells in infections is to provide help for the production of some antibody isotypes and for the generation of CTLs. In intracellular and extracellular infections, cytokines secreted by these cells, such as IFNγ and TNFα, activate macrophages so they are more efficient at disposing of antibody-coated infectious agents. They may have a similar role in intracellular infections. During HIV-1 infection, a predominance of Type 1 T cells characterizes cases in which the virus is better controlled, such as in long-term HIV survivors (reviewed elsewhere[431]). However, there may be too much of a good thing, because the results of some in vitro experiments suggest that type 1 T cells cytokines, such as IL-2, IFNγ, and TNFα, may upregulate a viral infection such as HIV.[432] Measles infections are also characterized by a period of immunosuppression from which, however, most infected children recover.[389] During this period, there is an increase in the production of IL-4 and IL-10, leading to strong antibody production and a functional impairment of CMI responses. This is generally self-limiting, but in some patients, the suppression of CMI responses persists, and the infection intensifies, resulting sometimes in death.[433]

CD4+ T1 cells are the main mediators of delayed-type hypersensitivity (DTH) reactions, and since the early work of Mackaness on bacterial infections,[434] this reaction has been regarded as indicating a protective response. In the sense that this reaction attracts effector T cells to the site of infection, this must be true. Much of this and subsequent work was done before the existence and potential activity of CTLs in intracellular bacterial infections was known. In murine listeriosis (a model system originally promoted by Mackaness), CD4+ T1 cells have since been shown to have a lesser role than CTLs,[435] because CTLs specific for a single nonamer determinant of the bacterial protein, listeriolysin, have been shown to be protective in vivo.[436] In contrast, in *Mycobacterium bovis* BCG and *Salmonella typhimurium* infections in mice, depletion of CD4+ T cells caused a large increase in bacterial numbers, but depletion of CD8+ T cells had only a small effect on the course of infection.[437] CD4+ and CD8+ T cells seem to be important for resistance of mice to infection by virulent *M. tuberculosis* organisms,[438] which reside in class II MHC–positive macrophages but are resistant to intracellular killing. Clearance therefore depends on activation of the macrophage and killing of the infected cell. However, β_2-microglobulin knockout mice were found to be very susceptible to *Listeria*[439] and tuberculosis[440] infections, showing that CTLs were important in controlling both these infections and that DTH reactions mediated by CD4 + T1 cells might not be a critically important protective response.

The importance of T1 and T2 responses in *Leishmania* infections in mice were mentioned in Section 2.2.3, but the relative contributions of CD4 + T cells or CTL responses in this situation have not been evaluated.

CD4 + T1 cells and not CD8 + CTLs were protective in one special viral system.[441] In a murine model of herpes simplex type 2 infection called the zosteriform spread model,[442] infection is initiated in the flank, and virus spreads by retrograde axonal transport to the spinal ganglia. After replication at this site, virus moves by anterograde axonal spread to the innervated dermatome, where lesions develop. In contrast to the cutaneous site, where CD4 + T1 type cells are protective, immunity in the nervous system may be mediated by CD8 + CTLs.[443]

3.1.4.2.5. Role of Effector γδ T Lymphocytes

Because of the diversity of this population, it may be difficult to define exact roles for different cell types and demonstrate their protective efficacy. The following three examples suggest that these cells may have a largely accessory or complementary function to αβ T cells:

1. Although a single clone of CTLs specific for listeriolysin can give protection against *Listeria monocytogenes* infection, γδ T cells can control inflammatory reactivity and prevent excessive liver damage during this infection.[444]
2. In experiments studying the role of γδ T cells in *Leishmania major* infections of resistant and susceptible mouse strains, the proportion of these cells in the spleen rose substantially but returned to normal in the resistant strain after resolution of the lesions. Depletion of the cells resulted in larger lesions and delayed healing.[445]
3. Successful adoptive transfer of contact sensitivity to mice was shown to require "cooperation" between αβ T cells and γδ T cells; it was suggested that the role of the latter was to counteract the activity of suppressor cells in the recipients.[446]

Mice deficient for the δ chain of the T-cell receptor (and therefore lacking functional γδ T cells) succumb rapidly when infected with *Mycobacterium tuberculosis* and develop large abscesses after *L. monocytogenes* infection, unlike mice lacking αβ T cells.[447] These findings suggest an independent role for γδ T cells, and the next few years should see a clarification of their role in various infectious situations.

3.1.5. Summary of Immune System Properties

Tables 3.1.4.1 and 3.1.4.2.1 summarize briefly properties of the different components of the two immune systems, innate and adaptive, and the roles they play at different stages of the immune response in naive and preexposed or immunized hosts. Table 3.1.4.1 summarizes the situation for extracellular infectious agents where CTLs are not involved and specific antibody is important at all stages. In the naive host, the components of the innate system have a more important role in limiting the infection until specific antibody is produced.

In the case of intracellular infections, our knowledge with viral, bacterial, and parasitic infections indicates that CTLs seem to be designed specifically for the purpose of controlling and clearing the infection. They achieve this by direct lysis of infected cells and by secretion of particular cytokines. Work with modified hosts, with added or subtracted cellular activities, indicates that the immune system is degenerate to the extent that, if the host is not stressed by a virulent infection, the activities of other components can lead to control and sometimes clearance of the infection in the absence of CD8 + $\alpha\beta$ CTLs. There is still much to learn about $\gamma\delta$ T cells. When interpreting many laboratory-based experiments, it should be remembered that the animals used in the experiments live in a particularly favorable and generally unstressed environment, quite unlike that in the outside world.

CHAPTER 3.2. EVASION, SUPPRESSION, AND SUBVERSION OF IMMUNE RESPONSES BY INFECTIOUS AGENTS

The last few years have seen a surge of interest in understanding the interaction between host and intracellular pathogens (reviewed elsewhere[448,449]). Both have co-evolved over prolonged periods, and if one believes in the concept of the selfish gene,[450] both host and pathogen aim to survive. The host has developed an effective but complex and degenerate system of controlling and destroying most infectious agents at three levels: innate immunity, humoral immunity, and CMI. Many agents have one chance per individual naive host to infect and replicate and for the progeny to escape to infect other naive hosts. There are two extremes. In an acute infection, such as influenza, the virus infects the respiratory tract and replicates, and some progeny escapes in droplets expelled from the infected lungs before the adaptive immune system is operative. In contrast, in a primitive society, a young female adolescent may become infected with HIV by sexual transmission. All the host's immune processes become activated, and the person may remain healthy for as long as 10 years before acquired immunodeficiency syndrome (AIDS) develops. By that time, the woman may have infected other adolescents and had several children, who may or may not be infected. It is important that some are not infected so that the host race does not die out. In either situation, the virus persists, and the cycle begins again.

3.2.1. Innate Immunity

Cells such as macrophages, NK, and neutrophils; complement; and some cytokines (IFNs) are rapidly mobilized. Some proteins secreted by bacteria are the source of small peptides containing formyl methionine as their N-terminal amino acid, which attracts neutrophils.[451] The major mortality during influenza A virus epidemics may result from a bacterial superinfection. Neutrophils and macrophages-monocytes participate in the early inflammatory response to such viral epidemics. Components of the influenza virus can interact with surface proteins of neutrophils, and this can result in deactivation of the neutrophil, thereby decreasing the inflammatory response but also facilitating a subsequent bacterial infection.[452] There is also evidence that infection of alveolar macrophages by RSV, although it enhanced the immunoregulatory functions of the cells such as secretion of lymphokines (eg, TNFα, IL-1, IL-6), results in a decrease of the microbicidal activity of the cells.[453]

Serpins are a superfamily of serine proteinase inhibitors that act as pseudosubstrates for specific proteinases. They have a variety of roles, including antiinflammatory activity. Poxviruses may contain several proteins that mimic serpin activity and therefore may help to downregulate inflammatory responses during the early stages of infection.[454]

3.2.1.1. Cytokines

Some large DNA viruses produce proteins that mimic host proteins, including cytokines and their receptors; these are called virokines and viroceptors. Cytokines can be important as part of the adaptive immune response, and some, especially IL-1 and TNFα, are also important in enhancing the activity of cells involved in innate immunity (see Table 2.1.1.2). If this activity of the cytokines could be subverted, the pathogen would doubly benefit. Poxviruses secrete a viroceptor, vIL-1βR, that is a homolog of the cellular receptor for IL-1β.[455] This could have several effects, including slowing the activation of these cells (see Table 2.1.1.2) and minimizing the fever induced by this cytokine.

Poxviruses may also produce three other distinct viroceptors that bind TNF,[456] IFNγ,[457] or type I IFNs.[458] Each of these cytokines have strong antiviral activities, and the possibility of subverting the early host response by these viruses increases the opportunity of the virus to replicate to higher levels in the host. Cytomegaloviruses (CMV) encode a functional receptor for a class of compounds called chemokines.[459] In this case, the class of chemokines involved, the C-C class, attracts monocytes. However, these compounds can react with a variety of cells, including lymphocytes, and they are also produced by different cell types.

Adenoviruses produce several products that can interfere with host early defenses. They include an RNA and several proteins that can interfere with the activities of IFNs and at least three proteins that can prevent TNF cytolysis. Two other proteins can prevent apoptosis of the infected cell, allowing continuing viral infection.[460]

Epstein-Barr virus (EBV) infection produces a protein, BCRF1, which is a homolog of IL-10 and can block the synthesis of cytokines such as IL-2 and IFNγ.[461]

3.2.1.2. Complement

Complement can interfere with viral activity by coating the surface of the virion, by enhancing phagocytosis, or by lysis of the virion (see Chapter 2.1). It would be an advantage for a virus if it could inhibit complement activation, and the poxviruses and herpesviruses can do this. Two proteins secreted by vaccinia virus, a 35-kD and a C4-BP protein, bind complement proteins and accelerate the decay of an enzyme involved in the complement cascade.[462] The gamma herpesvirus, *herpes saimiri*, contains nine viral gene products with striking homologies to known cellular proteins. Two of these are complement control proteins that act at different levels of complement activation, the formation and assembly of the convertases and on the terminal membrane attack complex.[463] They may act to protect infected cells.

3.2.2. Subversion of Humoral Immunity

Although subversion of innate immunity seems to be mainly a speciality of large viruses, evasion of the humoral immune response is a feature of many infectious agents. The major mechanism employed by representatives of viruses, bacteria, and parasites is antigenic variation, but many other strategies may be employed, including destruction of some antibodies, poor immunogenicity or accessibility of critical epitopes, and immune enhancement.

3.2.2.1. Antigenic Variation of RNA Viruses

3.2.2.1.1. Antigenic Drift

RNA viruses show high mutation frequencies, partly because of a lack of the proofreading and mismatch repair systems that ensure a much greater fidelity of DNA replication in mammalian cells.[464] This high mutation frequency is coupled with high rates of replication and is reflected in rates of RNA genome evolution, which can be more than 1 million-fold greater than the rates of DNA chromosome evolution of their hosts.[464] Such antigenic change is seen most markedly in the external viral antigens, which are usually the source of epitopes recognized by neutralizing antibodies and are often expressed on the plasma membrane of infected cells.

Retroviruses, especially HIV, demonstrate this high mutation rate most vividly. Errors occur during translation and transcription, and additional errors can occur during replication at the level of reverse transcription and integration into the host cell genome. As a result, the level of mutations in the gp120 of HIV-1 is much greater than that, for example, in the influenza virus, which was once the classic case of such antigenic drift. Up to 30% of the amino acid residues in gp120 are subject to mutation, and in the V3 loop of this molecule, commonly called the principal neutralizing domain, up to 12 different amino acids may be found at individual positions.[465] A population of such variants can be stored or "frozen" for some time in the form of provirus in an infected cell. The net result is that, after infection in vivo with HIV-1, a range of quasispecies of virus accumulates, and by the time antibody to virus of one specificity is made, many escape mutants may be present. A tetramer at the tip of the V3 loop is relatively conserved,[465] and this has given rise to the hope that this sequence could be targeted for vaccine development. A number of viral subtypes or clades has been defined based on the intact env and gag sequences. In the case of the V3 region, there is an intersubtype variance of about 20% to 30% and an intrasubtype variance of 7% to 15%.[466] Different subtypes dominate in different world regions, which potentially makes the task of formulating vaccines for global use much more difficult. Contrary to the situation with many other viruses, the internal proteins of HIV-1 also show a high but not as great a rate of mutation.

About 10% of the residues in the HA or the NA of the influenza virus are subject to change, but the internal proteins of the virus are much more constant in amino acid sequence.[467] The variation in amino acid sequence in the HA is particularly noticeable in the epitopes recognized by neutralizing antibody.

Most other RNA viruses show antigenic drift, although at a much lower level than the retroviruses and the influenza viruses. Poliovirus exists as three distinct subtypes and, although mutations occur in each subtype in the field, the vaccines are effective. Similarly, antigenic variants of measles virus have been detected in the HA but not in the fusion proteins, the two external antigens of the virus, and the measles vaccine is effective anywhere in the world.[468] The reasons why some RNA viruses (excluding retroviruses) show much greater antigenic variation than others is not clear. Perhaps with the external antigens of some viruses, there is a much greater constraint on the extent of mutations that can be tolerated without destroying the structural and conformational requirements.

3.2.2.1.2. Antigenic Shift

Influenza A viruses have a segmented genome, and this allows an interchange of those segments of RNA coding for different viral antigens.[467] The process is called genetic reassortment and has been observed and demonstrated mainly between human and animal influenza viruses. Figure 3.2.2.1.2 indicates the epidemiologic pattern seen since late last century. The recent shifts all occurred in China, and with the modernization of that country, perhaps future antigenic shifts will occur less frequently. Of the 8 genes in the virion, current vaccines strains are produced by varying only the genes for the HA and NA on an otherwise constant background of internal antigens.

HIV-1, HIV-2, and influenza viruses are two of the three cases mentioned under new and emerging diseases (see Table 1.4.2). Howard Temin[469] wrote about retroviruses in particular, but his comments apply to some other RNA viruses: "The ability of viruses to evolve rapidly and thus take advantage of new environmental niches is inherently unpredictable. Because these mutational and recombinational

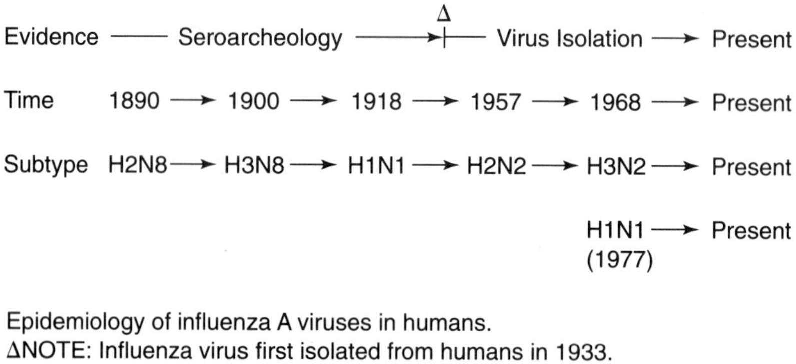

```
                                            Δ
Evidence ──── Seroarcheology ───────→├──── Virus Isolation ───→ Present

Time      1890 ──→ 1900 ──→ 1918 ──→ 1957 ──→ 1968 ──→ Present

Subtype  H2N8──→ H3N8 ──→ H1N1 ──→ H2N2 ──→ H3N2 ──→ Present

                                            H1N1 ──→ Present
                                            (1977)
```

Epidemiology of influenza A viruses in humans.
ΔNOTE: Influenza virus first isolated from humans in 1933.

FIG. 3.2.2.1.2. Epidemiology of influenza A viruses in humans. Influenza virus was first isolated from humans in 1933. (From Murphy BR, Webster RG. [1990] Orthomyxoviruses. In: Fields BN, Knipe DM, eds. Virology, 2nd ed. Raven Press, New York, 1091–1154.)

processes are random, novel combinations of characteristics ensure that new viral pathogens will appear when they have new opportunities to replicate."

3.2.2.2. Antigenic Variation of DNA Viruses and Other Infectious Agents

Some DNA viruses have mutation frequencies (and hence adaptability) greater than that of their host cells. The spontaneous mutation rates of all living organisms tend to be inversely proportional to the sizes of their DNA genomes. The increasing complexity of higher organisms requires an increase in the fidelity of their DNA genomes.[470] However, because of the greater stability of DNA-containing organisms, the term *serotype* is most often used. There are 47 known serotypes of human adenoviruses and 83 pneumococcal serotypes that cause invasive infections. Vaccines in the United States contain the commonest (and safest) serotypes that cause disease in that country, two in the case of the adenoviral and 23 for the pneumococcal vaccines. This choice of different serotypes for vaccine efficacy may vary for other countries.

The need to rapidly change the specificity of individual organisms is solved in a unique way by protozoan trypanosomes, the causative agent of Chagas disease in South America and sleeping sickness in Africa. They are transmitted to man by flies, and their life cycle is represented in Figure 3.2.2.2. The slender form in the bloodstream after transmission by flies replicates and finally changes to a nongrowing stage suitable for transmission back to a fly. The trypanosome genome contains multiple DNA genes coding for the major surface glycoprotein (SG) but of different antigenic specificities. As antibody to one SG specificity is made and prevents that organism from further proliferation, others can switch DNA expression and produce SG of another antigenic specificity. This is achieved through DNA rearrangements or alternative activation of the telomeric SG gene expression sites. Although the

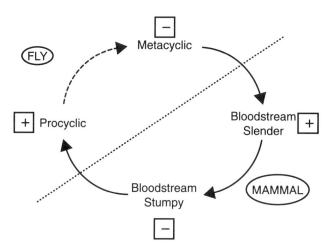

FIG. 3.2.2.2. The life cycle of African trypanosomes. This cycle alternates proliferative (+) and quiescent (−) stages. The differentiation intermediates between procyclic and metacyclic forms are not specified (*dotted line*). (From Vanhamme L, Pays E. [1995] Control of gene expression in trypanosomes. Microbiol Rev 59:223–240.)

number of possible SG specificities is limited, a sufficient number can be expressed over time to ensure that a population of the organisms will survive and be transmitted to other flies, because, as in HIV infections, the host's humoral immune response never catches up with the changes (reviewed elsewhere[471]). Because antibody is the main adaptive immune mechanism for control of infection and replication, this ability to change antigenic specificity makes vaccine development a major challenge.

3.2.2.3. Other Mechanisms

Although secretory IgA is designed to withstand the rigors of life in the gut, including resistance to proteases in general, *Neisseria gonorrhoeae* and *Neisseria meningitidis* secrete a protease that selectively cleaves human IgA1 but not IgA2.[472] It is possible that fragments of IgA may influence the synthesis of the secretory component.[473]

A second mechanism applies particularly to agents showing antigenic variation. Such variation often occurs in immunodominant regions of an antigen, but there may be conserved neutralization epitopes that are less accessible to antibody or poorly immunogenic. The linear V3 loop of HIV-1 gp120 is immunodominant, but it shows great variation. In contrast, the site that binds to CD4, the cell receptor, is conserved and is strongly conformational, but it is poorly immunogenic because prolonged immunization is required to raise neutralizing antibody to it.[474]

Antibody that neutralizes group A streptococci recognizes the M protein and some may cause rheumatic fever. Protective antibodies opsonize the bacteria in the presence of neutrophils. Immunity previously was thought to be essentially strain specific and dependent on antibodies to the variable serotype-specific regions of the protein. There are more than 100 such serotypes. However, people living in endemic regions have been found to have antibodies to a conserved region, a 20–amino acid sequence called peptide 145. Antibodies to this peptide (raised using Freund's complete adjuvant) were able to opsonize seven isolates representing five serotypes,[475] giving some hope that a vaccine based on this peptide might afford a significant amount of protection.

In an outbred population and even during a severe viral epidemic (against which none would be previously immune), not all individuals may respond to all major epitopes. The availability of panels of MAbs to three neutralizing epitopes of the HA of the Hong Kong strain of influenza virus (H3N2, 1969–71) enabled an assessment of the response of infected individuals to each epitope.[476] Thirty-three percent responded to all three, 50% to two epitopes, and 17% to only one (but not always the same one)—an example of *Ir* gene effects.

In contrast, a virus may use a specific immune response for its own ends. Antibody bound to the virus can enhance viral infectivity in cells such as monocyte-macrophages with Fc and/or C receptors. The classic example is dengue virus; sequential infection with different subtypes may cause a severe clinical disease, dengue hemorrhagic fever and shock syndrome.[477] In vitro, antibody may also enhance HIV infectivity, and this effect is more pronounced with antibody from AIDS patients.[223] Epitopes of HIV gp160 recognized by enhancing antibody have been identified.[478] Immune enhancement may occur with any agent that replicates in cells possessing such receptors.

Measles immune sera and MAbs to HA can modulate the measles antigens on the infected cell surface and downregulate the expression of internal structural antigens of the virus inside the cell, a process that protects infected cells from subsequent immune recognition.[479]

3.2.3. Subversion of the Cell-Mediated Immune Response

Many infectious agents can be placed in one of two groups: those that cause acute infections and those that induce persistent infections. Table 3.2.3 lists many agents that cause persistent infections. The distinction is not absolute. For example, some viruses (eg, influenza, measles, rubella) that usually cause acute infections may cause persistent infections in a small percentage of cases, especially if the brain or central nervous system becomes infected.

The mechanisms of subversion cited in the previous two sections are not major contributors to the development of a persistent infection. Production of factors such as viroceptors may contribute initially to an increased level of infection. Generally, the presence of specific antibody does not control many intracellular organisms, such as leishmaniasis in susceptible mice and lepromatous leprosy in humans. The major factor causing persistence is evasion of the CMI response mediated by T1

TABLE 3.2.3. *Agents that cause persistent infections*

Viruses	Adeno; cytomegalo; Epstein-Barr; hepatitis B, C, D; herpes simplex-1,2; human herpes-6; HIV-1,2; HTLV; measles; papilloma; parvo; polyoma; rubella; varicella-zoster
Bacteria	*Chlamydia trachomatis*; *Helicobacter pylori*; *Mycobacterium leprae, Mycobacterium tuberculosis, Neisseria gonorrhoeae*; *Steptococcus pyogenes*; *Treponema pallidum*
Parasites	Trypanosomes; *Leishmania*; *Plasmodium*; microfilariae; schistosomes; *Toxoplasma gondii*; *Trichomonas vaginalis*

HIV, human immunodeficiency virus; HTLV, human T-cell lymphotropic virus.

cells. The main contributing events include latency, privileged sites, factors that interfere with antigen processing and recognition by T1 cells and CTLs, and infection and destruction of important cells involved in the immune response.

3.2.3.1. Latency

Important examples of latency include herpesviruses, EBV, and retroviruses. Herpesviruses infect neurons, and gene expression does not occur except for one region of the genome. The infection may remain latent for long periods. Persons who had chickenpox during childhood may much later have a recurrence of viral replication, perhaps as their immunity wanes. Unusual stress may also result in an outbreak of herpes lesions. Latency is an efficient way for the virus to escape the immune system for long periods, but lateral spreading does not occur during this latency period. B cells latently infected with EBV express only one protein, called EBNA-1, and it has been a puzzle why such cells are not recognized, at least by the CTLs of some people. It now appears that the Gly-Ala amino acid repeats in EBNA-1 generate an inhibitory signal that interferes with antigen processing and class I MHC–restricted presentation (see Section 3.2.3.2).[480] Retrovirus cDNA is integrated by a reverse transcriptase and an integrase into the host cell genome, where it may remain unexpressed.

3.2.3.2. Sanctuary Sites

Several sites in the body are not easily accessible to components of the immune system. These protected sites include the brain and the epididymis, which are separated from the blood by a barrier, and the kidney. HIV, for example, replicates in the brain and is present in semen. The finding that many individuals infected with HIV have a very strong and persisting CTL response that fails to clear the virus suggests that there is a continuing source of virus to infect other cells, which induce new CTL production. It was postulated that there was a sanctuary of infected cells that was inaccessible to the CTLs and that this provided a constant source of new virus (Fig. 3.2.3.2).[481] There are also a few cell types that do not express class I or II MHC antigens, such as neurons, gametes, and red blood cells. Herpes and measles

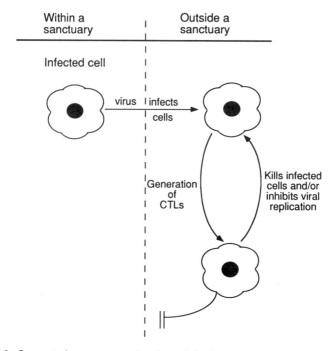

FIG. 3.2.3.2. Concept of a sanctuary, whereby an infectious agent, usually a virus, can escape immune surveillance. Infected cells within a sanctuary can liberate progeny virus, which may infect other cells outside the sanctuary. Some of the latter may act as antigen-presenting cells and induce the formation of cytotoxic T lymphocytes (CTLs,) which can kill virus or inhibit viral replication in all cells outside the sanctuary but not affect viral replication of cells inside the sanctuary. A sanctuary may be formed by a physical barrier, such as the blood-brain barrier, or an infected cell may not be recognized by effector CTLs (eg, downregulation of major histocompatibility complex expression, failure to produce appropriate peptides).

viruses infect neurons, and plasmodia infect red blood cells. Human polyomaviruses and CMV replicate in the kidney, and progeny is shed into the urine. Because lymphocytes traffic through the kidney, the mechanism of escape from surveillance is not clear. Other possibilities include downregulation of class I MHC or failure to produce correct peptides in infected cells. In some cases, the reason is unknown. It was early found that transfer of CTLs would completely clear a poxvirus infection in some strains of mice, but in another strain, the virus persisted in the spleen.[482]

3.2.3.3. Viral Effects on Cells of the Immune System

A variety of viruses infects cells of the immune system. Hepatitis B, adenovirus, EBV, and human herpesvirus-6 infect T or B lymphocytes. HIV infects or affects most critical cells of the immune system, especially CD4 + T cells, macrophages, and dendritic cells, the major antigen-presenting cells for CTL induction,[483] and it has been found in CD8 + T cells. It is present on follicular dendritic cells in lymphoid tissues, and attaches to M cells on Peyer's patches and to galactosyl-cerebroside–positive cells in the brain and gut.

3.2.3.4. Regulation of Class I Major Histocompatibility Complex Expression

Shortly after the description of MHC restriction, it was found that about 22 hours after infection of some target cells by ectromelia virus, the cells were less susceptible to lysis by virus-specific CTLs than at an earlier time.[484] A similar effect was later found to occur in CMV, herpesvirus, and adenovirus infections. Human CMV encodes a MHC-like protein that can bind β_2-microglobulin.[485] An early expressed protein of adenovirus infection, E3/19K, binds and forms a complex with MHC antigens, with the net result that expression of MHC antigen at the cell surface is greatly reduced.[486] Herpes simplex–infected cells express a cytoplasmic protein, ICP47, that has been shown to efficiently inhibit peptide transport across the endoplasmic reticulum membrane so that nascent class I MHC molecules fail to acquire antigenic peptides; the ICP47 binds to the peptide transporter, preventing peptide translocation into the endoplasmic reticulum.[487,488,493]

3.2.3.5. Mediation of Cytotoxic T Lymphocyte Recognition, Activity, and Production

Like antigenic drift in B-cell epitopes, a similar phenomenon in T-cell determinants could also be expected to occur, especially in persistent infections. Escape by a virus from CTL control was first shown with LCMV in a transgenic mouse model.[489] The pattern of HIV infection has many of the features that make it a good candidate for CTL escape mutants to occur during the infection. Many CTL determinants in HIV proteins have already been mapped.[430] Such escape mutants have been found in several determinants in the gag protein presented by HLA-B8, but the response restricted by HLA-B27 is more stable.[490] A rather similar situation has been found with the tax protein of HTLV-1. Substitutions occurred in infected HLA-A2 subjects, but the ability of the tax protein to transactivate three promoters was reduced in many of the variants.[491] In contrast, some determinants appear to remain constant. CTL escape mutants did not accumulate in vivo in 8 to 14 months for an HIV HLA-B27–restricted gag immunodominant determinant.[492] Similarly, CTLs did not appear to select for mutations in an immunodominant gag determinant of SIV.[493] Although escape mutants may contribute to the persistence of retroviral infections, they may not be a dominant factor.

A second potential escape mechanism is a type of antagonism whereby a virus can block CTL activity. In two systems, HIV-1[494] and hepatitis B,[495] naturally occurring variants of the determinants recognized by CTLs may act as antagonists in vivo, because the corresponding peptide was able to prevent a specific CTL response in vitro. In the HIV experiments, the effect was found with free peptides and with a recombinant virus containing DNA encoding the donor protein. It has been pointed out[496] that, in a sea of *agonistic* viruses, the infected cell might well escape destruction by CTLs; such an escape mechanism would only be effective if the viruses concerned were noncytopathic, which is the case with hepatitis B.

3.2.3.6. Epitope and Determinant Dominance

In Section 3.2.2.3, evidence was presented about the potential importance of a nondominant but conserved epitope in the search for a vaccine against group A streptococci.[475] A similar pattern is emerging concerning determinants recognized by CTLs. Weakly immunogenic determinants recognized by CTLs have been found in the conserved regions of the circumsporozoite protein of plasmodia, but the immunodominant determinant is in the variable region.[422,423] Typically, CTLs in an individual host recognize only one or a small number of the potential determinants in a protein.

One model based on preliminary data[497] proposes that, in an antigenically homogeneous pathogen, a dominant response against a single determinant is induced and that, if there is antigenic variation in this determinant, the pathogen may escape because of the antigenic weakness of other determinants, which may result in fluctuating responses to them. If these early reports hold up in other situations, a clear message for designers of a vaccine to a pathogen that shows great antigenic variation is to find ways of enhancing the immunogenicity of the weaker epitopes or determinants if they are in antigenically conserved regions. In the case of CTL determinants, one possible approach is the "string of beads" concept, in which linked "minigenes," each coding for different peptides, are incorporated into a live vector.[498]

3.2.3.7. Cellular Receptors for Viruses

Viruses usually recognize a surface-expressed antigen on a susceptible cell. The more critical the role of antigen is for a cell, the less likely there will be a deficiency of target cells. HIV uses CD4 as its target, and as virus progeny is secreted from the cells, gp120 is released, and it may attach to other CD4 + T cells. This may limit the opportunity for those cells to participate in immunologic reactions or to be infected by HIV. ICAM-1, a cell-surface ligand, is the cellular receptor for rhinoviruses on nucleated cells and for plasmodia on red blood cells.[499,500] ICAM-1 and its receptor, LFA-1, are important for lymphocyte adherence.

CHAPTER 3.3. THE IMMUNOLOGIC REQUIREMENTS FOR SUCCESSFUL VACCINATION

The ability to define these requirements is based on our increasing understanding of the mammalian immune system in general and the responses of the host, especially in model systems, to infectious agents. In this respect, viruses that induce an acute infection such as influenza virus have been particularly useful.

3.3.1. Four Requirements

Successful vaccination has four requirements:

1. The activation of antigen-presenting cells, involving the processing of antigens by the lysosomal or cytoplasmic routes, expression of co-stimulatory factors at the cell surface, and the secretion of appropriate cytokines
2. The activation, replication, and differentiation of T and B lymphocytes to generate large pools of memory cells of both types
3. The incorporation of sufficient epitopes and determinants that specifically bind to at least the major regional HLA haplotypes and the complex recognized by the receptors on B cells and T cells, respectively
4. The long-term persistence of conformationally intact antigen, preferably as aggregates of antigen complexed with antibody and held at the surface of follicular dendritic cells in lymphoid tissues, allowing the continuing formation of memory B cells, followed by their recruitment to form antibody-secreting cells, and ensuring continuing production of agent-specific antibody of increasingly higher affinity

The third and fourth items require further comment. An individual protein may contain a number of T-cell determinants, but an individual or mice of an inbred strain may respond to only a few or even one determinant. This finding led to the concept of *immunodominance* (see Section 3.2.3.6). Because this determinant may be subject to variation, there may be a strong case for inducing responses to less dominant determinants, especially if they are present in conserved regions of the antigen. Second, there is the possibility of peripheral tolerance to one MHC molecule that can affect the ability of the host to respond to a particular determinant in the context of another MHC molecule, an effect often referred to as *cross tolerance*.[501] The identification of a determinant as immunogenic in the presence of a particular MHC molecule does not automatically guarantee a response when that particular MHC-determinant complex is present. There remains the strong need for a vaccine to contain a variety of T-cell determinants to overcome these problems and MHC antigen polymorphism in an outbred population.

The evidence for long-lived antibody production that depends on the persistence of antigen was reviewed in Section 2.2.5.2. There are several other possible contributing factors. First is the persistence of the infectious agent. Because this has been shown not to occur in murine influenza infections,[502] it cannot be a general explanation. Second, although stimulation by crossreacting antigen, a form of original antigenic sin,[503] may occur sometimes, it may not offer a general explanation. Some volunteers for phase I trials of a recombinant vaccinia virus/HIVgp160 preparation were found to have anti–vaccinia virus antibody 15 years or more after having been vaccinated against smallpox,[504] and there was no evidence for long-term persistence of infectious vaccinia virus. General vaccination against smallpox stopped in 1971, well before these trials in 1991. In the case of vaccinia virus, the only other poxvirus that replicates in humans is monkeypox, and human infections by this virus are rare. Idiotypic or anti-idiotypic antibody networks are a third possible factor. There are many examples of such networks, but few reports of effects over periods of years. This effect may contribute to long-lived antibody production but is unlikely to be the main mechanism.

3.3.2. Factors Affecting the Development of Effective Vaccines

A study of the properties of successful vaccines (especially the live, attenuated viral vaccines), of the host's immune response to them, and of the disease process after natural infection allows a list of some of the factors that favor vaccine development (Table 3.3.2A). Some additional factors that were important or helpful in the smallpox eradication campaign are also given. The last two items are not critical requirements, as witnessed by the progress toward the eradication of poliomyelitis.

Two of these characteristics are especially important. First, most of the infections are acute; for most persons, the host's immune system can cope with a sublethal dose so that the infection is short-lived and recovery complete. Second, the agent shows little antigenic variation.

Another list can be compiled of factors that may make vaccine development more difficult, particularly if most of these points apply to one agent, as is the case with HIV (Table 3.3.2B).

TABLE 3.3.2A. *Factors favoring development of an effective vaccine to control or eradicate an infectious disease*

The infectious agent
1. Only one or a small number of important serotypes; little or no antigenic shift or drift
2. The agent is only moderately or poorly infectious.
3. Antigens that are sources of important B-cell epitopes or T-cell determinants are readily identified.
4. Route of immunization: long-lasting systemic immunity is more readily generated than immunity at some mucosal sites.

The infection
1. Infection by the wild-type agent produces protective immunity; this is usually the case with an acute infection.
2. There is available a relatively inexpensive animal model that mimics the infectious process, with onset of the characteristic disease.

Eradication
1. The infection is specific for humans; there is no animal or bird reservoir.
2. Infection causes a characteristic clinical disease; there are no subclinical infections or a carrier state.
3. There is a simple marker of successful vaccination.

TABLE 3.3.2B. *Factors obstructing development of an effective vaccine*

The infectious agent
1. Antigenic variation: there are many serotypes or, more important, there is marked antigenic drift (high mutation rate) or shift.*
2. The agent is highly infectious.
3. There is a potential for change in viral tropism.*

The infection and disease
1. Infection may be transmitted by infected cells that may or may not express viral antigen (eg, latency) that is recognized by the immune system.*
2. Viral DNA/cDNA integrates into the host cell genome.*
3. Protective immunity does not occur after natural infection; escape mutants (T and B cells) occur over time.*
4. Suppression of some responses may occur; antibody of an appropriate isotype (eg, C fixing) may not be formed.*
5. Antibodies may enhance infection of susceptible cells (eg, macrophages, monocytes).*
6. Crucial cells of the immune system are infected or affected.*
7. A readily available, affordable, and susceptible animal model that can mimic the human disease is not available.*

*These points apply to human immunodeficiency virus type 1 infections.

CHAPTER 3.4. THE IMMUNOLOGIC BENEFITS OF VACCINATION

3.4.1. Immunopathology of Infection Versus Vaccination

The hazards associated with infection by the measles virus or by *Bordetella pertussis* are illustrated in Tables 1.2.8 and 1.2.9, and immunopathology contributes to these hazards. Immunopathology associated with the use of several of the childhood vaccines is discussed in Section 1.2.6.[68]

Immunopathology associated with infection is more readily studied in model systems. Lymphocytic choriomeningitis (LCM) is an inflammatory disease of adult mice that occurs after direct infection of the brain with LCMV. The degree of inflammation corresponds to the level of virus-infected cells. The activation of NK, T cells, and macrophages contributes to inflammation, but CTLs are the only population essential for the development of disease.[505] Infection in neonatal or in adult immunosuppressed mice is relatively noncytopathic, even though the virus persists. It has been suggested that the immunosuppression observed during HIV infection is a result of HIV-specific CTL-mediated immunopathology rather than viral cytolytic effects.[506] The very high level of infected cells and of CTL activity in infected lymph nodes supports this proposal.

In a murine model of RSV infection, transfer of a small number of cloned virus-specific CTLs is well tolerated and clears the infection; transfer of a larger number of such cells induces disease in the infected mice.[507]

The complex balance between host and virus is exemplified by hepatitis B virus (reviewed elsewhere[498]). A low-dose infection in a mature host induces a rapid immune response sufficient to clear the virus.[508,509] If the T-cell response is delayed, a

TABLE 3.4.1. *Some responses of mice after intranasal inoculation with the parental or the cold-adapted (ca)-strain of influenza virus, A/Ann Arbor/6/60*

Virus	$TCID_{50}$ inoculum	Lung consolidation*	Lung weight[†]	^{51}Cr release[‡]	DTH[§]
Parent	5.0	35%	0.27 g	70.2 ± 3.4	16.4 ± 5.3
Ca-variant	5.0	< 5%	0.14 g	71 ± 3.1	14.8 ± 3.9[¶]

*At different times between 6–12 days after infection, the consolidation varied from 20–60% for parental virus, and <5–15% for the *ca* strain.

[†]Normal lung weight is c.0.15 g.

[‡]Measured at effector/target ratios of 100:1 and 50:1.

[§]Mean increase in footpad thickness. The same virus was used to both sensitize for and elicit DTH reactions in individual mice.

[¶]All responses quoted were measured at day 9 after virus administration. At day 6, the lung viral titers ($TCID_{50}$) were as follows: parental strain, $4.2 + 0.02$; *ca* strain, <2.0. At day 9, no virus was recovered from either group.

Data from Mak NK, Zhang Y-H, Ada GL, Tannock GA. (1982) The humoral and cellular response of mice to infection with a cold-adapted influenza A virus variant. Infect Immun 38: 218–225.

chronic infection may develop. A high-dose infection in an immature or immuno-suppressed host may lead to an apparently healthy carrier state, although other complications can occur at a later stage.

The availability of an attenuated, cold-adapted (*ca*) strain of influenza virus enabled a comparison to be made of the T-cell responses in mice infected with the *ca* or parental strain.[510] Mice were inoculated intranasally with an equal dose (5.0 $TICD_{50}$) of either strain. The degree of lung consolidation, the lung weights, the NK cell and macrophage cytotoxic activities, the DTH and CTL responses, and lung viral titers were measured at times between 6 and 12 days after infection. Some of this data is presented in Table 3.4.1. With this dose, the magnitude of the different immune responses were similar (DTH and CTL activities are given in Table 3.4.1), but the immunopathologic damage, as indicated by the extent of lung consolidation and the increase in lung weight, was very different. The extent of viral replication, that is a reflection of the number of infected cells, differed by up to 1 thousand-fold at day 6 after the initial infection. The important conclusion to be drawn from this experiment is that, although immunopathology in an infected host may be caused primarily by the effector T cells generated, the extent of infection is the critical factor. Effector T cells cause little damage if there are relatively few infected cells.

Although similar experiments do not seem to have been done with intracellular bacterial infections, it is likely that a similar situation could be demonstrated by comparing attenuated bacterial with wild-type bacterial preparations.

3.4.2. Applying the Benefits of Vaccination

The main benefits resulting from vaccination are the continuing presence of high-affinity, specific antibody to neutralize infectivity and a large pool of memory effector T cells. In the case of an agent that is antigenically constant, the level of specific antibody after vaccination is likely to be sufficiently high to decrease the infectious dose of the challenge virus by more than 99%; in such a case, the normal level of naive T cells may be sufficient to cope with the small portion of infectious agent that escaped antibody neutralization. However, if the agent shows great antigenic variation or antigenic shift, as can be the case with influenza virus, the presence of a pool of memory cells can result in a substantially quicker CTL response, which can prevent a build-up of infected cells and a high level of infectious virus.

An experiment demonstrating such a situation is shown in Figure 3.4.2.1, in which three antigenically distinct types of virus, A/WSN (H1N1), A/JAP (H2N2), and A/Port Chalmers (H3N2), were used.[511] One of two groups of mice was infected intranasally with A/WSN virus. Some weeks later, both groups of mice were inoculated intranasally with A/JAP virus. The levels of infectious A/JAP virus and of CTL activity (assayed on target cells infected with A/Port Chalmers virus) in the mouse lungs were measured on days 3, 4, 5, and 7 after infection with A/JAP virus. Although there is little cross-neutralization by antibodies to H1 and H2 molecules, the level of virus in the pre-primed mice is lower at 3 days compared with the controls, and this level decreases further by day 5, coinciding with the early and rapid increase in CTL activity in this group of mice. The CTL activity in the pre-primed mice occurs 1 to 2 days earlier and may reach a higher level of activity compared with the controls. In this experiment, the CTL activity measured was only to determinants shared between these three viral subtypes. The time difference in appearance of responses between pre-primed and naive mice may have been greater if target cells infected with A/JAP or A/WSN had been used (ie, expressing more shared determinants). This more rapid production of CTLs would at least have decreased the extent of immunopathology and may have prevented death had the strain of virus been highly virulent for mice.

Figure 3.4.2.2 demonstrates three different scenarios.[512] In a primary infection, a substantial CTL response occurs as a result of substantial virus replication. In a secondary response, the extent of a more rapid and possibly higher CTL response due to the recruitment of memory CTLs is proportional to the amount of virus that escapes antibody neutralization and hence replicates to provide an increasing stimulus (see Fig. 3.4.2.2*B* and *C*). Whether this more rapid CTL response is caused by qualitative rather than quantitative changes in memory cells compared with naive T cells is being investigated. Some findings indicate that memory alloreactive CTLs[513] and memory influenza virus–specific CTLs (A. Mullbacher, personal communication), compared with naive T cells, do not require co-stimulation for activation, suggesting in the latter case that any infected cells could act as antigen-presenting cells. This may be sufficient to explain the earlier response by memory cells.

Evidence suggests that CTLs may clear an HIV-1 infection under certain circumstances: in seronegative infants born of infected mothers,[407,408] in seronegative partners of infected men,[409] and in seronegative prostitutes in some African countries.[410] In a "normal" infection, HIV virus–infected cells at a mucosal surface may reach the draining lymph nodes within a short period and replicate to high titers there.

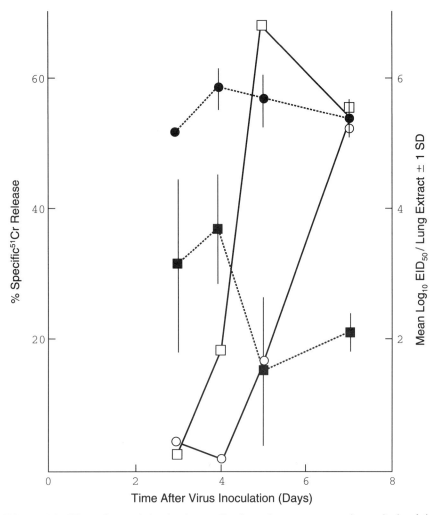

FIG. 3.4.2.1. Effect of pre-priming in vivo on the time of appearance and magnitude of the crossreactive cytotoxic T lymphocyte (CTL) response to influenza viruses. Crossreactive CTL activity recovered from the lungs of mice preinfected with A/JAP (H2N2) virus (□) and from naive (○) mice after a challenge infection with A/WSN (H1N1) virus. CTL activity was measured on target cells infected with A/Port Chalmers (H3N2) virus. Virus levels in the lungs of pre-primed (■) or naive mice (●) are indicated at different times after the challenge. Each point represents the mean $\log_{10}$ EID$_{50}$/lung extract ± 1 SD from three lungs.

This leads to viremia 2 to 3 weeks later, allowing wide dissemination of the virus to distant sites. HIV has been detected in the brain 2 weeks after infection occurred.[514] CTLs have been detected among white blood cells at the time of viremia, but neutralizing antibodies were not found until many weeks or months later. If the vaccine employed induced a high level of memory CTLs and these could be efficiently

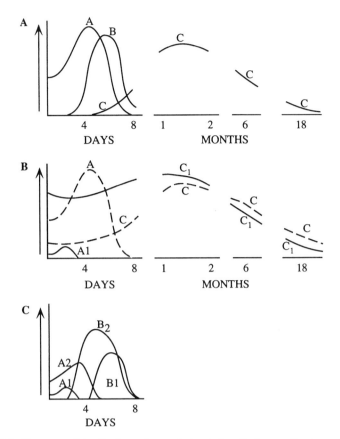

FIG. 3.4.2.2. Three possible situations demonstrate viral replication, antibody, and cytotoxic T lymphocyte (CTL) production in an acute infection in naive or pre-primed mice. Viral titer, curve A; CTL activity, curve B; antibody level, curve C. (**A**) Infectious viral levels, CTL activity, and antibody titers in a primary infection. (**B**) Infectious viral level (curve A1) and antibody level (curve C1) for pre-primed mice challenged with a virus of similar but not identical antigenic specificity to the priming virus, such that some virus escapes, replicates, and is sufficient to induce some CTL formation (curves, A1 in Fig **B** and A1, B1 in Fig. **C**). (**C**) If more virus escapes neutralization by antibody and replicates (curve A2), there will be a more rapid and larger CTL response (curve B2).

recruited at the relevant submucosal and regional lymph node sites within a few days of infection, the virus could be cleared and viremia avoided.[352] Such a scenario seems to offer the best chance of defeating this virus.

The most successful vaccines are those used against acute infections. When vaccinating against an agent causing an infection that persists because it subverts a CMI response, the aim of the vaccine should be to generate such a strong protective immune response that the challenge infection is effectively converted into an acute infection, as is proposed for HIV.

SECTION 4

Immunopotentiation and the Selective Induction of Immune Responses

CHAPTER 4.1. IMMUNOPOTENTIATION OF IMMUNE RESPONSES

The term *adjuvant* is widely used to describe a preparation that boosts the immune response to an antigen by increasing immunogenicity in a specific or nonspecific way. The term *adjuvanticity* strictly refers to the efficacy of the preparation but is sometimes used as an alternative to immunogenicity. The term *vehicle* describes the way in which the antigen is presented, as in mineral oil. The term *carrier* is used in the immunologic sense, as part of a hapten-carrier complex, and it is usually a protein. The final mode of presentation has been called the *adjuvant formulation*.[515]

A variety of materials has been shown to display adjuvanticity. Probably the first adjuvant widely used and the only one still registered for general medical use is alum. It was first used nearly 60 years ago. Glenny and colleagues[516] noticed that an injected antigen gave only a short-lived antibody response. It was reasoned that this was because the deposited antigen rapidly left the injection site. By mixing with alum, an antigen depot was formed, resulting in a more prolonged immune response. The introduction by Freund[517] of the technique of emulsifying antigen in

122

mineral oil with the addition of dead mycobacteria (Freund's complete adjuvant [FCA]) and a preparation not containing bacteria (Freund's incomplete adjuvant [FIA]) provided the means for greatly boosting an immune response. By using FCA, it was shown that strong delayed-type hypersensitivity (DTH) reactions to minute amounts of simple proteins could be obtained.[518] For many years, FCA was regarded as the standard that new formulations must meet to be competitive. FCA was found to form granulomas at the injection site. This was once thought to be desirable, but an adjuvant with this type of reaction is no longer considered acceptable for medical use, nor is it used in many animal experiments.

During the period when vaccines were composed mainly of whole organisms, live or inactivated, the main need for adjuvants was for use with toxoids or with diphtheria-pertussis-tetanus (DPT) vaccine and for experimental studies. With the advent of subunit preparations and of oligopeptide preparations, the need for adjuvants that were safe and highly effective became a high priority. However, there is always a trade-off between these two properties.

4.1.1. Desirable Properties and Different Roles of Adjuvants

Some of the properties and roles of adjuvants are listed in Table 4.1.1A. As with vaccines, the safety of adjuvant formulations became a top priority and led to some

TABLE 4.1.1A. *Some desirable general properties of adjuvants*

Safety
It must not be carcinogenic, teratogenic, or abortogenic.
The formation of granulomas, local necrosis, hypersensitivity, fever, or autoimmune effects should be avoided.
Nonspecific effects on cell activation, caused by perturbation of cell membranes by surfactants or oils, should be avoided.
It should be biodegradable and preferably have a short half-life.

Specificity
Because most activation signals may be transduced by membrane phospholipase activation, the activity should be targeted to specific cells of the immune system. Such cells may already possess specific receptors, especially if the adjuvant is derived from an infectious agent.
Having a known chemical structure is desirable.

Feasibility and formulation
The preparation should be stable, inexpensive, simple to (reproducibly) manufacture, and have a long storage life.
Presentation of the antigen with adjuvant as particles with multimeric arrays of antigen is advantageous.

Data from Myers KR, Gustafson GL. (1991) Adjuvants for human vaccine usage: a rational design. In: Cryz SJ Jr, ed. Vaccines and Immunotherapy. New York, Pergamon Press, pp. 404–411 and from Cooper PD. (1994) The selective induction of different immune responses by vaccine adjuvants. In: Ada GL, ed. Strategies in vaccine design. RG Landes, Austin, pp. 125–158.

guidelines about safety, specificity, feasibility, and formulations. It became clear over time that the final effector step of an adjuvant would be to enhance an already naturally occurring event, one that was most likely to involve specific interaction with a receptor at the cell surface. The adjuvant should be easy and inexpensive to manufacture.

The last decade has witnessed great activity in the field of adjuvant design, and a variety of studies point to a number of roles for adjuvants. Some are listed in Table 4.1.1B. There have been extensive reviews of candidate adjuvants.[519–521] The complete issue (1995;13) of *Vaccine* was reserved for such reports, and a group of candidate adjuvants was compared for activity and safety.[522] One of the pioneers of the study of adjuvants, Chedid,[523] proposed that the role of adjuvants could essentially be described by three concepts (which have been slightly modified):

1. The formation of a depot of antigen primarily at the site of application and from which the antigen was released over some period, which preferably could be predetermined
2. The presentation (or delivery) of antigen to cells involved in immune responses, principally antigen-presenting cells (APCs)
3. The induction of secretion of enhancing factors, such as lymphokines, which would act principally on cells of the immune system, especially T and B lymphocytes

With different preparations, there is some overlap between these stages. Nevertheless, this approach is followed in this presentation.

TABLE 4.1.1B. *Materials with adjuvant activity and possible sites of action*

Activities	Materials
Delayed release of antigen	Depot formers, water in oil; oil in water emulsions; controlled release devices; inert carriers (eg, alum)
Mobilization of T-cell help	Proteins as carriers
	Polyclonal activators of T cells: PPD, poly A:poly U
Modulate Ig receptors on B cells	B-cell mitogens, antigen-polymerizing factors
Localization of antigen in T-dependent areas	Hydrophobic antigens; addition of lipid tail to proteins
Stimulation of antigen-presenting cells	MDP and derivatives: LPS, lipid A
Facilitate cell-cell interaction	Surface-acting materials; saponin, lysolecithin, Quil A, liposomes, pluronic polymers
Focusing of antigen on leukocytes with Fc receptors	Alternate pathway of complement activators: inulin, zymosan, endotoxin

LPS, lipopolysaccharide; MDP, muramyl dipeptide; PPD, purified protein derivative.

4.1.2. Mechanism of Action of Adjuvants

4.1.2.1. Persistence and Controlled Delivery of Antigen

There are three main approaches to controlling the delivery of antigen: relatively insoluble mineral or other compounds, mineral oils for making mainly water-in-oil emulsions, and biodegradable, controlled-release formulations.

4.1.2.1.1. Alum

Alum is the only adjuvant universally registered for human use. (In this sense, all other adjuvants mentioned in the text should be regarded as candidate preparations.) The antigen solution usually is mixed with preformed aluminium hydroxide, aluminium phosphate, or both compounds. A specific preparation, Alhydrogel, was chosen as a scientific standard in 1988.[521] Cells involved in immune responses, particularly eosinophils, may be attracted to the antigen depot,[524] and complement may be activated, which could result in increased antigen localization of follicular dendritic cells and hence improved B-cell memory (see Section 2.2.5.2). Aluminium compounds are universally used as adjuvants for DPT vaccines, mainly because of the increased response to the toxoids.

Alum has given somewhat variable results when used with other vaccines such as inactivated poliovirus vaccine, cholera, a Hib-tetanus toxoid conjugate, and the influenza HA antigen.[521] Alum has been widely used in experimental work but is probably best used to stimulate a humoral (type 2) response to weak antigens. For example, it can produce up to a 100-fold increased antibody response to keyhole limpet hemocyanin (KLH).[525] Alum is neither pyrogenic nor antigenic and has a long record of safety for human use. Billions of doses of DPT have been administered.

4.1.2.1.2. Inulin and Algammulin

Inulin is a neutral storage carbohydrate of known structure of the plant, *Compositae*. It activates complement by an enzymatic cascade. At 37°C, a slowly soluble form, gamma inulin, is formed, and it is the basis of an adjuvant. When used with KLH, it enhanced immunologic memory, as shown by the finding that the secondary IgG response in mice was increased by up to 28-fold.[526] It enhances type 1 and type 2 T cell responses. It is nonpyrogenic and nonantigenic, and it has a low toxicity. Particles are probably digested by macrophages.[520] Gamma inulin has been co-crystallized with Alhydrogel to form a product, Algammulin,[520] that binds antigen and still activates complement. When used with KLH and a malaria peptide–diphtheria toxoid complex, the preparation produced specific IgG levels corresponding to those induced by using FCA. Not unexpectedly, this complex was no more toxic than either of the parent preparations.

4.1.2.1.3. Mineral Oils

A water-in-oil emulsion was first used to boost an immune response about 80 years ago,[521] but it was the studies of Freund that drew attention to this approach. Because of the multiple side effects of FCA, this preparation is no longer used. FIA is less toxic and has been widely used in model systems and in veterinary vaccines. In humans, it was used successfully with influenza and killed polio vaccines to enhance immunogenicity but had little effect with some other preparations.[521] The primary effect of FIA is to serve as a depot and in some cases, oil droplets have been found in lymph nodes distant from the injection site.[527] A variety of mineral oils has been used over time; Arlacel A (mannide monooleate) is a popular choice (eg, for human chorionic gonadotropin vaccine). Usually, an emulsifier such as squalene and a stabilizer is used to prepare the final product. Several side effects have been documented, and in the United States, mineral oil adjuvants are no longer recommended for general human use.[521] Arlacel A has been replaced with a purified mannide monooleate. Because of the effectiveness of this type of adjuvant for some antigens, the trend in research is toward the use of components that are readily metabolized, such as lecithin and glycerol. The use of biodegradable stearyl tyrosine has given some encouraging results in this way.[521]

Nonionic block copolymer surfactants have come into prominence as adjuvants.[528] The length of the chains of the hydrophobic polyoxypropylene and the hydrophilic polyoxyethylene chains influences the adjuvant activity and the antibody isotype produced. The substances can bind readily to lipid-soluble or water-soluble antigens, and different combinations of the chains can be prepared according to needs. The preparations have a low toxicity and have been widely used for other commercial biologic purposes. Two preparations, SAF-1 (Syntex Corp.) and TiterMax (CytRx Corp.) are widely promoted as adjuvants. The inclusion of other adjuvant preparations such as lipopolysaccharide (LPS) can give synergistic effects.

4.1.2.1.4. Controlled-Release Devices

Particulate antigens, such as polymeric structures (eg, flagella), or infectious agents are usually more immunogenic than soluble antigens, and association of the latter with microparticles may lead to increased immunogenicity.[529,530] The importance of size is shown by experiments in which a soluble antigen, linked to synthetic beads and in the absence of added adjuvant, induces a strong T-cell response. In such situations, macrophages are important for presentation of the antigen.[531]

These particles have been used to provide a reservoir from which the antigen may be released, often at a predetermined rate. A variety of such particles has been used over the years, including polymethylmethacrylate, polyacrylstarch, crystallized dextran nanospheres, and biodegradable glass. Gelatin crosslinked with glutaraldehyde has been tried,[532] but most work has been with mixtures of microparticles composed of polylactide-coglycolide. These polymers have been used in alternative biomedical applications for many years without evidence of significant side effects. The components dissolve to form lactic and glycolic acids, which are normal metabolites.

Adjusting the proportions of each polymer varies the rate of release of the entrapped antigens. Entrapped antigens can be released at predetermined rates or intervals after a single immunization and so may obviate the need for booster doses of a vaccine. The size of the microparticle is critical. Particles with a diameter of less than 10 microns are taken up by macrophages and transported to the draining lymph node, and produce a more rapid rise in antibody levels compared with larger ($>$10 microns) particles that remain at the injection site.[530]

After subcutaneous primary and secondary immunization of mice with ovalbumin (OVA) in microparticles (5.3 microns), the antibody titers reached were comparable to those reached by immunization with OVA in FCA over a 12-week period.[533] A single injection of tetanus toxoid in microparticles to mice gave long-lasting antibody responses to the toxoid, equivalent in length of time to those elicited by three injections of the toxoid in alum.[534] In another case,[535] staphylococcal enterotoxin B toxoid entrapped in microparticles induced antibody responses in mice that were comparable to those induced by FCA. Microparticles ($<$10 microns) were taken up by macrophages and transported to the draining lymph nodes. The researchers also demonstrated that different sizes of microparticles could be administered in combination to provide a biphasic antibody response. After a single injection to rabbits of a conjugate of a human chorionic gonadotrophin hormone peptide linked to diphtheria toxoid, the antibody titer to the peptide at 50 weeks was approximately 10% of the peak level at about 5 weeks after administration.[536] In this case, a muramyl dipeptide (MDP)–type adjuvant was incorporated with the antigen into the microparticles. Production of antipeptide antibody persisted much longer than when only the conjugate with adjuvant was injected.

A major interest in these preparations is their possible use for the oral delivery of vaccines. A range of infectious agents, including bacteria, viruses and parasites as well as macromolecules and synthetic particles, has been shown to be transported into Peyer's patches through M cells after oral administration.[530] According to many reports, antigens encapsulated in microparticles have been given orally, with or without parenteral administration. Eldridge and colleagues early showed that the microparticles delivered orally targeted the M cells and that those smaller than 5 microns were transported to the Peyer's patches.[537] They induced a rise in serum antibody and secretory IgA. Oral immunization with staphylococcal enterotoxin B encapsulated in this way induced a pulmonary antibody response.[538] Encapsulated, inactivated influenza virus delivered orally was shown in primed animals to induce improved levels of antibodies in saliva compared with parenteral immunization.[539]

Five of six female macaque monkeys, when given microencapsulated, inactivated simian immunodeficiency virus (SIV) intramuscularly and orally, were protected against a vaginal challenge with the virus. Oral administration alone was ineffective.[540]

Several aspects of the immune response under these conditions are of general interest:

1. The length of the mucosal immune response after oral administration is frequently quite short (see Section 2.3.5).
2. The cost of production of such preparations is relatively high and may become a consideration for their use in developing countries. It has been argued, however, that the savings in the overall cost of delivery of vaccines would more than compensate for the extra expense.[530]
3. The uptake of the microparticles in the gut is rather low, and this could affect the extent of their use in this way. Attempts are being made to increase this uptake by the use of bioadhesive polymers.[530]
4. During the microencapsulating process, antigens are usually exposed to potentially damaging conditions, such as an organic solvent. Many antigens lose their native conformation under these circumstances, and minimizing such effects has been one reason for the development of other formulations.

4.1.2.2. Presentation and Delivery of Antigen to Immune System Cells

Various ways have been devised for the delivery of antigens to immune cells. Some have a degree of specificity. Anti-mouse Ig has been coupled to ferritin, and the immunogenicity of the conjugate compared with ferritin alone in vitro and in vivo. The conjugate was more immunogenic in vitro and at low doses in vivo. Although the data were not conclusive, it was proposed that the conjugate enhanced B-cell presentation of the ferritin.[541] In an analogous approach, anti–class II major histocompatibility complex (MHC) antigen monoclonal antibodies (MAbs) were coupled to antigens and injected into mice. Under the experimental conditions used, the conjugate, but not the free antigen and MAb, was immunogenic. Focusing the conjugate on cells expressing class II MHC was proposed as the explanation of the findings.[542]

Adhesive antigens, such as pili from strains of enterotoxic *Escherichia coli*, are effectively taken up by cells in the gut lumen, and they induce good antibody titers. Co-feeding galactose, lactose, or sorbitol abolished the attachment to the mucosa,[543] and it has been proposed that pili could act as vectors for other antigens.

Cholera toxin (CT) is a potent enteric immunogen, mainly because of its ability to bind avidly to the GM_1 ganglioside on the surface of cells, including M cells. CT is composed of A and B chains, and this adjuvant property is ascribed to the B chain. Oral administration of soluble proteins frequently results in tolerance, as shown by a diminished immune response on subsequent challenging by a parenteral route. Coupling the B chain of CT (CTB) to a soluble protein or even co-administration of

CTB with the protein induces a high mucosal antibody response.[326,544] A subclinical dose of the CT also acts as a powerful adjuvant and greatly promotes the priming of CD4+ T cells but not CD8+ T cells by antigen; both T1 and T2 CD4+ T cells were primed.[545] It was therefore a major surprise to find that, when proteins were conjugated to CTB made by DNA-transfected cells (ie, free of any intact CT) and a single dose administered orally, systemic immune responses were subsequently suppressed in naive and primed animals (see Section 2.3.7).[325] In many previous experiments, the CTB used as the adjuvant probably was contaminated with subclinical amounts of CT. The finding has cast some doubt on the future use of CT as an adjuvant and has important implications for the future development of vaccines to prevent unwanted responses such as autoimmunity that might lead to autoimmune disease (see Chapter 6.2).

The well-known interaction between complement and antibody has led to a new approach to make use of the binding of complement to cellular receptors. If the C3 component of complement is missing, less antibody is made. To make use of this knowledge, three copies of a C3 fragment, C3d, were bound to hen egg lysozyme. This reduced the amount of lysozyme required to induce an antibody response by up to 10,000 times, compared with the amount of free lysozyme needed.[546]

Liposomes have concentric lipid membranes containing biodegradable lipids such as phospholipids in two layers that are separated by an aqueous compartment.[521] They were developed as carriers of biologically active substances such as therapeutic drugs and have a history of safe application. Several factors, such as the composition, the charge, the number of layers, and the method of preparation, affect their adjuvanticity. Depending on their nature, antigens may be adsorbed onto the liposome or incorporated into the particle. A variety of antigens, including saccharides, has been delivered in this way, and there is usually an increase in the antibody and cell-mediated immune (CMI) responses.

Other adjuvants such as lipid A can be readily incorporated into the preparation, and this approach may increase the immune response.[547] One mechanism of action enhanced by the inclusion of lipid A is the recruitment of macrophages that may act as APCs in the activation of T cells. It would be of interest to know if there was a similar effect on dendritic cells.

Liposomes are being evaluated as orally delivered adjuvants.[521] Inclusion of MDP into the preparation enhanced the mucosal immune response. Drawbacks to the wide use of liposomes include the reproducibility of their manufacture on a large scale, their instability during storage, and the relatively high cost of their manufacture, compared with, for example, oil-in-water emulsions.

4.1.2.3. Stimulation of the Immune Response

The increase in adjuvanticity gained by adding dead mycobacteria to mineral oils (ie, FCA), and by adding dead *Bordetella pertussis* to the tetanus and diphtheria toxoids indicated that these organisms must contain factors that were especially active in this respect and that might be present in the conserved parts of bacterial envelopes. The LPS, particularly the lipid A component, and the MDP portion of the peptidoglycans have been examined most extensively. MDP is the smallest unit that has immunomodulatory activity. Many derivatives of MDP have been made and analyzed, and several have been found that display enhanced beneficial and reduced harmful effects.[548] Hydrophilic analogs induce mainly a humoral response, but their incorporation into a hydrophobic vehicle also induces CMI responses. Promising MDP derivatives include murametide, threonyl-MDP, and murabutide.[521] The Syntex Adjuvant Formulation-1 (SAF-1) contains threonyl-MDP in a squalene-pluronic polymer emulsion. It induces humoral and CMI responses in animals and is said to be as effective as FCA but without FCA's toxicity.[521]

Succinylated or phthalylinated LPS is much less toxic than LPS while retaining adjuvanticity.[521] Removal of the terminal phosphate group from lipid A to form monophosphoryl lipid A maintains the adjuvanticity while reducing the toxicity.[549] Incorporation of these products into liposomes also reduces their toxicity. The product DETOX contains monophosphoryl lipid A and the purified mycobacterial cell-wall skeleton. When used in a clinical trial with a polyvalent melanoma vaccine, the adjuvant potentiated the antibody response but not the DTH response. However, it did not appear to improve disease-free survival compared with a control group using alum as adjuvant.[550]

The adjuvanticity and reactogenicity of *B. pertussis* are due to the pertussis toxin and LPS components. The toxin potentiates the humoral and CMI responses, including DTH.[521] Like CT, it is too toxic to be administered directly to humans, although it is present in the vaccine. A particulate fraction, P40, composed of the peptidoglycan and glycoprotein, has been isolated from *Corynebacterium granulosum*. It enhances the humoral and CMI responses and induces the formation of interleukin-2 (IL-2), tumor necrosis factor, interferon-α, and interferon-γ.[521]

In 1995, 24 candidate adjuvant preparations were compared in mice for their ability to enhance antibody production to whole human immunodeficiency virus (HIV) type 2, as measured by levels against five viral antigens, and for their toxicity.[522] FCA, FIA, liposomes, and several other well-known preparations were included. Three main conclusions were drawn from the results:

1. In line with earlier observations, hydrophobic preparations gave the best results, probably because increasing hydrophobicity favors cell adhesion and phagocytosis.
2. Particle size was also critical. Polymethylmethacrylate was the most effective preparation but only when the particle size was in the range 60 to 200 nm. Generally, larger particle sizes of any preparation were less effective.
3. Only one preparation, FCA, induced antibody production against all five antigens; gp120 and gp41, the surface antigens of HIV-2, were the most refractory, but most candidate preparations induced antibodies to p17 and p24, subunits of the internal gag antigen.

The investigators suggested that future vaccines might include two or more different adjuvants, though their data give little support to this proposal, and it could be technically difficult.

4.1.3. Antigen Delivery Systems

It has already been stressed that the size of an antigenic construct or package can markedly influence the effectiveness of inducing the desired immune response. The experience with the controlled-release microspheres and to a lesser extent with liposomes demonstrated this principle. Similarly, multimeric particulate antigens are commonly more immunogenic than monomeric antigens. The flagella of *Salmonella* were more impressive as immunogens than the monomeric molecule, flagellin.[253] A similar effect is seen with the surface[551] and core antigens[552] of hepatitis B virus.

The precise conformation of the protein multimers may also be important. Antibody induced by monomeric preparations of HIV-1 gp120 (env) neutralize to some extent the infectivity of laboratory-grown homologous virus, but not field strains of the virus. The evidence (reviewed elsewhere[553]) indicates that MAbs to monomeric env do not predict the efficacy of neutralization, even of homologous laboratory strains of HIV-1; this is reminiscent of findings with other viruses (see Section 3.1.2). The evidence also demonstrates that MAbs to oligomeric env from laboratory strains correlates with the efficacy of neutralization of laboratory strains, but not of field strains, suggesting that in vitro passage of a field strain of HIV causes a subtle conformational change in the surface glycoprotein.

It seems likely that the immune system is fashioned to respond to multimeric rather than to monomeric structures. The B cell must process and present antigen to the T cell to receive help to differentiate and replicate. Because the B-cell IgM receptor is bivalent, a polymeric structure binds more avidly to adjacent receptors and possibly is endocytosed more readily. Studies[554,555] have shown that 100 to 200 peptide-MHC complexes per presenting B cell are needed for the T cell to respond, and this density on the B cell is more likely to be achieved if multimeric particles are endocytosed.

Several approaches have made use of this structural effect by making a construct whereby a mosaic of adjacent, identical molecules is presented to the immune system. Immunostimulatory complexes (ISCOMS) consist of antigen incorporated into a matrix of cholesterol and Quil A to form 35-nm structures. ISCOMS are potent inducers of antibody production[556] and cytotoxic T lymphocyte (CTL) formation.[557,558] A less toxic preparation than Quil A, possibly a component of the mixture, is being sought.

The p1 protein of the yeast retrotransposon Ty spontaneously assembles into multimeric virus-like particles, called Ty-VLP, and there has been considerable interest in inserting DNA sequences coding for epitopes into the p1 protein, which can reassemble in this fashion. The entire capsid protein p27 of SIV, as well as the V3 loop of HIV-1, has been inserted into the 3' end, and the modified protein was found to assemble into a multimeric virus-like particle of about 50 nm.[559] When administered with alum, high HIV antibody neutralizing titers were obtained. This sort of approach to enhance the immunogenicity of an oligopeptide is being increasingly applied to benefit from the final multimeric structure that can be obtained. In other examples, sequences from the V3 loop of HIV-1 have been incorporated into the surface antigen[560] and core antigen[552] of the hepatitis B virus and into the VP1 capsid protein of poliovirus.[561] In each case, the hybrid proteins self-assembled into multimeric particles and induced strong antibody responses.

CHAPTER 4.2. SELECTIVE INDUCTION OF IMMUNE RESPONSES

The options available to induce particular immune responses such as different Ig isotypes or the types of CMI responses desired were quite restricted until recently. A secretory IgA response was likely to occur if an antigen was administered at a mucosal surface, but there were restrictions and unknowns even in this case. A soluble and medium-molecular-weight protein given orally could induce tolerance rather than immunity, and the same preparation given intravaginally was likely to induce no response or a very poor and short-lived immune response. Polymeric antigens were better at inducing IgM responses than the monomeric form,[253] and the body tended to produce strong IgE responses to some parasite proteins. Some adjuvants such as dextran sulfate, in contrast to FCA, preferably induced an IgG2 response to a bacterial antigen.[371]

In the late 1950s and early 1960s, a series of reports indicated that antigen might be administered in ways that stimulated or suppressed antibody or DTH reactions (reviewed elsewhere[562]). The phenomena were referred to as immune deviation, split tolerance, or preimmunization tolerance. There were reports that low doses of antigen preferentially induced CMI.[563] Strong evidence for a dichotomy in the responses of T cells was provided by the use of a chemically modified antigen, acetoacetylated flagellin. Three approaches[562] gave important findings:

1. As the antigenic activity of the flagellin was progressively reduced by this modification, there was a rapid decline in the ability of the host to produce antiflagellin antibody, but an enhanced ability to induce flagellin-specific DTH (ie, the reaction was elicited by flagellin).
2. The modified flagellins efficiently induced flagellin-specific antibody tolerance.
3. Flagellin had previously been shown to induce high- and low-zone antibody tolerance and high antibody production at intermediate doses. Using the acetylated derivative, suppression of DTH responses occurred at doses that induced good antibody production, and conversely, high DTH responses occurred at doses that resulted in antibody tolerance.[564]

The suggestion[562] that humoral and cell-mediated responses might evolve from separate T-cell lineages was fully vindicated a decade later, when the ability to clone T cells led to the description of CD4+ TH1 and CD4+ TH2 cells (see Section 2.2.3.1).

Class I MHC–restricted lysis of virus-infected target cells was first demonstrated using infectious lymphocytic choriomeningitis virus[19] and was soon shown to be a general phenomenon with viruses. One of the questions that soon arose was whether exposure of cells to noninfectious virus, in vitro or in vivo, would also sensitize cells to lysis by CTLs. A spectrum of findings with a range of virus preparations was obtained (reviewed elsewhere[565]). Some inactivated viral preparations were effective, and other than the observation that virions that fused with a cell membrane were active, no other correlation was found. For several years, the fact that some inactivated viruses could sensitize the cell for lysis in the complete absence of protein synthesis was seen as favoring the idea of intact viral antigen complexing with the MHC antigen to form the ligand recognized by the CTL. Much later, when the importance of the cytoplasmic pathway for the interaction of peptides with class I MHC molecules was understood, it became clear that "leakage" of foreign antigen from a lysosome into the cytoplasm might occur under certain conditions. Although the use of infectious virus remains an effective way to generate CTL activity, the critical requirement is introduction of the preparation into the cytoplasmic pathway, and a variety of methods is now available to achieve this effect, frequently by enhancing fusion of the antigen preparation with the cell membrane.

4.2.1. T-Cell Responses and Antibody Isotypes

T cells are major producers of cytokines, and many of these determine the nature of the immune response.[305,566,567] Table 4.2.1 lists some cytokines that have been shown to influence the production in mice of various immunoglobulin isotypes. Not

TABLE 4.2.1. *Cytokines that influence different immunoglobulin isotype production in mice*

Cytokine	Effect on immunoglobulin production and secretion
IL-2	General increase in Ig production
IL-4	Increase in IgG1, IgE
	Suppression of IgG2a, IgG2b, IgG3
IL-5	Increase in IgM, IgG, IgA
IL-6	Important for mucosal IgA, IgG responses
IL-10	Increase in IgM and IgG
IFNγ	Increases IgG2a
	Decreases IgG1, IgG2b, IgG3, IgE

Data from Fitch FW, Lancki DW, Gajewski TF. (1993) T-cell mediated immune regulation. In: Paul WE, ed. Fundamental immunology, 3rd ed. Raven Press, New York, pp. 733–761; from Pike BL. (1992) Cytokines acting on B lymphocytes. In: Roitt IM, Delves PJ, eds. Encyclopedia of immunology. Academic Press, New York, pp. 440–441; and from Ramsay AJ, Husband AJ, Ramshaw IA, et al. (1994) The role of interleukin 6 in mucosal IgA antibody responses in vivo. Science 264:561–564.

unexpectedly, IL-2 has an overall enhancing effect on antibody production. Of particular interest is the rather dominant effect IL-6 has on secretory IgA production.[305] This is consistent with the broad distribution of cells containing IL-6 mRNA in intestinal mucosa.[568]

4.2.2. Selective Induction of T-Cell Responses and Cytotoxic T Lymphocyte Formation

Approaches that lead to the selective induction of type 1 T-cell responses, and particularly of CTL responses, are of special interest. In the case of intracellular infectious agents (eg, viruses, bacteria, parasites, chimeric infectious agents), it is easy to see how such responses are produced if the agent infects a "professional" APC or a cell that can be induced to become an APC by expression of co-stimulator molecules. However, in the absence of such conditions, are there more general approaches for induction of CTL responses? Can endogenous antigens induce a CTL response, or foreign proteins from an infected or mutant cell be introduced into the class I pathway of an APC? There is progress in understanding how this may happen.

Proteins can be delivered into the cytosol by osmotic lysis of pinosomes,[569] through electrophoration,[570] or in liposomes that may fuse with the cell membrane. Some adjuvants such as FCA[571] or QS21[572] also facilitate such responses. After an early suggestion[573] that only particulate antigens, in the form of damaged cells, would be processed by phagocytic APCs for class I presentation, there is increasing evidence that antigen in particulate form primes more efficiently than soluble antigen for class I presentation.[574] Lipid-encapsulated antigens,[575] antigens on beads,[576] or aggregated antigens[577] can prime such responses. Compromising macrophage or dendritic cell function can reduce the effectiveness of these approaches, implicating a role for these cells.[578] Nair and colleagues[578] presented some evidence that macrophages could pass on antigen to dendritic cells, although there is also evidence that at least some dendritic cells can be phagocytic.[579]

A clue to a mechanism by which immune information might be transferred from a particular cell to APCs came from a series of investigations following a rather surprising original observation, that tumor-specific immunity could be induced by immunization with irradiated tumor cells.[580] Such studies have led to the discovery that heat shock proteins (HSPs) could act as carriers of peptides,[581,582] which after translocation might be further processed by the macrophages' class I processing machinery so that the peptides complexed with class I MHC molecules. This finding led to the possibility of immunization with HSPs from malignant or infected cells to induce specific CTL formation.[583]

The ability to sensitize target cells with virus-specific peptides for recognition and lysis by effector T cells led to the possibility of immunization with such preparations to induce CTL formation. It was first shown that immunization of mice of an appropriate MHC haplotype with a virally derived free peptide in FIA would induce

CTL formation[584] and that such mice were protected in vivo from the virus.[585] In another report, immunization of mice with a virus-specific free synthetic peptide primed for CTL activity, and the mice were protected against a lethal dose of Sendai virus.[586] Immunization of mice once with polypeptides in FIA from the *Plasmodium falciparum* circumsporozoite protein induced helper T cell and CTL responses.[587] Others have reported less success,[588] and it was found that repeated injection of peptide without the adjuvant could cause temporary T-cell tolerance,[589] demonstrating that the method of presentation of the peptide to the immune system is critical. Attaching a lipid tail to a peptide enhances the ability to induce a CTL response,[590] and in a modification of this approach, a lipopeptide construct containing a CTL determinant was modified to contain three influenza virus nucleoprotein CD8 T cell determinants, each restricted to a different H-2 haplotype.[591] A CTL response was obtained to the construct in all three mouse strains.

An alternative approach is to present CTL determinants in a chimeric vector. In one case,[498] three discrete CTL determinants were expressed from "minigenes" encoding peptides as short as 12 amino acids in a vaccinia virus construct. The minigenes were fused to form a "string of beads." Each was effectively expressed, and antiviral protection was achieved on the two MHC haplotypes chosen. CTLs to different determinants could act synergistically on the same MHC background.

Following early successful experiments, immunization with tumor-specific peptides is being more widely explored as a possible approach to tumor therapy. This work is discussed in more detail in Chapter 6.1.

A novel method of inducing a predominantly type 1 response to antigen is to conjugate the protein to mannan under oxidizing conditions.[592] Immunization of mice with such a construct containing the MUC-1 antigen, a heavily glycosylated polypeptide with tandem repeats and produced by many epithelial cells and tumors, induced the formation of CTLs, DTH activity that was mainly mediated by CD4 + T cells, and little antibody. Immunization with such a construct made under different conditions led to a type 2 response (see Section 6.1.7).

The feasibility of immunization with a small dose of antigen to induce preferentially a type 1 T-cell response and therefore favoring CTL formation (see Section 2.2.3.2; reviewed elsewhere[183]) has yet to be explored in detail. A series of "experiments of nature" reported mainly in 1994 and 1995 do raise an exciting prospect. In an acute viral infection such as influenza in the mouse, specific CTLs are detected in infected lungs only a few days before specific antibody-secreting cells are detected.[350] In contrast, in human HIV infections, specific CTLs have been reported[353,354] at the time of viremia and up to several months before specific antibody, especially neutralizing antibody, is detected; CTLs are clearly implicated in the early control of viremia.

The finding of memory CTLs specific for one or more HIV proteins in the blood of individuals who have been exposed to HIV was described in Section 3.1.4.2. These groups included infants born of infected mothers[407,408] (although it is not known how frequently this may occur); long-term partners of infected men or women[409]; a small proportion of long-term female sex workers in two African countries[410]; and 7 of 20 health care workers exposed once to body fluids of HIV-infected individuals. The test results for all 20 control health care workers were negative.[411] The relevance of these findings to this discussion depends on the widely accepted dogma that CTL formation to HIV only occurs if host cells are infected and at least some virally encoded proteins are synthesized. As four separate observations, these reports cannot be ignored, but it is the last that may be of special relevance. First, the CTL activity was assessed only against one viral antigen, the env protein. Because other antigens, especially gag and pol, contain many CTL determinants, it is reasonable to propose that, if activity had been measured against a cocktail of viral antigens, a majority (>10) of those exposed would be found to be CTL positive. Based on epidemiologic data on seroconversion rates in Western societies, the efficacy of transmission of HIV has been considered to be 1% or less,[593] which is much lower than infection rates of other sexually transmitted diseases. The implications of the findings for health care workers is that an infectious dose, albeit low, may be transmitted far more frequently than at an exposure rate of 1% and that seroconversion results from the transmission of a larger dose of HIV than the dose that can induce CTL activity.

The way is open to test whether a similar result can be seen with the SIV model after exposure of monkeys to graded doses of infectious virus.[594] Because most workers in these areas do not quantitate CTL data (eg, by expression of results as lytic units/given cell number), it is difficult to compare findings from different groups. Until recently, it seemed that use of intracellular infectious agents or chimeric live vectors expressing many other foreign antigens would remain the most effective means to induce CTL responses, but the number of other approaches that have been described means that there are many possibilities to choose from.

SECTION 5

Newer Approaches to Vaccine Development

CHAPTER 5.1. PEPTIDE-BASED CANDIDATE VACCINES

Molecular approaches to vaccine development began in the 1950s with work on synthetic oligopeptides, and this trend has blossomed with developments in recombinant DNA (rDNA) technology. A major incentive to devise new approaches has been the need to make vaccines against the many agents, such as human immunodeficiency virus (HIV), *Mycobacterium leprae* (ie, leprosy), *Chlamydia*, and plasmodia, for which traditional approaches are unavailable or do not work. As time went by, it seemed likely that, using one or more of these new approaches, it might be possible to immunize against some self-like antigens and possibly control fertility and malignancy. There are three main approaches: to make synthetic oligopeptides and polypeptides, to make anti-idiotypic antibodies, and to manipulate DNA in one of several ways. Most progress has been made with the last approach; the use of naked DNA is of particular interest.

5.1.1. Use of Epitopes and Determinants

Initially, the development of oligopeptides as the basis of possible vaccines was entirely directed to the production of an antibody response by the provision of an epitope that would be recognized by B-cell receptors.[595,596] The concept was to identify and then to isolate or synthesize the "essential" sequences of proteins of an infectious agent that could form the candidate vaccine. The use of such products was thought to have a number of distinct advantages, as indicated in Table 5.1.1. It was soon found, however, that such oligomers were very poorly immunogenic. It was necessary to attach several copies of the putative B-cell epitope to a carrier protein, which acted as a source of T-cell determinants. Initially, products such as the tetanus or diphtheria toxoids were used because they were highly immunogenic and because most recipients would have been preimmunized, ensuring a secondary T-cell response. One example is the coupling of the C-terminal 37–amino acid

TABLE 5.1.1. *Perceived advantages of peptide-based vaccines*

- Chemically defined product
- High temperature, chemical, and (probably) biologic stability
- Easy to sterilize and could be stored freeze-dried, if required
- No infectious agent (or nucleic acid genome) in the final product or used during production
- Only sequences representing protective B-cell epitopes and T-cell determinants need be present
- Epitopes or determinants with undesirable properties, such as suppressor activity, showing molecular mimicry with host sequences (ie, risk of autoimmune disease) or inducing infection-enhancing antibody responses, usually can be eliminated
- Can link together peptides with different properties, such as B-cell epitopes with T-cell determinants
- Class I and class II MHC-restricted T-cell responses can be generated by the same preparation
- Multivalent constructs can be made, gaining the benefits of polymeric structures for B-cell activation together with "universal T-cell determinants" for use in an outbred population

sequence of the β chain of human chorionic gonadotropin hormone to diphtheria toxoid in about a 50:50 ratio (by weight).[597] This preparation has been shown to be safe and immunogenic in nonfertile women in phase I trials. In this case, a T-cell response to a self protein was to be avoided. Bacterial toxoids are used as the carrier in some of the newer bacterial subunit vaccines (see Table 1.2.4).

Keyhole limpet hemocyanin has been used frequently as a carrier because it is a large, immunogenic molecule. It could also be predicted that the internal antigens of viruses would be highly immunogenic. The influenza virus nucleoprotein (NP)[598] and the core antigen of hepatitis B virus (HBcAg)[599] are now favored for this purpose. Even with attached peptides, HBcAg may assemble into a virus-like particle. It was reported[599] that the antibody response to a peptide representing a neutralizing epitope of rhinovirus and conjugated to HBcAg was much higher when the complex was in particulate form compared with the monomeric form.

It can be argued that another protein of the organism from which the peptide B-cell epitope is derived should be used as the carrier, because subsequent exposure to the agent will result in activation of T- and B-cell memory responses specific to that agent. The outer membrane protein (OMP) of meningococcus has been successfully used as a carrier in a vaccine. The polysaccharide of *Haemophilus influenzae*, when coupled to the OMP, has been shown to be immunogenic in young children.[600]

Increasing the number of the haptenic groups in a conjugate can substantially increase immunogenicity, particularly if the peptide epitopes are presented as a tandem array. A well tried approach is to form multiple antigenic peptides (MAPS). Up to eight copies of a peptide are synthesized on a dendritic matrix of lysine residues,[601] an approach that is reminiscent of the much earlier work of Michael Sela with artificial antigens.[602] A construct having this general structure with repeats of oligopeptides from the HIV gp120 was highly immunogenic.[603] Using the amino acid sequence 115–131 from the *Schistosoma mansoni* antigen rSm28-GST, which is known to contain a B-cell epitope and a T-cell determinant, a comparison was made of the immunogenicity of five preparations: the single peptide, a tandem repeat, a copolymer made with glutaraldehyde and two MAP constructs (2 and 8 residues). The MAP (8 residues) was found to be the most immunogenic.[604] This technology has recently been reviewed.[605]

A further refinement was to replace the protein carrier with helper T (TH) cell determinants. There were several unknowns. How many TH cell determinants would be needed so the majority of members in an outbred population would respond? How should the epitope and determinant be linked? Complete answers to questions such as these are still being sought, but substantial progress has been made. A candidate vaccine for HIV was constructed by combining a peptide from the V3 loop that induced neutralizing antibody activity with different TH determinants from the gp120 to form a construct called T1-SP10.[606] A cocktail approach was subsequently adopted to generate antibody responses that would be broadly reactive. Sequential administration of these induced some interference in the antibody response, similar in some respects to the concept of "original antigenic sin."[607] This problem was overcome by simultaneous administration of the components of the mixture. The inclusion of a cytotoxic T lymphocyte (CTL) determinant together with a fusion sequence to facilitate entry of the construct into the cytoplasmic pathway induced, rather unexpectedly, a state of tolerance to the B-cell epitope, for reasons that are unclear.[608]

There are many studies on the most favorable orientation of epitopes and determinants with each other,[609] and there are still some unknowns about the way amino acid sequences adjacent to a B-cell epitope can interfere with or enhance the response to the epitope.[610] Nevertheless, progress continues to be made in preparing oligopeptides containing B-cell epitopes and T-cell determinants, especially if "universal TH determinants" are used; these are determinants that interact with several class II major histocompatibility complex (MHC) haplotypes within and even between species. For example, a sequence, 181–210, from the envelope protein gp41 of the type 1 human T-cell leukemia virus, when prepared as a MAP on a branched polylysine backbone, produced high titers of neutralizing antibody in rats. T cells from infected humans of different human leukocyte antigen haplotypes responded to the construct.[611] In another example, a polypeptide construct from the repeat region of the circumsporozoite protein of *Plasmodium yoelii*, PyCSP, was used to make a MAP containing universal T-cell epitopes from tetanus toxin. Immunization with an adjuvant protected 100% of outbred mice, and passive transfer of purified immunoglobulin (Ig) from immunized mice protected naive recipients from challenge with the parasite.[612] Great progress has also been made in inducing CTL formation with peptides, as is described in Sections 4.2.3, 6.1, and 6.2.

5.1.2. Approaches to Overcome Drawbacks to the Use of Peptides

A list of some perceived deficiencies in a peptide-based vaccine approach is presented in Table 5.1.2. If an important epitope is composed of sequences from

---

TABLE 5.1.2. *Perceived deficiencies in a peptide-based vaccine approach*

- In the case of some viruses, such as influenza virus, poliovirus, and human immunodeficiency virus, neutralizing B-cell epitopes are discontinuous, and adjacent molecules contribute to the epitope
- The conformation of a B-cell epitope in a protein may differ markedly from its adopted shape as a free peptide
- Carbohydrates may contribute to the conformation of an important viral glycoprotein
- One or more peptide bonds, which in the parent protein may be protected by conformational constraints or sugar side chains, may, as the corresponding peptide, also be very susceptible to proteolytic degradation
- Even when a B-cell epitope is clearly linear, a single amino acid mutation outside this sequence can affect the antigenic specificity of the epitope, presumably by conformational changes
- If there is a need for a vaccine to include several B-cell epitopes and T-cell determinants, the manufacturing costs may become prohibitively expensive. The cost of making even a simple construct may be too high for its use in developing countries, unless it is made in the country itself

---

adjacent molecules, there is no easy approach to constructing a peptide analog unless the three-dimensional structure of the packaged proteins is known. Even then, it would be a considerable achievement to design an effective linear peptide. Of the points listed in Table 5.1.2, the one most amenable to study is the question of conformational differences between the shapes of sequences in a native protein and their shapes after isolation or synthesis.

On the five occasions when crystals of a complex of a monoclonal Fab with its intact antigen have been examined by x-ray crystallography, it was found that the epitopes occupy large areas composed of 15 to 22 amino acid residues that are present on several surface loops.[613] This suggests that linear (continuous) peptides may not reflect the native conformation within the intact protein antigen. An extension of this argument is that peptide-based preparations may not be a uniformly suitable way to induce high-affinity antibodies to many B-cell epitopes. In contrast, the synthesis of short peptides is a most appropriate way to induce T-cell responses.

Although most short linear peptides are unstructured in water, some peptides of known immunogenicity prefer a conformational structure. By using mainly nuclear magnetic resonance and circular dichromism spectroscopy, β turns and helical and nascent helical conformations have been detected. A preference for folded forms has been found in peptide sequences derived from the influenza virus hemagglutinin (HA), from the gD-1 antigenic domain in herpes simplex virus, the transmembrane protein of simian immunodeficiency virus, and the repeating tetrapeptide of the *Plasmodium* circumsporozoite protein (reviewed elsewhere[614]). The V3 loop of HIV gp120 has two antiparallel β strands and a short COOH-terminal α helix. In solution, only a small section of peptide fragments from this loop show a preference for a structured form. When bound to Fabs from neutralizing monoclonal antibodies, there is evidence for a β turn at the short sequence, GPRG, as predicted.

There is considerable interest in developing a set of rules that can be used to design a peptide able to fold in a predictable manner, one that mimics the secondary structure of the parent protein.[615] Some progress has been made,[616,617] but much more needs to be done. Some T-cell all-stimulating peptides appear to show preferences for a helix conformation in solution, and an extended conformation is seen when the peptide is bound to the MHC molecule.[614]

5.1.3. Improving on Nature

A major difficulty facing the development of many vaccines is the great antigenic variation seen in important (neutralizing) B-cell epitopes that are also immunodominant, such as the V3 loop of HIV gp120. Several examples of conserved epitopes have been identified, but they are poorly immunogenic; one is the CD4-binding region of HIV gp 120. As discussed in Section 3.2.3.4, a conserved 20–amino acid peptide from the M protein of group A streptococci has been used to immunize mice and produce antibody that lysed the organism.[475] Antibody in sera from most residents in endemic areas bound to the peptide, and this peptide may form the basis of a vaccine against the organism. This example suggests similar approaches could be made in other situations in which antigenic variation in important B-cell epitopes makes effective vaccine development difficult.

Although some residues are important as anchor sites, the relative unimportance of conformation requirements for T-cell determinants opens the way to varying the sequence at other residue positions.[618] By changing the amino acid residues at certain positions, it has been possible to increase the affinity of binding of the peptide to the relevant MHC molecule for TH and CTL determinants (reviewed elsewhere[618]). One potential result is that the modified peptide may bind to other MHC molecules with an increased affinity (ie, the peptide is more crossreactive).

An alternative approach may also be useful in certain cases. A peptide sequence in the HIV env antigen contains several overlapping TH determinants that bind to MHC antigens of different haplotypes. Rather than use a mixture of several individual determinants, a longer peptide (ie, cluster peptide) that included the sequences of all determinants was made. Three such cluster peptides were recognized by four strains of mice and also by humans with different HLA specificities.[619]

5.1.4. Prospects for Peptide-Based Vaccines

Although it is doubtful that peptide-based vaccines will become a general approach to vaccine development, it is virtually certain that they will find suitable niches. For antibody production, there should be opportunities especially with bacteria and parasites. No peptide-based vaccine is licensed for general use, but a candidate malaria vaccine has undergone and is undergoing several phase III clinical trials.

In 1987, Patarroyo and colleagues[620] published data indicating that a mixture of three peptides from plasmodia proteins isolated at the schizont and merozoite stages of infection partially protected infected monkeys from disease. Encouraged by this partial success, a synthetic protein (ie, SPf66) was made. It was composed of sequences from three merozoite proteins and one from the circumsporozoite protein of *Plasmodium falciparum*.[621] It was shown to be safe and immunogenic in a large field trial. In Columbian volunteers, it was found to have an overall protective efficacy against *P. falciparum* malaria of 39%.[622] In a trial in Tanzania, which was a more severe test because transmission of infection is intense there, the protective efficacy was 31%,[623] a value considered by some to be a borderline result. In an equally well-conducted trial in Gambia with very young children, however, no protection against clinical attacks of malaria during the rainy season after immunization was found.[624] Although other field trials are in progress, more work must be done to develop a better vaccine.

For some infectious agents, peptide-based preparations seem to offer the best hope for vaccine development. The OMP of *Chlamydia* contains the epitopes recognized by infectivity-neutralizing antibody. These variable epitopes occur between hydrophobic sequences that span the bacterial cell wall.[625] It is very difficult to isolate the intact protein without using detergents that would affect the native conformation.

An important future application for this approach is the induction of T-cell responses, particularly CTL formation to control intracellular infections and perhaps as immunotherapy against tumors.

CHAPTER 5.2. ANTI-IDIOTYPIC ANTIBODIES AS CANDIDATE VACCINES

5.2.1. General Requirements

The number of hypervariable regions generated by humans is about 10^8, a range of specificities that allows recognition of virtually all possible shapes. It was argued that the shapes of the hypervariable regions of Ig receptors on B cells or Ig molecules should similarly be recognized by other antibodies, promoting the concept of a network in which there was at any one time a dynamic equilibrium mediated by these idiotypic interactions. The introduction of a "foreign" antigen temporarily disturbs this equilibrium. The first step is the formation of antibodies, Ab_1, that recognize epitopes on the introduced antigen. Antibodies are then generated that recognize the idiotypes of Ab_1 molecules. Because the latter have multiple idiotypes, the complementary antibodies are structurally and functionally heterogeneous, but it is standard practice to divide these into several categories[626,627]:

1. Ab_2 *a* recognizes framework-associated and regulatory idiotypes.
2. Ab_2 *b* recognizes the paratope idiotype (ie, the antigen binding site); it has an "internal image" of the original antigen.
3. Ab_2E recognizes idiotypes of autoantibodies and epitopes of antigens that bind to autoantibodies.
4. Ab_2g recognizes combining site–associated idiotypes, but does not carry the internal image of the antigen.

Because Ab_2b antibodies carry the internal image of the antigen, they should be able to function as surrogate antigens in vaccines against infectious agents, to combat cancer by induction of a tumoricidal immune response, or to induce remission of an autoimmune disease. Certain criteria have been proposed to identify Ab_2b antibodies. Structural criteria include shared sequences between the antibody and the antigen; these have been found, although rarely.[627–629] Functional criteria include the binding to Ab_1 molecules of different species, inhibition of specific antibody to the antigen, and the induction of humoral and cell-mediated immune responses.

The study of anti-idiotypic antibodies was particularly popular during the 1980s, and the antigens studied comprised viruses, bacteria, parasites, fungi, toxins, and ligands of receptors and hormones. There are many examples of immunization with an idiotypic antibody preparation resulting in protection or partial protection when the host was later challenged with the infectious agent. Table 5.2.1 gives a partial list of the infectious agents studied in this way. Several factors favored this ap-

TABLE 5.2.1. *Anti-idiotypic antibodies isolated and studied for their protective activity against different infectious agents*

Type of agent	Antibodies
Viruses	Tobacco mosaic, Venezualan equine encephalitis, polio, hepatitis B, rabies (glycoprotein), influenza (hemagglutinin), herpes simplex, reo type 3 (hemagglutinin), bluetongue, human immunodeficiency virus (env protein).
Bacteria	*Escherichia coli* (polysaccharide), pneumococcus (polysaccharide), *Pseudomonas* (LPS side chain), *Streptococcus* group A (carbohydrate)
Parasites	Schistosomes, trypanosomes
Fungi	Trichothecene mycotoxin

Data from Ada GL. (1989) Vaccines. In: Paul WE, ed. Fundamental immunology, 2nd ed. Raven Press, New York, p. 1015.

proach. First, as a product, antibodies should be safe. Second, it should be relatively easy and safe to mass produce a given antibody (see Section 5.5). Third, Ab_2b preparations could be particularly valuable in certain situations, as when Ab_1 recognized a quaternary structure, such as epitopes formed by adjacent molecules, and when the epitope was oligosaccharide in nature (all the bacterial examples in Table 5.2.1 were anti-idiotypes directed against oligosaccharides). In the latter two cases, developing a peptide-based vaccine would be difficult. Despite the apparent attractions of this approach and the many experimental systems in which significant protection was achieved by prior immunization, there is little evidence that it will lead to an effective vaccine against an infectious agent in the foreseeable future.

5.2.2. Antibodies to Cellular Receptors

Many viruses bind to susceptible cells by attaching to a specific receptor. Because such receptors are likely to be antigenically homogeneous, it should be possible to make an antibody that binds so strongly to the receptor that it prevents infection or make an anti-idiotypic antibody to the receptor that mimics the receptor so closely that the antibody will bind to the virus and prevent infection of the cell. The first of these methods was seen as an attractive approach in the case of rhinoviruses, which show such great antigenic variation that it is extraordinarily difficult to develop an effective vaccine. Although monoclonal antibodies specific for the main cellular receptor blocked virus attachment to the cells in vitro and a small clinical trial showed that administration of the antibody could lessen the severity of a challenge infection,[630] this approach was considered to be impractical as a public health measure.

CHAPTER 5.3. SITE-DIRECTED REPLACEMENT OF NUCLEOTIDE SEQUENCES

The ability to attenuate virulent infectious agents by selective mutation techniques was demonstrated by Germanier and colleagues in the early 1970s, when they generated Ty21a, a nitrosoguanidine-induced *gal-E* mutant of *Salmonella typhi* strain Ty2.[631] In the absence of galactose, this mutant becomes more susceptible to destruction by the host's immune response. Ty21a vaccine is licensed for oral administration in many parts of the world. This approach has not been as successful with other bacteria, and it is now known[632] that this treatment results in additional mutations in *S. typhi*. This approach using whole organisms is being replaced by the selective deletion of DNA sequences (see Section 5.4.5.1).

However, this technique is being used to produce a new generation of nontoxic bacterial toxins that are superior in safety and immunogenicity to the chemically inactivated toxoids (reviewed elsewhere[633]). Using nitrosoguanidine mutagenesis and classic genetic methods to isolate the gene coding for a nontoxic derivative of diphtheria toxin, the preparation CRM197 was isolated and characterized.[634] Similar approaches have been used to mutate and isolate the genes for pertussis, cholera, and *Escherichia coli* heat-labile enterotoxins.[635-637] Studies show that, in contrast to chemically treated products, the genetically detoxified molecules retain defined B-cell epitopes and T-cell determinants and the ability to bind to cellular receptors.[633] One product, LT-K63 (from *E. coli* enterotoxin), has been found to be a strong mucosal immunogen and an effective adjuvant for several different antigens that alone are poorly immunogenic.[633] Clinical trials of this product are expected to begin shortly.

CHAPTER 5.4. APPROACHES USING RECOMBINANT DNA TECHNOLOGY

The elucidation of the structure of DNA and the demonstration that the structure was universal constitute perhaps the most seminal biologic discovery made in this century. This knowledge led in the early 1970s to the formation of chimeric DNA molecules, cloning of segments of DNA in transfected cells, and production by those cells of proteins coded for by the inserted DNA. Equally interesting was the ability to selectively delete DNA sequences from the genome of a virus or bacterium. A related development was insertion into the DNA of foreign DNA segments coding for highly immunogenic proteins of viruses or bacteria, causing hosts immunized with the chimeric protein to respond to the inserted foreign sequence. Similar or larger DNA sequences could be inserted into the genomes (or cDNA copies of RNA genomes) of existing or potential live attenuated viral or bacterial vaccines. Cells infected by the chimeric vectors produced the foreign and the vector-coded proteins.

This approach took a fascinating turn when it was shown to be possible to immunize with DNA itself to obtain immune responses. The concept of using transfected plants for the production and as a possible source of immunogens for oral delivery of vaccines also became the subject of investigations (see Sections 5.4.9 and 5.4.10).

TABLE 5.4.1. *Selective deletion of nucleic acid base sequences from* Salmonella *and* Vibrio cholerae *to render the agent less virulent while retaining immunogenicity*

Agent	Deletion or designation	Properties of modified agent
Salmonella	Δaro A	Requires *p*-aminobenzoic acid[638]
	Daro A,C,D	Effective as single-dose immunogens[639]
	Δcya Δcrp	Genes for adenylate cyclase and cAMP receptor protein[638]
	ΔphoP	Genes that regulate genes necessary for intracellular survival[638]
	Δcdt	Genes which control ability to colonize deep tissues[638]
Cholera	CVD103HGR (Inaba strain)	Produces B toxin subunit, is mercury resistant[640]
	Peru 14 (El Tor strain)	Deletion that encodes virulence factors, RSI; inclusion of B subunit of toxin[641]
	Bengal-15 (0139 strain)	Deletion of multiple copies of toxin DNA; inclusion of DNA for B subunit of toxin[642]

RSI is the target site for the insertion of other genetic elements.

5.4.1. Attenuation by Selective Deletion of Nucleic Acid Base Sequences

The ability to delete specific segments of DNA from genomes has transformed the practice of making attenuated strains of infectious agents. Table 5.4.1 lists some of the gene deletions in the DNA of *Salmonella* and *Cholera* bacteria that have resulted in attenuated preparations, some of which are in clinical trials.

The results with some viruses have been equally exciting. To make a safe but immunogenic strain of vaccinia virus, the entire sequence of the Copenhagen strain was determined. The DNA was shown to contain 191,636 base pairs encoding 198 potential open reading frames (ORFs) of 65 or more amino acids.[643] A total of 18 ORFs were precisely deleted, including two that were required for replication in certain cell lines, including human but not vero cells. The final product, NYVAC, was found to retain good immunogenicity but to demonstrate remarkably low levels of pathogenicity, including that resulting from intracerebral inoculation into baby mice or into immunocompromised or immunodeficient mice.[644]

Other research groups have deleted or inactivated genes in vaccinia virus coding for thymidine kinase, growth factor, HA, ribonucleotide reductase, envelope proteins, steroid dehydrogenase, complement control protein, and host range genes (reviewed elsewhere[645]). The effects of individual and multiple gene deletions in vaccinia virus have been documented.[646]

A major advantage of this approach of attenuating an infectious agent is the precise knowledge of changes made to the agent, the reproducibility of the technique, and the relative ease of performance compared with the traditional approach of multiple passages in different hosts or cells in culture.

5.4.2. Transfection of Cells with DNA and cDNA

Three types of cell substrates are used: prokaryotic cells such as *E. coli*; lower eukaryotic cells such as yeast; and mammalian cells in the form of primary cells, cell strains, or cell lines. The general procedure is to insert the selected DNA sequence into an autonomously replicating vector such as a retrovirus or into a plasmid with a selectable marker. These are introduced into the cell using special techniques, and the cell is thus transformed or transfected.

5.4.2.1. Transfection of Prokaryotic Cells

Several plasmid and viral systems have been used for cloning DNA of different sizes and origins into *E. coli*. A promoter sequence and ribosome binding site are required to ensure that transcription and translation occur. Two modes of expression are used.[647] The first is as fusion proteins, in which existing bacterial transcription and translation initiation signals are retained so that a hybrid product is formed, consisting of the "new" polypeptide joined to the amino terminus of a bacterial protein, such as β-galactosidase. The second is as a "native" protein with an amino-terminal methionine residue, because the 5′ end of the gene was inserted adjacent to the bacterial promoter.

Some fusion proteins made in this way have proved to be immunogenic and have been obtained in high yields. DNA coding for the pilus protein antigens of enterotoxigenic *E. coli* have been successfully cloned into nonpathogenic *E. coli* strains. In contrast, successful expression of the hemagglutinin gene of influenza virus in *E. coli* has not been obtained,[648] and early attempts to make a satisfactory HBsAg by this method were also unsuccessful.[649]

Producing nonbacterial proteins in bacterial vectors has been generally disappointing. For example, glycosylation of proteins in bacteria usually does not occur. With glycoproteins made in eukaryotic cells, the carbohydrate moiety may be antigenic, may contribute to the protein's conformation, or may protect protease-susceptible bonds from cleavage. The hydrophobic domains in some proteins appear to be toxic for *E. coli*. Some fusion proteins, once formed in the bacterial cell, may be insoluble and therefore be protected from proteolytic degradation. Although they may be solubilized by denaturants such as guanidine hydrochloride, this action is likely to result in undesirable conformational changes to the protein.

5.4.2.2. Transfection of Lower Eukaryotic Cells

Yeast (*Saccharomyces cerevisiae*) is an obvious choice as an expression system for foreign DNA for several reasons. Much is known about the genetics of yeast, offering many opportunities for manipulation. Virtually everyone is exposed to yeast products in food and drink, and if the product from transfected yeast contained some yeast-derived contaminants, they would probably not be a safety hazard. Large-scale fermentation for bulk production of a yeast-grown product should be readily achieved.

The desire to avoid using the blood from HBV-infected humans as a source of the viral surface antigen, HBsAg, initiated research to find an alternative source of the antigen. Its production by transfected yeast cells heralded the new era of genetically engineered vaccines.[649] The antigen exists in glycosylated and nonglycosylated forms, and it can be produced in high yields using different yeast promoters.[650] This product, isolated from the disrupted yeast cells, has the same chemical properties as the human product. Clinical trials[651] showed the safety and acceptability of the new product, and vaccines from several producers are now available for human use.

Other viral antigens have been produced in yeast. Complete and anchor-deficient influenza virus HA molecules in a glycosylated form have been made. The products reacted with polyclonal and monoclonal antibodies made to the native glycoprotein.[652] Some HIV antigens have also been made in transfected yeast cells. However, gp120, the envelope glycoprotein, prepared in this way failed to bind to CD4, the cellular receptor for this viral protein, and it was referred to as a denatured form of the protein.[653]

The simple eukaryote, *Dictyostelium discoideum*, that normally feeds on dead bacteria is under examination for use as an expression system for producing recombinant subunit vaccines. Genes of human, parasitic, bacterial, and viral origin have been expressed in high yield, and the produced proteins may be glycosylated and may react well with monoclonal antibodies against the product produced in mammalian cells.[654] In the case of viral antigens, there seems to be a lack of immunogenicity data comparing the antigen produced by these cells with that made in mammalian cells.

5.4.2.3. Transfection of Mammalian Cells

Cultured human and animal cells have been classified into three groups, as shown in Table 5.4.2.3. Vaccines for human and for veterinary use are made in all three cell substrates. They include poliomyelitis viral vaccines in monkey kidney cells,

TABLE 5.4.2.3. *Classification of human and animal cells*

Cell groups	Classification criteria
Primary cells	Cells used directly after isolation from intact tissues without further subculture
Cell strains	Cells that have a finite capacity to replicate, have the karyotype of the tissue of origin, are anchorage dependent, and do not produce tumors when inoculated into experimental animals
Cell lines	Cells that replicate indefinitely, may produce tumors when inoculated into experimental animals, may not have the karyotype of the tissue of origin, and are anchorage independent

rubella and rabies viral vaccines in cell strains, and a rabies viral vaccine in a cell line.

The potential of cell strains and of cell lines as substrates for vaccine production (and other biologics) would be considerably enhanced if they could be transfected successfully with DNA coding for specific antigens. DNA is normally taken up very poorly by mammalian cells, and special techniques are required to facilitate the process. Even under optimal conditions, less than 10% of the DNA may enter the cell, and much of this is degraded in the cell. One consequence is that cellular DNA, which may be a contaminant in products of a transfected cell, is unlikely to be a serious safety concern. Retroviruses have proved to be effective vectors of foreign DNA, because part of the normal replication cycle is integration of a DNA copy of their RNA into the host cell genome.

5.4.2.3.1. Use of Primary Cells

Monkey kidney cells have been transfected with DNA coding for influenza virus.[655,656] The two research groups used SV40 early and late gene replacement vectors. Both approaches resulted in the synthesis of viral HA, which was glycosylated, expressed at the cell surface, and appeared to be immunologically identical to the protein made by virus-infected cells. The amounts of viral antigen produced were comparable in the two systems. Clearly, this technique could be used to produce viral antigens commercially.

5.4.2.3.2. Use of Cell Strains or Continuous Cell Lines

The use of cell strains or continuous cell lines has several advantages compared with primary cells, including the relative or complete independence from a live host source and the ease of continuous culture. There is however, concern about the neoplastic origin of continuous cell lines because of the possibility of heterogeneous contaminating DNA, of endogenous or latent viruses, and of transforming proteins. A study group[657] concluded that the risk of each of these possibilities could be assessed and was in most cases very small or negligible. Conditions for their use as substrates for vaccine production were recommended, based on methods for the treatment of biologic products to decrease these risks.

Two examples drawn from HIV studies indicate the utility of this approach. Both used genetically modified Chinese hamster ovary (CHO) cells. In the first example,[658] the cells were transfected with modified DNA constructs of HIV-IIIB strain gp120 or gp160, the latter lacking a transmembrane segment. Both proteins were secreted from the transfected cells. They also differed in that the V3 loop, the principal neutralizing domain, was intact in the gp120. Both preparations were glycosylated. Chimpanzees immunized with the gp120, but not with the gp160, were protected against challenge with the homologous virus. There was a correlation between protection and the antibody titer against the intact V3 loop in the gp120. In the second example,[653] gp120 preparations (HIV-1 SF$_2$ strain) were made in genetically modified CHO cells and in yeast. On prolonged immunization, only the CHO cell preparation yielded antibodies that neutralized antigenically distinct HIV strains. The data were interpreted as showing that only the mammalian cell preparation possessed epitopes of the correct conformation for neutralization.

5.4.3. Recombinant Live Vectors

5.4.3.1. General Requirements

The discovery of bacteriophage-mediated transduction in 1952[659] indicated the potential of viruses as tools for moving foreign genetic material from one cell to another. Rous sarcoma virus was the first animal transducing virus recognized. With the advent of rDNA technology, it became clear that infectious vectors could be engineered to have properties that would help to answer particular questions. Initially, viruses seemed to offer special advantages in this respect, because there were several attenuated live vaccines that might be suitable vectors. Such chimeric vectors might be useful in several ways: as a means of producing large amounts of particular gene products; as a means of determining the importance of individual gene products of disease agents in protective immune responses; and as a means for studying the specific roles of individual cytokines. By using existing or newly developed vaccine strains of infectious agents, the potential exists for making recombinant or chimeric preparations to use as vaccines to control diseases for which there were no existing vaccines.

5.4.3.2. Expectations of a Live Vector Vaccine

A number of desirable attributes nominate chimeric live vectors for useful and acceptable vaccines, particularly on a global scale. They are listed in Table 5.4.3.2 under five headings: safety, efficacy, immune response, molecular biology, and utility.[660] Many of the points made are applicable to a new vaccine developed using any technology, but taken together, they all apply to the development and use of chimeric live vectors. It is likely that no single preparation will have all of these attributes, but all should be borne in mind when a project is planned.

5.4.4. Recombinant Live Viruses as Candidate Vaccines

In 1982, two publications[661,662] appeared almost at the same time and showed that recombinant viral particles could be recovered from cells infected simultaneously with vaccinia virus and a source of foreign DNA contained in a plasmid. Both research groups recognized that the DNA could come from any source, including other infectious agents. In this case, the recombinant virus could act as a vector of the foreign DNA, which would be transcribed and translated, leading to the induc-

TABLE 5.4.3.2. *Desirable attributes of a live vector for global use as a vaccine*

Safety
Acceptably low level of side effects
Safe to administer to immunodeficient or immunocompromised hosts
Infectious only for the target population
Agent not contagious (passed from vaccinee to contact) or tumorogenic (or capability can be deleted)
Infection is acute; infectious agent does not persist
No integration into host cell genome; no persistence of provirus or a state of latency
Does not induce autoimmune disease

Efficacy
Long-term protection from disease, after one or two or infrequent administrations (may vary with route of administration)
Effective herd immunity induced in target population
Potential for the inclusion of DNA coding for several antigens (and cytokines if required)
Induces immunity to the nominated antigen in the presence of specific antibody (maternal, preexisting) to that antigen

Immune response
Induction of humoral and cell-mediated immune responses to nominated antigens
Generation of a large pool of memory T and B cells
Favorable kinetics of antigen accumulation and kinetics
Appropriate immune response when administered mucosally (if required)
No interference with the response to other vaccines given at a similar time
No polyclonal activation of T or B cells

Molecular biology
Construct should be genetically stable
A suitable promoter for early expression after infection is available
High yield of expressed protein
Product is secreted (especially in the case of a bacterial vector) or expressed appropriately (cell associated) in infected cell
Expressed protein has the same properties (eg, conformation, amino acid sequence, glycosylation pattern, antigenicity) as occurs naturally

Utility
Heat stable (ie, provision of a cold chain unnecessary)
Can be administered orally
Affordable in countries where the need is great
Can be administered by paramedical personnel
Readily incorporated into national and international vaccination programs
Successful vaccination can be readily assessed (ie, simple diagnostic test)

From Ada GL. (1991) Strategies for exploiting the immune system. Elsevier Science, Kidlington, UK, pp. 228–229.

tion of an immune response that might protect against infection by the agent that was the source of the foreign DNA or cDNA. Further experiments soon showed that this could be the case. The technology was seen as combining the effectiveness of live attenuated viral vaccines with the increasing desire to immunize with a subunit preparation of another infectious agent. The method should overcome the need for several injections of a subunit protein with a strong adjuvant to induce a comprehensive and lasting immune response. Table 5.4.4 lists some viral preparations, including some existing human vaccines, that are being used or are proposed as vectors for foreign antigens.

TABLE 5.4.4. *Viruses used or proposed as vectors of nucleic acids from other sources*

Vector	Virus
Human infections	Vaccinia, ORF, poliovirus, herpesvirus, varicella, adenovirus, influenza, bovine papilloma, Epstein-Barr, mengo, SV40, retroviruses
Avipox	Fowlpox, canarypox
Insects	Baculovirus

5.4.4.1. Poxviruses

Far more experimental work has been carried out with poxviruses, especially vaccinia, than with any other vector because of the ease of working with this virus and because of its properties. These include the susceptibility of many cell types to infection, the ease of growing virus to a high titer, the thermostability of the virion, the large capacity for insertion of foreign DNA, and the high level of gene expression that can be initiated early or late in the infectious cycle.

The commonly used strains of vaccinia include Copenhagen, Wyeth, Lister, and Western Reserve. The latter was derived from the New York City Board of Health vaccine strain by passage in mouse brains.

5.4.4.1.1. Construction of Recombinants

Because the viral DNA is noninfectious, chimeric genomes are formed by homologous recombination within infected cells by a two-stage process. One method uses plasmids, called insertion vectors, that possess a vaccinia virus promoter with downstream cloning sites and flanking sequences of nonessential viral DNA. The foreign gene is cloned into the vector, and the plasmid is then transfected into the vaccinia virus–infected cells. Recombination occurs between the sequences of viral origin flanking the promoter or foreign gene construct and the corresponding sequences of the infecting viral genome. Because the process is relatively inefficient, suitable markers are used to identify and select the resulting chimeric virus.[663] Figure 5.4.4.1 illustrates the way a recombinant poxvirus vector is constructed.

Many sites have been used for insertion of the foreign DNA into the virus genome and of different promoters. Many genes coded for at either terminus of the viral genome are nonessential for viral growth. For example, a total of 55 ORFs have been deleted from the Copenhagen strain without loss of infectivity for cells in culture. Different types of vaccinia virus promoters have been described, including early, intermediate, and late. Whereas neither the level of antigen expression nor its temporal regulation appeared to affect antibody titers, there were selective effects on CTL activity. In the case of influenza virus NP determinants, CTLs specific for the sequence 50–63 but not for the sequence 365–379 could recognize late-expressed NP.[664] This defect in late presentation could be overcome by increasing the rate of degradation of the expressed antigen in the cell. Similarly in another report,[665] delayed-type hypersensitivity reaction (DTH) and T-cell proliferation in response

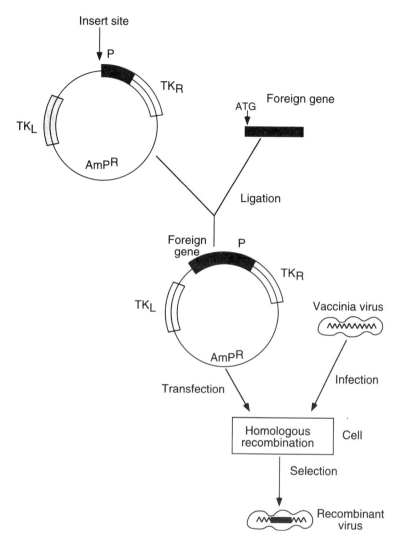

FIG. 5.4.4.1. Construction of recombinant vaccinia viruses. The foreign gene is ligated into a unique insert site in the plasmid, which is then transfected into cells that have been infected with vaccinia virus. The plasmid sequence lying between the flanking thymidine kinase (TK) sequences is then inserted by means of homologous recombination of these TK sequences at the appropriate site in the viral genome. Recombinant viruses are selected by plaquing on TK-positive cells in the presence of bromodeoxyuridine.

to the late-expressed antigen were reduced, but antibody levels to early and late-expressed herpesvirus glycoprotein D were indistinguishable. It can be argued that if, after infection, viral replication is to be controlled by CTLs, the early production of determinants would optimize the chances of recognition and control by the CTLs before infectious progeny was assembled and secreted or released.

One of the uses of chimeric vaccinia viruses has been to produce large quantities of a given foreign protein, sometimes for use as a vaccine candidate. One elegant method was to use the bacteriophage T7 RNA polymerase gene expressed behind a promoter within vaccinia virus. High levels of expression of a target gene could be obtained if it was regulated by a T7 promoter in another vaccinia virus, and other cells were then co-infected by the two viruses.[666]

5.4.4.1.2. Experimental Models

There is a wealth of information on the use of vaccinia viruses as vectors to make candidate vaccines (reviewed elsewhere[667,668]). For example, the list of viruses that are important human pathogens and that have been sources of DNA and cDNA coding for different antigens includes rabies virus, hepatitis B virus, herpesvirus, cytomegalovirus, Epstein-Barr virus, influenza virus, parainfluenza virus, measles virus, dengue virus, Japanese encephalitis virus, HIV, Lassa fever virus, and respiratory syncytial virus (RSV).[669] Where tested adequately, immunization of various mammals with most of the preparations has resulted in antibody formation, T-cell proliferation, and at least CTL memory. Protection against a challenge infection has not always been achieved when primates such as chimpanzees have been immunized, as against hepatitis B[670] and RSV.[671] This may indicate the importance of the chimpanzee as an animal model for testing vaccines designed for human use.[672]

There are many examples of successful vaccination, and two are cited here. First is the use of a vaccinia/rabies glycoprotein construct to protect foxes from rabies infection.[673] The vaccine is administered as bait for oral consumption and has undergone very successful field trials. Local eradication of environmental (eg, foxes) rabies should be achievable if a vaccine is potent, safe, and thermostable and if there is an efficient bait system, a practical and sure method of bait dispersal, and an effective spatial and temporal pattern of bait distribution.

The second example is a construct containing DNA coding for the HA or fusion glycoproteins of rinderpest virus, a pathogen of major importance for cattle, especially in Africa; it has elicited neutralizing antibodies and protected cattle from a severe challenge.[674] This protection was sufficiently impressive to prompt the suggestion that this vaccine might offer the prospect of rinderpest eradication.[675]

Vaccinia constructs containing genes coding for the HIV-1 env antigen or including, in addition, other viral antigens, are undergoing clinical trials to assess safety and immunogenicity.[676] The initial immune responses have only been moderate, but one interesting point emerged. In some experiments, recipients of the vaccinia/env construct who had previously been vaccinated against smallpox (ie, before 1977) gave a poorer response than vaccinia-naive recipients,[677] and this was considered to be caused by the long-term persistence of antibody after earlier vaccination.

Viruses, such as measles and RSV, cause high morbidity and mortality in young children, particularly in developing countries. One desirable attribute of a vaccine specific for such infections is efficacy in the presence of maternal antibody to these viruses (see Table 5.4.3.2.). Unfortunately, there are reports that polyclonal antibodies to the surface antigens of these two viruses[678,679] inhibit the replication of the recombinant vaccinia viruses in mice (measles recombinant) or in cotton rats (RSV recombinant).

5.4.4.1.3. Overcoming Disadvantages Associated with Vaccinia Virus

Despite the success of the vaccinia vaccine in the smallpox eradication campaign, concerns about the possibility of its continued use in human vaccination programs were widespread because of the high level of side reactions.[680,681] Three approaches are directed at reducing the level of complications.

The first approach is to produce vaccinia virus recombinants expressing additional genes coding for certain cytokines, such as interleukin-2 (IL-2). Depending on the cytokine used, this can have the effect of further attenuation of the virus itself. This approach is discussed in more detail in Section 5.4.6.

A second approach involves reproducible attenuation of the virus by deletion of certain DNA sequences so that the virus replicates very poorly in mammalian cells but remains immunogenic. The preparation called NYVAC (see Section 5.4.1) is in this category. DNA sequences from a number of antigens of other infectious agents, including equine influenza virus, pseudorabies virus, Japanese encephalitis virus, and HIV, have been inserted into the NYVAC genome and the recombinants tested successfully in different animal models.[682]

A third approach is the use of attenuated virus that does not replicate in mammalian cell lines, such as the modified vaccinia virus Ankara produced by extensive passaging in chick embryo fibroblasts. The block is at a step in virion assembly, and when used as a vector, recombinant proteins are produced at levels comparable to infection with the wild-type virus.[683] An alternative is to use the Jennerian approach, in which a strain of virus is virulent for a different host. Avipox viruses have been shown to be effective vectors in mammalian cells, even though they undergo only an abortive infection. Fowlpox and canarypox viruses are being used as vectors, with the latter (ie, ALVAC) in particular being highly effective.[684] A recombinant preparation expressing the rabies virus glycoprotein is as effective as a vaccinia construct in affording protection against rabies. Encouragingly, protective immunity could be induced in very young dogs in the presence of maternal antibody.[684] A variety of other constructs using this vector and including HIV and cytomegalovirus antigens have been made.[685] A potential additional bonus of this vector is that the DNA behind early and intermediate promoters seems to be preferentially expressed. Because genes coding for proteins containing some B-cell epitopes are behind late promoters, abortive infection does not lead to strong antiviral antibody production, and it may be possible to use sequential vaccination with this vector.

5.4.4.2. Adenoviruses

Although poxviruses are usually administered parenterally, there is a great need for chimeric vectors that could be given by a mucosal route. The adenovirus vaccine composed of the 4 and 7 serotypes is given orally and has proved to be safe and effective in military recruits in the United States. The virus is readily grown in tissue culture, a high copy number of the viral DNA is present within the cell during replication, the viral genome possesses strong promoters, and up to 7 kbp of foreign DNA can be inserted.

Owing to the lack of an in vitro system for growing HBV, an initial effort was to develop recombinant constructs expressing the surface antigen, HBsAg. Chimpanzees infected with the construct were protected when challenged. Several other constructs have been made, including the DNA coding for surface glycoproteins from other viruses, such as that causing vesicular stomatitis, herpes simplex virus, cytomegalovirus, RSV, parainfluenza virus, and rabies virus, and the constructs have been tested in different host animals. In most cases, protection was obtained against a challenge infection (reviewed elsewhere[686,687]). Adeno-HIV constructs have been made, containing the env or gag proteins, and used to infect chimpanzees (permissive infection) or beagles (abortive infection). The availability of various adenovirus serotypes allowed effective boosting to be done with a different serotype. Intranasal administration was much more effective than oral administration at inducing antibody responses in different mucosal secretions, including vaginal and rectal sites. Replication-defective preparations of adenoviruses have been made, and these may prove to be useful as vectors for human use (see Section 6.1).

5.4.4.3. Polioviruses

The great success of the oral polio vaccine in providing effective protection at a mucosal surface stimulated interest in the possibility that it might be used as a vector for foreign genes.[688] Initially, intertypic hybrid viral particles were constructed in which short amino acid sequences from type 2 or type 3 polio viruses were grafted into a short segment (about 15 amino acids long) at the highly exposed B-C loop of VP1 (the antigenic site 1) of the very safe type 1 Sabin strain. It then became feasible to graft amino acid sequences (principally known B-cell epitopes) from other sources (mainly viral) into this site.[688] Although some success was achieved, it was inevitable that this approach was severely limited, especially for B-cell epitopes, by the smallness of the fragment that could be successfully inserted and enable the virus to retain its infectivity and the inserted sequence to maintain its correct conformation.

Another approach has been to replace the VP2 and VP3 genes within the capsid precursor protein, P1, by the in-frame insertion of foreign DNA. This recombinant virus can be successfully encapsidated if P1 is provided in *trans* by a recombinant vaccinia helper virus.[689] On infection, the minireplicons so formed express HIV-1 gag and pol. Because these structures do not productively replicate, it remains to be seen whether they are sufficiently immunogenic when given by a mucosal or parenteral route to induce a good humoral response to the insert.

5.4.4.4. Herpesviruses

Sexually transmitted diseases are becoming increasingly important globally as causes of great morbidity and, in the case of HIV, mortality. It is difficult, however, to induce long-lived immune responses in the reproductive tracts, as discussed in Section 6.2. One possibility would be to use an attenuated recombinant herpesvirus for local infection that might induce persisting immunity because of latency. Herpes simplex virus can tolerate insertions of at least 8 kbp, and presumably, some nonessential viral DNA could be replaced. Some progress has been made toward the development of vectors that might allow gene transfer to the brain,[690] but no construct has been shown to overexpress foreign genes.[691]

5.4.5. Recombinant Live Bacteria as Candidate Vaccines

5.4.5.1. Salmonella

Most work has been done with *S. typhimurium* strains because of the ease of testing in mice. After passage across the intestinal epithelium and the lamina propria, *S. typhimurium* replicates in the gut-associated lymphoid tissue and in Peyer's patches and enters the blood stream through the lymphatics. It replicates in the spleen and liver, and a disseminated infection occurs that may lead to death. It has been reported that clearance of the infection is mediated mainly by CD4 + T cells,[692] but it would be useful to extend such studies using class I MHC antigen knockout mice, perforin-negative mice, or both.

Several approaches have been used to develop *S. typhimurium* recombinants that would express foreign antigens or epitopes of those antigens:

1. A standard experiment is to use high-copy-number plasmids carrying antibiotic resistance markers and a constitutively active promoter element. One problem has been plasmid segregation in vivo with loss of expression of the foreign gene.
2. Systems for the chromosomal integration of expression cassettes by homologous recombination have been described.[693]
3. Another way is to make recombinant bacterial proteins by using the bacterial protein as a carrier of foreign epitopes. For example, *Salmonella* flagellin, the monomeric unit of flagella, has highly conserved amino and carboxy termini but a hypervariable central region. When existing or prepared as a polymer, the important B-cell epitopes are present in this central section, which is exposed to

the medium.[694] Relatively large foreign sequences have been inserted as a replacement sequence into this central region. Some constructs were reported to be immunogenic after repeated oral administration of the recombinant organism.[695] Other secreted bacterial proteins have been used similarly.

4. Another approach is to use the HBcAg protein as a carrier protein in *Salmonella* and to insert other B-cell epitopes into this carrier, which can assemble into particles.

A variety of viral, bacterial, or parasite antigens have been expressed in this vector,[696] but immunologic data are unavailable for some. Five examples illustrate these approaches:

1. The nucleoprotein gene of influenza virus was inserted into an Aro A *S. typhimurium* strain and fed orally to mice.[697] The mice produced specific IgG antibodies and demonstrated CD4 + T-cell proliferation. The CD4 + T cells became cytolytic only after further in vitro culture. No cytolytic CD8 + T cells were detected. This immunization did not protect against an influenza virus challenge.

2. The DNA coding for the *Streptococcus pyogenes* M protein was put into an Aro A *S. typhimurium*, and mice were immunized by the oral route.[698] The mice developed serum IgA, IgG, and IgM antibodies and salivary sIgA that opsonized *S. pyogenes* in vitro. The mice were protected against a lethal *S. pyogenes* (given intranasally or intraperitoneally) and a wild-type *S. typhimurium* (given intraperitoneally) challenge.

3. The circumsporozoite (CS) antigen of *Plasmodium berghei* was expressed in an attenuated *S. typhimurium* strain and fed orally to mice.[699] CS-specific CD8 + CTLs, but no anti-CS antibody, was detected, and the mice were partially protected against challenge, a result attributed to the CTL response.[700] A similar experiment carried out by another group[701] also showed CD8 + CTL formation, but no protection against challenge was found.

4. Using the carrier HBcAg approach, an internal insertion site was found that greatly enhanced the immunogenicity of the inserted B-cell epitope,[702] as demonstrated with epitopes from the HBV surface antigen and from the CS protein of different malaria parasites. The HBcAg/epitope/*Salmonella* construct was immunogenic after a single oral administration to mice. A similar construct in *S. typhi* is to undergo clinical trials.

5. A well-defined MHC class II–restricted determinant was inserted into the central domain of the flagellin of attenuated (ΔAroA) *Salmonella dublin*. The flagella subsequently expressed multiple copies of the determinant. When flanked by Lys-Lys cathepsin B cleavage sites to facilitate its subsequent release, the determinant was efficiently processed in macrophages. The chimeric bacteria were cleared more rapidly from the organs of T-cell receptor-positive transgenic mice than were control bacteria.[703] Similarly, a significant decrease in the number of *Listeria* organisms was found in mice immunized with *Salmonella* expressing flagella containing class I and class II MHC determinants from the listeriolysin

of *Listeria monocytogenes*.[704] Spleen cells from the immunized mice had listeriolysin-specific CTL activity.

An expression cassette containing a bacterial promoter and sequences from the HIV-1 env antigen has been inserted into the chromosome of an attenuated *S. typhi*. The construct was stable and clinical trials are planned.[705]

5.4.5.2. Bacille Calmette-Guérin

BCG seems to offer many advantages as a vector. It has been administered to billions of persons, particularly to infants, as part of the World Health Organization (WHO) Expanded Programme of Immunization. It has an impressive safety record. Occasionally, a vaccine batch is less attenuated than is optimum, but the availability of antibacterial drugs helps to avert serious effects. Because the organism persists, a chimeric construct is likely to give long-lasting immune responses, but this will also depend on the expressed foreign antigen. When administered with other antigens, it frequently demonstrates strong adjuvant activity.

There were several early reports on the expression of foreign genes in BCG. In one report,[706] the bacterial heat shock protein promoters were used to drive expression of DNA coding for the env, gag, and pol antigens of HIV-1. A second group[707] developed a multicopy plasmid system for extrachromosomal replication of the foreign DNA, as well as a method for achieving a site-specific integration into the bacterial chromosome. Bacterial antigens such as β-galactosidase and a fragment of tetanus toxin were used. Good CD4 + and CD8 + T-cell responses were obtained, as were persisting antibody responses, to the two bacterial proteins, but the antibody response to the HIV antigens was quite low.

Vector systems that export or secrete the expressed foreign antigens have been developed.[708] Expression of the OspA antigen of *Borrelia burgdorferi* as a chimeric membrane-associated lipoprotein resulted in high-titer protective responses after administration. In contrast, expression of the PspA antigen of *Streptococcus pneumoniae* as a secreted or membrane-associated lipoprotein did not result in higher titer antibody responses compared with cytoplasmic expression, but the quality of protective antibody appeared to be improved. Mice immunized with the OspA BCG construct by a single nasopharyngeal administration elicited high-titer systemic and mucosal (upper respiratory tract) antibody responses. Clinical trials are planned in response to these encouraging results.

5.4.6. Insertion of Genes Coding for Cytokines

An obstacle to the use of vectors such as vaccinia virus for vaccination is the danger of serious side effects if the vaccine is inadvertently given to immunodeficient individuals, particularly because of the substantial current rate of disease and other conditions affecting immunocompetence. The expression of genes encoding cytokines in a range of different recombinant vaccine vectors has become widely used in attempts to provide suitable attenuation of the vector with retention of immunogenicity.

In 1987, three publications reported results of experiments in which genes coding for cytokines interferon-γ (IFNγ) or IL-2 were incorporated into vaccinia virus and shown to be expressed when cells were infected with the construct.[709–711] In two publications,[710,711] infection of nude mice with the control vaccinia resulted in death. Mice infected with recombinant vaccinia expressing IL-2 survived, suggesting that it would be safe to use such constructs in immunocompromised hosts. The extensive virus growth and resultant tissue destruction that normally occurs after infection with vaccinia virus was absent, with the reduction in pathogenicity depending on cytokine expression and not simply the expression of a foreign gene. Despite the reduced levels of virus replication, specific serum antibody responses in mice and primates immunized with the IL-2/vaccinia virus were of similar magnitude to control responses.[710,712] When immunodeficient mice were infected with a construct encoding IL-2 and the HA gene of influenza virus (strain A/PR8/34), they were rendered resistant to challenge with the type-specific influenza virus.[713] The genomic configuration of this recombinant vaccinia is outlined in Figure 5.4.6.

Investigation of the mechanisms of activity of the encoded cytokines in these

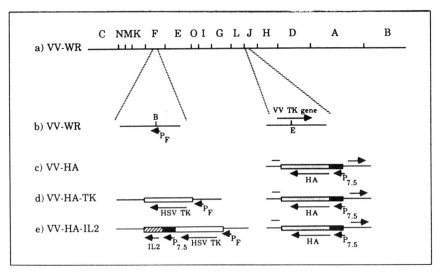

FIG. 5.4.6. Genomic configuration of VV-HA-IL-2. A *Hind*III map of vaccinia virus, strain VV-WR, is shown with insertion points at the *Eco*RI (E) and *Bam*HI (B) sites on the J and F fragments, respectively. Arrows indicate orientations of the vaccinia virus thymidine kinase: TK gene, vaccinia promoters P_F and $P_{7.5}$, the influenza virus HA gene, the herpes simplex virus (HSV) TK gene (as a selectable marker), and the murine IL-2 coding sequences. (Courtesy of Dr. G. Karupiah, John Curtin School of Medical Research, The Australian National University, Canberra, ACT, 2601.)

systems showed that infection by the IL-2–expressing virus led to enhancement of host cellular cytotoxic activities, particularly natural killer cell activity,[714] and that the antiviral effector function of the IL-2–activated cells was mediated by IFNγ.[715] A major component of this effect of IFNγ was a direct antiviral activity, in that vaccinia encoding IFNγ also exhibited markedly reduced pathogenicity without enhancing host immunity.[716] The enhanced production of tumor necrosis factor-α, like IFNγ, through expression in recombinant vaccina virus also resolved the virus infection rapidly, probably by direct antiviral activity, but in this case, specific antibody responses were depressed.[717]

The expression of type 2 cytokines in vaccinia virus, unlike the previously mentioned type 1 factors, apparently had no attenuation effects on virus pathogenicity. However, they were able to selectively modulate antibody responses to co-expressed vaccine antigens. Infection of mice with vaccinia virus expressing IL-5[718] or IL-6[305,719] led to enhanced production of different isotypes of immunoglobulins, such as sIgA, and different subclasses of IgG. In particular, when inoculated onto a mucosal surface, virus-encoded IL-5 elicited anti-HA sIgA-secreting cells at much greater levels than those induced by a control virus.[718] IL-6 also induced enhanced anti-viral mucosal IgA reactivity, with strong evidence of synergistic interaction between virus-encoded and host-derived factors in the development of this response.[719] These findings may be of particular importance for improvement of mucosal vaccination strategies, because responses at mucosae are often difficult to induce and are notoriously short lived. A wide range of cytokine genes has been encoded in vaccinia virus vectors, and their effects on antiviral immune responses have been monitored, as exhibited in Table 5.4.6.

The expression of IL-6 in recombinant fowlpox virus also led to a significant enhancement of primary and secondary systemic and mucosal antibody responses to co-expressed vaccine antigen in mice.[720] This virus undergoes only an abortive infection in mammalian cells and therefore represents a potentially safer vector than vaccinia virus. Fowlpox virus–encoded IL-6 also primed for enhanced recall mucosal antibody responses to sublethal challenge with the infectious wild-type agent, indicating the potential importance of this approach for enhancing resistance to infection. Several alternative vaccine vectors, including adenovirus and *Salmonella*, have been engineered to express cytokine genes in attempts to induce selectively desired vaccination responses. Mice immunized intranasally with adenoviruses encoding IL-6 induced lymphocytic hyperplasia in the lungs, but the effects on local antibody production were not reported.[722] Recombinant *S. typhimurium* encoding IL-6 elicited levels of systemic and mucosal antibody similar to those of the control bacteria, but the recombinants displayed reduced invasiveness in mice.[723] However, it was not clear whether cytokine expression led to the failure to invade M cells or to accelerated clearance of bacteria in the Peyer's patches before reaching the spleen. No similar decrease in virulence or enhancement of immunogenicity was recorded for *Salmonella* vectors encoding other cytokines, including IL-1β[724] or IL-4.[725] The latter displayed increased virulence in mice, probably because of an inhibitory effect of IL-4 on antibacterial macrophage activity.

TABLE 5.4.6. *Functions of cytokines and their effects in vivo when expressed by recombinant vaccinia viruses*

Cytokine	Major known function	Effects on immunity when expressed by rVV
Type 1 factors		
IL-2	T-cell growth factor, activates B cells, monocytes, and NK cells	Attenuates growth of virus, stimulates natural killer cells to produce IFNγ[710–712]
TNFα	Antiviral activity in vitro, activates CTLs	Limits growth of rVV, allowing T-cell–deficient mice to resolve infection[717]
IFNγ	Upregulates MHC molecules on antigen presenting cells, antiviral activity	Limits growth of rVV, allowing T-cell–deficient mice to resolve infection[716]
IL-12	Helps initiate type 1 responses, promotes IFNγ production	Limits growth of rVV, stimulates IFNγ secretion, downregulates type 2 responses (AJ Ramsay, unpublished observations)
Type 2 factors		
IL-4	Regulates antibody responses, especially IgE, downregulates type 1 responses	Increases pathogenicity of rVV, downregulates CTL responses[351]
IL-5	Regulates antibody production	Stimulates antigen-specific mucosal IgA responses[718]
IL-6	Involved in the maturation of B cells to ASCs	Stimulates antigen-specific systemic IgG and mucosal IgA responses[305]
Other factors		
IL-1α	Activates T cells	Enhances memory antibody responses[721]
IL-7	Early activator of T and B cells	Stimulates T-cell and nonspecific antiviral immunity (AJ Ramsay, unpublished observations)

ASCs, antibody-secreting cells; CTL, cytotoxic T lymphocytes; IFN, interferon; Ig, immunoglobulin; IL, interleukin; MHC, major histocompatibility complex; NK, natural killer; rVV, recombinant vaccinia virus; TNF, tumor necrosis factor.

This approach has also been applied to direct nucleic acid vaccination (see Section 5.4.9). As with the more established vector systems, cytokines encoded in cDNA expression vectors have produced biologically significant systemic effects. After injection of recombinant plasmids into murine skeletal muscle, encoded IL-2 augmented antibody and DTH responses to protein immunogens administered several days later, but transforming growth factor-β inhibited these IL-2–induced immunostimulatory effects.[726] IL-4 or IL-6 encoded in plasmids elicited marked enhancement of serum IgG antibody responses against co-expressed HA antigen. These effects were prolonged, probably because of the sustained expression of these genes in immunized animals (IA Ramshaw, AJ Ramsay, unpublished observations).

The encoding of cytokine genes in recombinant candidate vaccines enhances vector attenuation and immunogenicity. Future studies should yield more data concerning the protective nature of such enhanced responses.

5.4.7. Synthetic Recombinant Approaches

An additional approach to using the live agent as a vector is to construct the live chimeric agent so that the foreign DNA is inserted into the DNA coding for a highly immunogenic protein and to use the expressed and then isolated chimeric protein instead of the live agent as the vector. Such a product has been called a *synthetic recombinant vaccine*.[727] The flagellin molecule of *Salmonella* is being used for this purpose. It is readily polymerized to form a large polymer, polymerized flagellin,[728] that, like the parent flagella and in the absence of added adjuvant, gave long-lasting immunity after a single administration to rats.[253] When a small dose (5 μg) was injected subcutaneously into humans, flagellin subsequently induced a long-lasting antibody response.[729] Most recipients had specific IgM before the administration, but both IgM and IgG were produced after immunization.

Three separate chimeric flagella were prepared[727] containing amino acid sequences corresponding to a conserved neutralizing epitope from a subtype 3 influenza HA (HA 91-108) and from the conserved nucleoprotein, a TH determinant (aa 55-69) and a CTL determinant (aa 147-158). Administration of all three chimeric flagella intranasally to BALB/c mice provided cross-protection from death but not infection after a lethal challenge of influenza virus (most control mice died). Although it was stressed that this protection was only seen if all three preparations were administered, the data suggest that protection resulted largely if not entirely from enhanced crossreactive CTL activity. Experiments in which mice were immunized with the CTL, TH flagella, or both constructs were not reported.

It is possible to insert foreign sequences into the neuraminidase[730] and HA[731] of influenza virus while retaining the infectivity of the virus. An in-frame fusion construct has been made with a characterized foreign epitope in the influenza HA.[732] The chimeric protein was said to induce a sustained immune response in immunized hosts, but to achieve this required administration with a strong adjuvant and up to five doses over 35 weeks—a rather impractical approach compared with the previous report using bacterial chimeric flagella.

5.4.8. A Commentary on Recombinant Vaccines

A comparison of the different approaches to develop vaccines using recombinant DNA technology reveals the emergence of particular patterns. The conformational requirements for generating responses to T-cell determinants and B-cell epitopes are usually very different. The final conformation of T-cell determinants is determined by binding in the groove in the MHC antigen in which the peptide is held. The conformation of that sequence in the donor protein is largely irrelevant.

Some B-cell epitopes can also be represented by linear peptides, but these have at least a secondary conformation, as seen particularly in some bacterial (eg, *Chlamydia*, *Streptococcus*) and parasitic (eg, malaria) proteins, and these can be represented by oligopeptides. Other epitopes may have a tertiary conformation that, unless it is formed in part by a crosslinking disulfide bond to form a loop, may not be well represented by a synthetic peptide. Other epitopes, formed by contacting sequences of adjacent proteins, have a quaternary conformation, as is seen with many viruses and some bacterial structures such as flagella. These cannot readily be represented by oligopeptides. Carbohydrate side chains may also affect protein conformation. Because of this, mammalian viral proteins, especially glycoproteins, are likely to have the more correct conformation if produced in mammalian cells, whether these are DNA transfected or infected by a chimeric virus, because during synthesis in the cytoplasm, they undergo correct posttranslational processing. This concept applies particularly to an infectious agent's proteins or glycoproteins that are exposed to the environment for some time. It appears to be not so critical for many bacterial or parasite proteins. Nevertheless, an important general rule would be to produce protective proteins (antibody) in the cell type that is the natural source of that protein.

In contrast, internal antigens, particularly of viruses, are often good sources of T-cell determinants, in part because such proteins need not be designed to be protease resistant. Examples are the HBcAg (HBV) and the NP (influenza virus). The best sources of T-cell determinants in bacteria and parasites are not so well known. The method of fusing foreign epitopes and determinants into highly immunogenic proteins, especially to generate T-cell responses, rather than using the whole foreign protein, looks promising. Such sequences need to be released intact. Because it is known that flanking residues can impose constraints,[733] more information on the influence of neighboring residues is needed. Perhaps having a short protease-susceptible sequence at each end of the insert[703] may become a general approach. Most work has been done using inbred mice of known MHC haplotype. The number of T-cell determinants (TH and CTL) needed to obtain good protective responses for most in an outbred human population is unknown and may need to be determined on a region by region basis.

5.4.9. Naked DNA Preparations

Few announcements of a new approach to vaccination have been greeted with such enthusiasm as the use of DNA for this purpose. It is called naked DNA or genetic vaccination. Within a remarkably short time, a complete issue of a prominent journal was devoted solely to preliminary reports on its application to a variety of problems and the nature of concerns that regulatory authorities might have about its use in humans.[734]

The technique of administering DNA for different purposes is not new (reviewed elsewhere[735]), but its resurrection a few years ago came at an opportune time, when the other techniques for making vaccines against difficult diseases such as acquired immunodeficiency syndrome and malaria seemed to be making little headway.

The technique itself is remarkably simple. The DNA coding for the antigens concerned is placed behind a suitable (often a viral) promoter in a plasmid, which is then injected into muscle, where it is taken up into myofibrils. An alternative approach that has gained considerable favor is to coat the plasmids onto microscopic gold beads (about 600 copies per bead). A "gene gun" is used to ballistically accelerate the particles so they penetrate the cell membrane. When used on shaved skin, cells in the dermis and epidermis are transduced. The amount of DNA required to induce an immune response by this technique is much less than the amount used to inject into muscle.

5.4.9.1. Immunization with DNA Versus Immunization with Viruses or Bacteria

Essentially, the DNA is transcribed and translated principally in the cytoplasmic pathway so that all the major components of a specific immune response—specific antibody, CD4+ TH, and CD8+ CTLs—are generated. In this respect, they can be directly compared with a live attenuated virus or bacteria, whether used as such or as a live vector, because both induce these responses, which are usually long lasting. Table 5.4.9.1 documents some comparisons under the headings of immune responses generated, safety, preparation, and properties. With an acute infection, effector T cells (eg, CTLs) are usually present in an infected organ for a short time, but they decrease in number and disappear a few days after the infectious agent can

TABLE 5.4.9.1. *Immunization with DNA compared with immunization with a live, attenuated virus or a chimeric live vector*

Immune response
Each induces the long-lasting formation of specific antibody, CD4+ TH cells, and CD8+ cytotoxic T lymphocytes (CTLs). It is sometimes said that a DNA preparation is superior at inducing a CTL response, but this needs more documentation.[736,737] For example, DNA coding for the influenza virus nucleoprotein gene can cross-protect against disease (but not infection) caused by different influenza A strains, as can a live attenuated influenza virus.
With DNA, the immune response is directed almost solely against the particular antigen. With a live viral or bacterial vector, much of the immune response is against the vector, which may be undesirable. For example, the presence of specific antibody interferes with initial immunization with a viral construct,[678,679] but it should not interfere with initial or repeated immunizations with a DNA preparation. Local immunization remains more straightforward with some viruses or bacteria than with DNA.

Safety
The main theoretical concern (there is no direct evidence) with DNA is the insertion of the DNA into the host cell genome, resulting in the possibility of transformation or tumorogenic events and including the formation of anti-DNA antibodies.[734] With a live, attenuated agent or chimeric vector, there is often a risk of significant side reactions, including reversion to virulence, which is especially hazardous for immunocompromised recipients. There frequently is some immunopathologic response after immunization.

Preparation and Properties
DNA has distinct advantages. It is easy and inexpensive to prepare reproducibly in pure form and in quantity. It is heat stable and physically robust.

no longer be detected. In contrast, because the DNA persists after genetic immunization, there is the opportunity for effector CTLs to be continually generated, but this has not yet been described.[736] If this is the case, it will be a great advantage in situations such as influenza and HIV infection, in which antigenic specificity for neutralizing antibody is constantly changing but many CTL determinants on internal antigens are conserved. In such a situation, the very first infected cells would be susceptible to CTL attack. However, knowing the mode of action of the injected DNA should indicate the likelihood of this possibility. Another interesting possibility is the early induction of high-affinity antibodies due to the expression of relatively small amounts of antigen after DNA vaccination. Table 5.4.9.1 shows that genetic immunization has clear advantages in the areas of preparation and general properties.

5.4.9.2. Mode of Action of Injected DNA

Most experiments with injected DNA have been carried out in mice. The mode of action is as yet unclear, but three possibilities have been suggested.[736] The first is direct presentation by injected muscle cells. The cells should process the foreign DNA so that a viral antigen might be expressed at the cell surface or secreted, and class I MHC–associated foreign peptides would be expressed at the cell surface. However, efficient presentation of this complex to and activation of the T cell requires the antigen-presenting cell (APC) to express co-stimulator molecules. Because myofibrils are not known to have this capability, they are unlikely to act as APCs for T-cell stimulation.

A second possible mechanism is the transfer of protein antigens from the muscle cells to bone marrow–derived APCs, with crossover into the MHC class I processing pathway. This concept is supported by the finding that co-injection of DNA coding for granulocyte-macrophage colony-stimulating factor (GM-CSF) and DNA coding for the rabies glycoprotein enhanced humoral and cellular responses to the protein, and this enhanced response correlated with increased protection against a rabies virus challenge.[738] GM-CSF is known to induce the differentiation of hematopoietic progenitors in bone marrow into "professional" APCs that express co-stimulators (including dendritic cells). The extent to which crossover of protein into the class I MHC pathway may occur in such cells is not clear.

A third possibility is that dendritic cells are much more effective APCs than macrophages at activating naive T cells, including CTLs, at least in vitro. It may be that dendritic cells directly pick up small amounts of the injected DNA that persists in the cell. If plasmids slowly "leak out" of the myofibrils over time, dendritic cells, being very motile, could pick this up also. Some DNA-coated gold beads introduced into the skin by a gene gun are rapidly taken up by local dendritic cells, such as Langerhans cells, and transported to local lymphoid tissue. This may in part explain the higher efficiency of this technique. The second and third options are the more attractive and it may turn out that they are identical.

5.4.9.3. The Future of DNA Immunization

The prospects for DNA immunization look remarkably bright, provided no adverse findings about safety emerge. In a very short time, this approach has been tried experimentally with preparations against viral, bacterial, and parasitic agents.[735] With further information about the precise mechanisms involved, it may be possible to increase efficacy and direct responses to particular sites of infection, such as the respiratory tract and the lung for respiratory infections.

One of the most striking and important aspects of murine experiments is the longevity of the immune response after a single injection of DNA. There are a few reports of experiments using hosts other than mice, including ferrets and nonhuman primates,[735] but it will be critical to establish the most effective way to immunize man, the size of the inoculum, and the length of the response. Phase I and II clinical trials administering HIV DNA into HIV-infected persons,[735] and phase I clinical trials of HIV DNA and influenza virus DNA into uninfected persons are underway. A contribution[739] to a recent meeting on DNA vaccines expresses the feeling of many: "DNA is the thing!"

5.4.10. Plant-Derived Preparations

5.4.10.1. Vaccines

For generations, plants have been a rich source of medicinal compounds. As a result of initiatives started several years ago by Arntzen and colleagues, plants may have a still brighter future as inexpensive sources of antigens for some vaccines and possibly of antibodies for prophylactic or therapeutic use.[740] There are two scenarios. The first is to produce the biologics in a plant and then to isolate the product in a pure form for administration in the usual way. The second is to produce the biologics in plants that could be safely fed orally to humans (or to domesticated or farm animals) to induce an appropriate immune response. For vaccines, the long-term aim was to produce initially bacterial products that could protect against infections that are a major cause of diarrhea in developing countries.

After initial experiments using HBsAg as a model antigen, Arntzen's group has made transgenic tobacco and potato plants using DNA coding for a subunit LT-B of the *E. coli* heat-labile enterotoxin that binds to the GM_1 ganglioside on the gut epithelial surface. In oral feeding experiments in which mice were given four doses over 25 days of extracts from the transgenic tobacco plants, antibodies in the serum and mucosal extracts were tested for their ability to neutralize 50 ng of toxin. Control mice were fed bacterially expressed bacterial toxin. Mice fed the plant extract produced the same level of antibody as the controls. Similarly, mice fed raw transgenic potato tubers produced specific serum IgG and mucosal IgA.[741]

Generally, recipients of food proteins can become tolerant to the smaller proteins, and this mechanism could apply to foreign proteins fed in this way. One potential way to minimize this risk would be to express the protein as a particle (1 to 10 μm) to encourage uptake by M cells. It is of interest that a chimeric plant virus is being used in ongoing experiments.[740] Transgenic bananas rather than potatoes are suggested as an ideal source and vehicle for oral feeding.

5.4.10.2. Antibodies

An even more interesting experiment has been the synthesis of four separate components of a monoclonal antibody (ie, the light and heavy chains, the J chain, and the secretory component) in separate tobacco plants. Sexual crosses and filial recombinants resulted in plants that expressed all four components simultaneously. These components were assembled into a functional secretory Ig molecule with the correct antigen-binding specificity.[742] A fascinating aspect of this work is that, in mammals, sIgA manufacture depends on the interaction between two cells. In vitro synthesis is performed with some difficulty. In the tobacco plant experiment, the four components are assembled in the one plant cell, which adds to the attraction of using this approach for the large-scale manufacture of the antibody.

Specific sIgA represents a very early line of defense against mucosal infections, and, in this respect, plant-derived preparations may prove valuable for prophylactic use.

CHAPTER 5.5. ANTIBODY COMBINATORIAL LIBRARIES
EXPRESSED ON PHAGES

Murine monoclonal antibodies (MAbs) can be made against many antigens. It is more difficult to make human MAbs, but the murine version can be "humanized" to some extent and used for prophylactic or therapeutic purposes (see Section 1.2.9). However, it is difficult to make high-affinity antibodies against many self or self-like antigens and less ethical to make them against toxic materials. It would be useful to be able to make antibodies of any required specificity in vitro and perhaps avoid in vivo immunization completely. In 1990, a paper[743] indicated how this might be achieved—by displaying antibody V domains on the surface of filamentous bacteriophages. The concept was reviewed and expanded,[744] and there are now two groups in particular (The Medical Research Council Centre for Protein Engineering in Cambridge [UK] and a group at the Scripps Research Institute in La Jolla[745]) who have contributed significantly to this field.

Details of the different steps involved in generating antibody Fabs of great specificity have been described,[746] but briefly, the aim has been to learn from the way the immune system works and mimic it closely (reviewed elsewhere[747]). It was known that DNA coding for small peptides could be inserted into the gene encoding the proteins, pIII or pVIII, of filamentous phage, and the peptide fused to either of these two proteins would then be displayed at the tip of each phage. This could be repeated using the DNA coding for a single chain Fv fragment of an antibody. The phage particles so formed bound specifically to antigen. Dimeric Fab fragments could also be made by a modification of this approach.

The antigen-driven proliferation of B cells that takes place in lymphoid germinal centers involves affinity maturation and selection of those cells with the highest affinity receptors by selection with antigen bound to follicular dendritic cells (see Section 2.2.5.2). This is mimicked in vitro by the isolation of phages with high-affinity Fabs using antigen immobilized on columns, "panning" on antigen-coated plates, or interaction with soluble biotinylated antigen followed by capture with streptavidin-coated paramagnetic beads. With sequential rounds of selection, very high enrichments can be obtained, usually on the order of 10^6.

This approach is simplest if the Ig variable genes from an immunized donor are used so that the need to make hybridomas is bypassed. The approach has also been used to make constructs against a variety of antigens using peripheral blood lymphocytes from humans and combining the VH and VL genes at random (ie, starting off with a naive population of V genes). Additional diversity can be introduced by site-directed mutagenesis, followed by further rounds of selection. Antibodies with binding affinities of 10^8 to 10^9 M^{-1} with high specificity against foreign and self antigens have been made, and this compares well with the affinity of many hybridomas.

There seems to be no reason why products made by this technology should not have a ready use for in vitro diagnostic application. There could be even greater in vivo applications. Specific antibodies can prevent or greatly limit infection by viruses, most bacteria, and parasites. There are several examples of viral infections in which antibody can have a therapeutic effect[748] (see Section 1.2.9), and there could be a considerable demand for products made by this technology. It has already been shown that an anti-RSV–Fab preparation made in this way, if instilled intranasally into the lungs of infected mice daily for 3 days, can control the virus infection.[748]

There is one possible hurdle. Antibody given systemically for either of these purposes should preferably have a long half-life in the circulation. To judge from earlier work that compared Fabs with intact IgG,[749] Fabs made by this technology may have a short half-life because, apart from conformation, the product is not glycosylated. To be effectively used for many in vivo applications, DNA coding for an intact Ig may need to be transfected into a mammalian cell line and a glycosylated version produced.

CHAPTER 5.6. NEW POSSIBILITIES FOR COMBINATION AND SEQUENTIAL VACCINES

5.6.1. Combination Vaccines

The major cost in vaccination programs is delivery to the recipients, because the costs of delivery are usually much greater than the cost of the vaccines. One way of overcoming this and of increasing convenience, compliance, and coverage of vac-

TABLE 5.6.1. *Combinations of vaccines for childhood immunization*

Status	Vaccine
Inactivated candidates	
Current	Diphtheria-tetanus toxoid-pertussis (DTP)
Generally agreed	DTPa, *Haemophilus influenzae* b, hepatitis B
Uncertain	Addition of inactivated poliovirus vaccine
Other candidates	Meningococci, pneumococci
Live candidates	
Current	Measles-mumps-rubella
Other candidate	Varicella

Adapted from Conclusions of Workshop III. Vaccination Policy. (1994) Second European Conference on Vaccinology. Biologicals 22:435–436.

cines is the development of combination vaccines.[750] Fewer administrations would be needed to protect against more diseases. This has been recognized for many years with the development of measles-mumps-rubella and diphtheria-pertussis-tetanus combinations. With the increasing number of vaccines that will be licensed in the years to come, the immediate approach is to see whether additional individual vaccines can be added to the existing combinations. A list of preferred combinations was discussed at a European workshop held in 1994 (Table 5.6.1).[751]

The guiding principles in making combinations of vaccines are compatibility in their physical, chemical, and biologic properties. Each component should be safe and effective and not interfere with the "take" of others. However, as the number of components to be mixed increases, there is a greater risk of some interference through antigenic competition, the effects of different adjuvants and sites of administration, and interference with the replication of different infectious agents.

Antigenic competition may arise if the peptides from different protein antigens compete with binding to a particular MHC molecule, as well as differential recognition of the complexes by a T-cell receptor.[750] It is usually not possible to predict such interference in advance. Time-consuming and expensive testing is required each time a candidate is added to an existing mixture.

Various adjuvants and sites of administration can have different effects. There may be examples in which a mucosal response (type 2 response) to one component and a systemic response to another (type 1 or 2 response) is desired.

It is possible to interfere with the replication of infectious agents. Adjustments to the amount of each type of poliovirus in the OPV have been made, in part according to the host factors (eg, nutrition, extent of existing infections) in different regions.

5.6.2. Minimizing Interference Between Components in a Cocktail of Vaccines

There are a number of ways to help overcome the difficulties arising from a cocktail of vaccines. First, a common protein carrier can be used. This would be appropriate in the case of vaccines against encapsulated bacteria because antigenic competition should be avoided. Second, common live vectors can be employed. The use of the same viral or bacterial vector for systemic or mucosal administration should minimize the interference previously described. DNA may in the long run prove to be the ideal vector for protein-based antigens, because it should largely overcome the described constraints.

Provided the efforts of the Children's Vaccine Initiative and the WHO Global Programme on Vaccines and Immunization can be maintained and there is strong collaboration between such groups and industry, the prospects for improving and simplifying childhood immunization programs are bright.[752] If DNA immunization can be shown to be safe and the encouraging results obtained in murine systems can be reproduced in humans, DNA vaccination may progressively be used to immunize against virtually all protein antigens in the future.

5.6.3. Sequential Vaccines

The traditional procedure for repeated immunizations or vaccinations is to administer the same preparation on successive occasions. There have been isolated reports of different preparations being used, but to our knowledge, this has not been done in a systematic manner. It was of considerable interest when reports[677,753] appeared showing that, when volunteers were immunized with a vaccinia virus/HIV-1 gp160 construct and later challenged with a recombinant gp160 prepared in baculovirus-transfected cells (rgp160), the subsequent antibody titers were substantially greater than those seen after two successive immunizations with either of the preparations.

The reasons for this result are unknown, but subsequent work has demonstrated a similar phenomenon.[754] Mice were injected intramuscularly with 1, 10, or 100 μg of plasmids containing influenza virus HA DNA or with 100 μg of a control plasmid. Four weeks later, they were intravenously administered 10^7 PFU of a fowlpox/HA construct, and anti-HA antibody titers were measured at intervals thereafter. Three weeks after the challenge, mice injected with 10 or 100 μg of the HA plasmid had antibody titers (IgG2a) 25 to 50 times higher than those of the control mice. Titers remained elevated relative to controls for more than 15 weeks after the challenge.

It has been suggested that foreign DNA residing in cells might play a particular role in immunologic memory,[755] and the previously described findings seem to agree with this. A clue to possible mechanisms might be obtained if the reverse experiment were done: prime mice with the poxvirus construct, and then challenge with the plasmid. Although preliminary, findings such as these open up an otherwise largely unexplored area of immunology that may be of considerable importance in vaccinology.

SECTION 6

Vaccination Against Self and Self-Like Molecules

CHAPTER 6.1. VACCINATION AND IMMUNOTHERAPY TO PREVENT OR CONTROL TUMORS

The emphasis in preceding sections has been on immunization mainly as a form of prophylaxis to protect against infectious diseases. In that situation, there are unambiguous target molecules belonging to the infectious agent. A second category of situations for which there is opportunity or need to intervene is considered in this section: prophylaxis and immunotherapy to control tumors, immunotherapy to control autoimmune diseases, and immunocontraception to control human and wildlife fertility.

With one exception—tumors arising after a viral infection—the target antigens are self molecules, self molecules that have mutated, or self-like molecules (eg, in females exposed to male sperm). Some autoimmune diseases appear to be associated with particular viral infections. In most cases, however, there is no direct association between carcinogenesis and viral or other infections. There may be indirect associations such as the induction of a state of immunodeficiency by the infection.

The concept of developing cancer vaccines was based initially on the premise that there are quantitative and/or qualitative differences between tumor cells and most normal cells. The hypothesis that the immune system might be an effective way to detect these differences and deal with the tumor arose from the ideas of two great scientists. In 1959, Lewis Thomas[756] suggested that "perhaps, in short, the phenomenon of homograft rejection will turn out to represent a primary mechanism for natural defense against neoplasia." In 1957, Macfarlane Burnet[757] had proposed that "small accumulations of tumor cells may develop and, because of their possession of new antigenic potentialities, provoke an effective immunologic reaction with regression of the tumor and no clinical hint of its existence." With his ideas reinforced by Thomas' comment, Burnet coined the term *immunosurveillance* to describe the role of the immune system. He went on to popularize the concept, but it met with considerable resistance. For example, the incidence of tumors in nude mice, at least for a considerable period of their lives, was of the same order of magnitude as in control mice, despite the fact that such mice had defective immune systems. Nevertheless, the idea stimulated much research, and over time, it became clear that a tumor that might be controlled or cleared in normal mice would on transfer progress in immunodeficient mice, indicating that the concept of immunosurveillance had some validity.

As our understanding of the basis of immune recognition by the immune system and the steps leading to activation, especially of cell-mediated immune (CMI) reactions, expanded, it was realized that tumors arise and progress because they evade the immune system in one way or another. If this idea was correct, it should be possible to identify and then perhaps supply the missing components so the immune system could be activated and destroy the tumor. During the last decade, much experimental work has confirmed the essential correctness of this approach.

Tumors are initiated by alterations in the expression of one or several genes that regulate cell growth, differentiation, or both processes. Such changes can be caused by chemical or physical agents and by some viruses.

6.1.1. Viral Tumorigenesis

Viruses are known to be involved in the initiation of about 15% of all human cancers. Table 6.1.1 lists viruses associated with certain human tumors and viral infections leading to tumor development in some animals.

TABLE 6.1.1. *Viral infections associated with malignant tumors*

Virus	Kind of tumor
In humans	
Epstein-Barr	Burkitt's lymphoma
	Nasopharyngeal carcinoma
Hepatitis B, C	Hepatocellular carcinoma
Hepatitis A, D, E (others?)	
HIV-1	Kaposi's sarcoma
	B-cell lymphomas
HTLV-1, 2	Adult T-cell leukemia
Human papilloma 5, 8*	Squamous cell carcinoma
Human papilloma 16, 18*	Genital carcinomas
In animals	
SV40	
Adeno	
Marek's disease	
Feline leukemia	
Simian immunodeficiency	

*Types most commonly involved.

The development of the hepatitis B virus (HBV) vaccine is one of the great success stories of vaccinology. After infection by HBV at birth, it takes 20 to 40 years before liver cancer may appear. Most such infections occur in developing countries, particularly in southeast Asia, and this vaccine has only become available in most of these areas relatively recently. Although it is confidently expected that successful vaccination will prevent the cancer from occurring, it will take many years before this outcome is completely documented. A similar situation occurs with human T-cell leukemia viruses. It is transmitted from mother to baby or by sexual intercourse. The virus persists, especially in close-knit societies, but it can be 20 to 40 years before the cancer occurs in a small proportion of the infected persons.

Human papillomaviruses (HPVs) generally produce benign warts (papillomas) that regress in time. Infection by certain strains of the virus induce changes in the infected cell that may lead to cancer; HPV types 5 and 18 lead to squamous cell carcinomas, and HPV types 16 and 18 lead to genital carcinomas. Considerable success has been obtained in animal models by prophylactic vaccination with virus-like particles to prevent HPV-induced disease. Analysis of the viral antigens in the tumors has revealed that neutralizing antibody recognizes conformational epitopes. Although HPV is a DNA virus, there are many serotypes or genotypes, and a study of prostitutes in Copenhagen showed that with repeated exposure there was sequential infection, first with the more common genotypes, then with the rarer ones, and later with the untyped and unknown genotypes (reviewed elsewhere[758]). A prophylactic vaccine may have to contain virus-like particles of several genotypes. There are at least three phase I clinical trials in progress, with a recombinant E7 protein (Australia), with synthetic peptides (Netherlands), and with a chimeric vaccinia virus (United Kingdom).[758]

Human immunodeficiency virus (HIV) infections only indirectly result in the development of Kaposi's sarcoma or B-cell lymphomas. The infection in most cases induces severe immunodeficiency that allows the tumors to develop in some persons, usually about 8 or more years after the initial infection. Only a minority of HIV patients develop either of these tumors.

In each of the described cases, the most effective solution would be to prevent the initial viral infection. The HBV vaccine induces neutralizing antibody, and it is presumed that a human T-cell lymphotropic virus type I vaccine would depend on a similar effect, hoping that reducing the infectious dose by more than 95% would greatly decrease the risk of developing cancer. The great antigenic variation of HIV-1 substantially lessens the opportunity of developing a vaccine that would, because of neutralizing antibody, greatly lessen the infectious load. It is now thought that a vaccine, to be successful, would need to rapidly initiate a CMI response based on cytotoxic T lymphocyte (CTL) formation, which would at least curtail and perhaps clear the infection shortly after it had been initiated.

Infection with the Epstein-Barr virus (EBV) can result in the induction of various tumors. Infection very early in life in some African countries (ie, those with a high exposure to malaria infection) predisposes to Burkitt's lymphoma. In other ethnic populations, particularly in southeast Asia, a proportion of those infected with EBV develop nasopharyngeal carcinoma. In many other societies, delayed infection may lead to infectious mononucleosis (ie, glandular fever). There are good reasons for developing a vaccine to prevent or control this infection. Current experiments are aimed at inducing a CTL response to peptides from the nuclear antigen 3 of EBV.[759]

With EBV and HPV, there is encouraging progress in the generation of CTL responses specific for certain viral antigens. Similar approaches are being made toward the control of non–virus-associated tumors, and they are considered in a later section.

Noncytopathic viruses have been used to help induce an immune response to a tumor. In one example, injection of irradiated tumor cells (ie, a metastatic murine lymphoma) infected with Newcastle disease virus had a therapeutic effect against micrometastases and produced long-term survival of about 50% of the mice (reviewed elsewhere[760]). The injection caused the influx of lymphocytes to the injection site and a secondary CTL response.

6.1.2. Poor Immunogenicity of Tumor Cells

There are two theories about the poor immunogenicity of tumor cells. First, tumor cells are inefficient at inducing an appropriate protective immune response. It is generally accepted that tumor cells do not have the properties of "professional" antigen-presenting cells (APCs). It was established quite early that conditions for recognition and lysis of target cells were less stringent than the requirements for T-cell activation.[761] It is most fortunate that tumor cells that are poorly immunogenic can still be good targets for effector CTLs, provided a tumor-associated antigen

(TAA) is expressed by the cell. A second possibility is that T cells in tumor-bearing hosts are adversely affected by the tumor. Frequently, the immune response of patients and animals with cancer is suppressed. Possible explanations (reviewed elsewhere[762]) for the poor immunogenicity of tumor cells include

- Induction by many tumors of "peripheral tolerance" so that T cells exhibit abnormalities in signal transduction
- Suppressor cell effects due to secretion of certain cytokines
- Appearance of variants lacking TAAs
- Downregulation (sometimes quite selective) of major histocompatibility complex (MHC) expression, preventing presentation of peptides from cellular antigens to T cells

Examples of these effects are given in the following sections.

6.1.3. Approaches to Immunotherapy Using Antibodies

The ability to make monoclonal antibodies (MAbs) greatly facilitated the search for and identification of antigens that were largely specific for particular tumors or were present in substantially larger amounts on a particular tumor. Such antigens were given names such as tumor-specific transplantation antigens (TSTAs) and TAAs. For convenience, TAA will be used in the following discussions.

MAbs are being used in several different ways as candidates for immunotherapy, as outlined in Table 6.1.3. Using TAA-specific MAbs made radioactive or preferably carrying a cellular toxin such as the α subunit of ricin, it has been possible to kill tumor cells in vitro, but in vivo experiments have had mixed success.[763] One requirement is that the antibody should enter the cell so that the toxin can work, and this can be achieved. Moreover, the antibody-toxin complex should not be immunogenic, but frequently it is, and clearance of residual conjugate in the liver can

TABLE 6.1.3. *Constructs of monoclonal antibodies for immunotherapy*

Particular construct	Reference
MAb specific for TSA Made radioactive (eg, ^{125}I) or complexed with a cell poison, such as the α subunit of ricin	763

Bispecific MAbs
 Drug delivery
   One arm specific for TAA and the other arm specific for drug
   A mechanism for selective delivery of drug to tumor
   One arm specific tor TAA and the other arm specific for an enzyme that converts a tumor prodrug to the active form
	764

Effector cell delivery
   One arm specific for TSA and the other arm specific for effector T cell
   A mechanism for the selective delivery of effector cells to tumor cells
	764

MAb, monoclonal antibody; TAA, tumor-associated antigen; TSA, tumor-specific antigen.

cause toxic effects. The target antigen may mutate so that it is no longer recognized by the conjugate. Some clinical trials are underway.[763]

Another approach has been to construct bispecific antibodies. One arm of the molecule has specificity for the nominated TAA, and the other arm has specificity for an antitumor drug or an enzyme that converts a prodrug to the active form. In contrast, if the specificity of the second arm is directed to a suitable marker on the surface of a precursor or effector T cell or a natural killer (NK) cell, the construct acts as a vector to direct the cell to the tumor cell.[764] In vivo, the use of such constructs has resulted in an enriched population of the effector cells in the tumor, and in animal models such as severe combined immunodeficiency mice, a well-established tumor has been cleared in this way. Although CD4+ T cells assist in the activation of CD8+ T cells, the latter as well as NK cells have been mainly responsible for the destruction of the tumor.

This approach has advantages and disadvantages. One advantage is that the same construct (without the attached cell) should be effective for all individuals; there should be no difficulty with MHC incompatibility. However, this approach is limited to cell-surface–expressed antigens that focus the bound effector cell onto the tumor. Because most MAbs are of murine origin, repeated use of a construct in humans must overcome the immunogenicity of the murine protein. It seems likely that this may be achievable.[764]

6.1.4. Overcoming T-Cell Anergy and Immunosuppression: Recognition of Tumor Antigens

Interleukin-2 (IL-2) activates freshly isolated lymphocytes from the peripheral blood of a cancer patient to form lymphokine-activated killer cells that have the ability to recognize and destroy the cancer cells after infusion back to the cancer patient.[765,766] Sometimes with the additional direct infusion of IL-2, this approach has become a standard treatment for patients with malignant melanoma and renal cancers.

After intensive research,[767,768] at least seven human melanoma antigens known to be recognized by CTLs have been isolated. More are being identified, and CTL determinants are being characterized. Some findings are summarized in Table 6.1.4. There are two reasons for seeking multiple TAAs. The first is the MHC polymorphism in the outbred human population. For most of a tumor-bearing population to benefit from such an immunization protocol, several T-cell determinants are needed, and the best chance of achieving wide coverage of a population would be to have a number of TAAs as sources of such determinants. Second, not all tumors of a given type express a given antigen. For example, in the case of MAGE-1, MAGE-3, and BAGE antigens, the proportion of melanomas that express one antigen may be considerably less than 50%, although expression was found to be higher when metastatic lesions were examined.[768] If MAGE-1 was expressed, MAGE-3 was likely to be expressed as well. Some tumors did not express

TABLE 6.1.4. *Human melanoma antigens recognized by cytotoxic T lymphocytes*

Antigen	CTL determinants (number)	Present in normal tissues	Present on other tumors
MAGE-1	2	Testis	6/10
MAGE-3	2	Testis	7/10
BAGE	1	Testis	5/10
GAGE		Testis	6/10
Tyrosinase	3	Melanocytes	Melanoma
MART-1/melan-A	1	Melanocytes	Melanoma
gp100	5	Melanocytes	Melanoma

Data from Kawakami Y, Eliyahu S, Jennings C et al. (1995) Recognition of multiple epitopes in the human melanoma antigen gp100 by tumor-infiltrating T lymphocytes associated with in vivo tumor regression. J Immunol 154:3961–3968; and from Van Pel A, Van Der Bruggen P, Coule PG et al. (1995) Genes coding for tumor antigens by cytolytic T lymphocytes. Immunol Rev 145:229–250.

The tumors examined included melanomas, bladder carcinomas, mammary carcinomas, head and neck squamous cell carcinomas, non–small cell lung carcinomas, sarcomas, prostatic carcinomas, colorectal carcinomas, rectal carcinomas, leukemias and lymphomas.

any of these antigens, not all cells in a tumor seem to express the antigen, and the level of expression could vary.[768]

There is little information on the expression of these antigens by fetal tissues. However, for cancer patients, there is encouraging evidence that tumor regression can correlate with the recognition of a particular tumor antigen when the transferred autologous CTLs (with IL-2) are specific for that antigen.[767]

One benefit of working with a virus-associated tumor is that most and perhaps all tumor cells are likely to express a viral antigen. The E6 and E7 oncoproteins of HPV type 16 are constitutively expressed in most cervical tumor cells and are attractive targets for immunotherapy. Nine peptides from these proteins recognized in association with a human leukocyte antigen (HLA) haplotype were analyzed in HLA-transgenic mice. CTL clones raised to these peptides lysed appropriate cervical carcinoma cells. Peptides with a high binding affinity for the HLA were the most immunogenic.[769] In a comparable study, nonapeptides from HPV-16 E7 were used to raise CTLs that were able to eradicate established HPV-16–induced tumors in mice. A subdominant CTL determinant was used successfully in this study.[770]

Pancreatic and breast tumors express an antigen, MUC-1, which is recognized by effector CD8+ T cells, which can lyse the tumor cell. The unusual finding by one group is that these effector cells are not MHC restricted. This antigen is also present on normal cells, but on tumor cells it occurs in greater amounts and is less glycosylated. Because of this it was thought that the polypeptide core in the cell might be more readily available for degradation to appropriate peptides that could bind to class I MHC antigens, resulting in their recognition by CTLs.[771] It was found that, although antibodies against the T-cell receptor blocked tumor cell lysis, anti-MHC antibodies did not. A tumor-specific anti-mucin antibody also blocked tumor lysis. MHC-unrestricted T-cell lysis, by cells with $\alpha\beta$ or $\gamma\delta$ receptors, has been described previously, particularly if the target had a highly multivalent antigen (reviewed elsewhere[771]). This was confirmed by making tandem repeats of oligopeptides. In this sense, the MUC-1 peptide antigen on these tumors is considered to be a tumor-specific antigen, because on normal cells, the polypeptide component is hidden from the immune system by extensive glycosylation. However, in a subsequent paper, the same group identified a nonapeptide from this antigen that was class I MHC restricted, binding well to HLA-A11. A secondary CTL response was obtained with lymph node cells from a HLA-A11 breast cancer patient, and CTLs could be generated from the peripheral blood lymphocytes from healthy donors.[772]

Another group only induced class I MHC-restricted CTLs to MUC-1.[773] They used a novel technique, in which the peptide was conjugated to mannan under oxidizing conditions that, in many experiments, has only induced a T1 type response (see Section 4.2.3).

These combined findings suggest that as far as the host's CTL repertoire is concerned, MUC-1 is not a tumor-specific antigen. This may be a common situation, because CTLs recognizing the antigen tyrosinase on melanoma cells can be generated from healthy persons' blood. These CTLs can lyse melanoma cells.[774]

6.1.5. Transfection of Tumor Cells With Co-stimulators and Cytokines

Two possible reasons why successful tumors fail to induce a protective immune response are that the tumor cell does not express an appropriate co-stimulator molecule that could enhance its immunogenicity and that it does not secrete cytokines that could attract professional APCs or more directly help to activate local specific T cells. Most tumors examined do not express a member or members of the B7 family of co-stimulators,[775] and those that do still seem to be deficient as APCs.[776] However, if mice were given a tumor cell line that produced micrometastases and later cells of same lineage that had been transfected with DNA coding for B7, about one half of the mice cleared the initial tumor,[777] an effect mediated mainly by effector CD8 + CTLs. Results like this have been obtained with several different tumors that clearly express TAA peptides in the appropriate manner.

Interferon-α (IFNα) was the first cytokine to be used in clinical trials that showed some efficacy against certain types of human cancers.[778] Subsequently, transduced Freund leukemia cells expressing IFN-α1, when injected into mice, suffered a loss of their tumorigenic potential but induced an antitumor immunity shown when the mice were challenged with the metastatic parental cells.[779] Tumor cells of different types have been transduced with a range of cytokines, including IL-1, -2, -4, -6, and -7; IFNγ; tumor necrosis factor-α (TNFα); and granulocyte colony-stimulating factor (GM-CSF). Vaccination with many of these transduced cells, but not all of them (eg, IFNγ), induced some tumor immunity, mainly mediated by CD8 + T cells. The use of colony-stimulating factors can greatly enhance the immune effect by inducing the influx of cells that can act as effective APCs.[738] Tumor cells engineered to express GM-CSF markedly enhance systemic immunity against challenge with lethal doses of untransfected tumor cells.[780] It was proposed that GM-CSF mediated this antigen-specific effect by stimulating the differentiation of hemopoietic precursors into APCs such as dendritic cells (DCs).

6.1.6. Transfer of Dendritic Cells Pulsed With Cytotoxic T Lymphocyte Peptide Determinants

It is possible to generate large numbers of DCs by culture of the bone marrow-derived cells present in peripheral blood mononuclear cell populations with GM-CSF plus TNFα or with GM-CSF plus IL-4.[781] DCs derived by the second method in particular expressed high levels of class II MHC antigens, as well as B7.1 and 7.2, and they were potent stimulators of mixed lymphocyte reactions. This approach has made more feasible experiments to assess the use of DCs pulsed with CTL peptide determinants to develop tumor immunity. In three different murine tumor models, DCs pulsed with CTL peptide determinants were injected into mice that were then challenged with a lethal dose of tumor cells. Protection was achieved in each case. The treatment of mice already bearing macroscopic tumors with such preparations resulted in sustained tumor regression and a tumor-free status for more than 80% of cases.[781]

In a second example,[782] DCs obtained by a similar protocol from healthy human donors and pulsed with CTL determinants from tyrosinase, gp100, and melan A/MART-1 were used to generate melanoma specific CTLs, which lysed peptide-loaded target cells of the appropriate HLA haplotype. These CTLs were active against melanoma tumor cell lines. The results showed that healthy donors possessed precursor T cells of these specificities.

6.1.7. Direct Immunization to Achieve Tumor Control

In many ways, the simplest procedure to control cancer and perhaps to prevent a cancer from occurring would be direct immunization, as with vaccination against infectious diseases. Perhaps the most fascinating approach has been direct immunization with peptides that are known CTL determinants. MUT-1 and MUT-2, which were derived from a gap-junction protein produced by a murine lung carcinoma, are two such peptides.[783] Mice were immunized with the peptides in Freund's incomplete adjuvant (FIA) or with RMA-S cells pulsed with the peptides. The mice were protected from spontaneous tumor metastases, and immunization reduced metastatic loads in mice carrying preestablished micrometastases. The protection was largely mediated by CD8 + T cells.

Similarly, mice immunized with an oxidized mannan–MUC-1 fusion protein were completely protected against a tumor challenge.[773,784] High levels of CTL precursors and CTLs were generated.

Another approach is to use a live vector containing DNA coding for the tumor antigen. A recombinant replication-defective adenovirus containing the DNA coding for two melanoma cancer proteins, MART-1 and gp100, was used to infect murine cell lines expressing HLA-A2.[785] These cells were lysed by antigen-specific CTLs. Because of the suspected homology between the human antigens and their murine counterparts, mice were immunized with these recombinant viruses, which were found to protect them from a murine melanoma B16 challenge given intradermally. Depletion of CD8+ T cells, but not CD4+ T cells, from the mice eliminated the protective effect.

Tumors could be treated with selected cytokines by incorporation of the cytokine DNA into a live vector, as described previously, or into a DNA plasmid. Using gene gun delivery of recombinant DNA (see Section 5.4.9), cytokine genes such as those for IL-6, IL-2, and IFNγ were shown to inhibit the growth of a renal carcinoma in mice and to prolong the survival of other tumor-bearing mice.[786]

6.1.8. Comment

During the last few years, the field of immunotherapy for tumors has been revolutionized by the rapid progress made. Beginning in the early 1970s with the description of the co-stimulator effect[161] and the discovery of MHC restriction with the analysis of T-cell cytotoxicity for virus-infected target cells,[19] our understanding of antigen presentation and T-cell activation has grown very greatly. The immune system can be manipulated to a degree previously not thought possible. It is this knowledge that has made possible the progress in cancer vaccine research. In experimental models, prophylactic immunization to generate mainly CTL formation can prevent a cancer occurring after challenge and can greatly decrease the burden of an existing tumor.

However, there are still unknowns. Do tumor-specific antigens really exist? Presumably, mutations in CTL determinants in tumor antigens would fulfill this criteria, but would immune pressure favor the emergence of other mutations? Probably the greatest challenge is to translate the continuing progress at the laboratory bench into success in the clinic with cancer patients. Some of the potential difficulties, such as downregulation of MHC antigens or allele-specific loss, have already been mentioned, and one report suffices to illustrate this situation.[787] From a patient with melanoma, a large number of autologous CTL clones were obtained that recognized at least five tumor antigens. Four were found to be presented by HLA-A28, B13, B44, and Cw6. A few years later, metastases occurred, and a new tumor cell line was developed from them. This line was resistant to all of the previous CTL clones, and the only HLA class I molecule specificity expressed was HLA-A24. It seems possible that the melanoma cells may have lost the expression of HLA molecules of several specificities under immune pressure.

As Jack Strominger[788] commented, "The road ahead is unpaved and full of potholes, but the journey could be rewarding." Thierry Boon[789] is also cautiously optimistic: "Our advice to the general public, to the funding agencies, and to our industrial partners ought to be that they should not believe anyone who claims to be certain of success and that they should believe even less those who affirm that specific antitumor immunization will never work."

CHAPTER 6.2. IMMUNOTHERAPY TO CONTROL AUTOIMMUNE DISEASES

Autoimmune diseases are controlled by suppression of the host's immune responses using drugs such as corticosteroids, which tend to be toxic and are nonselective. Extensive research has revealed some of the immunologic mechanisms involved in these disease processes, and some very promising leads have been obtained.

6.2.1. Genetic and Environmental Associations of Autoimmune Diseases

Specific immune responses directed against self can result in an autoimmune disease. Environmental factors such as viral or bacterial infections and genetic factors, especially the MHC genotype, are important. Some diseases are mediated by antibody and others by T cells. Table 6.2.1.1 gives examples of known and possible associations between these factors and various autoimmune diseases. In the case of genotype associations, there is an extraordinarily strong association between ankylosing spondylitis and the HLA allele (85%) at one end of the spectrum, and at the other end, there is a weak association (3%) in the case of insulin-dependent diabetes mellitus.

Table 6.2.1.1 also indicates that the self target antigen is known in some cases. The disease that is best studied is experimental autoimmune encephalomyelitis (EAE), and some of this work is reported here. In other cases, the target autoantigen remains elusive despite extensive research.

A well-studied relationship between an infection and the occurrence of autoimmune disease is streptococcal infection in which antibodies to the bacterial cell wall antigens crossreact with cardiac muscle. There are major efforts to develop peptide-based vaccines so that the crossreactive peptide sequences can be eliminated from the candidate vaccine.

The extent to which a severe viral infection such as HIV can result in the broad manifestation of autoimmune syndromes has only become apparent in the last few years. Table 6.2.1.2 lists some of the autoimmune syndromes that are mediated by antibody or by T cells.[793] These autoimmune syndromes occur in HIV-infected persons long before a state of immunodeficiency is found. Two mechanisms likely to play major roles in autoantibody production are dysregulated activation of B cells and molecular mimicry. In contrast to the situation with most CMI-mediated autoimmune diseases, in which CD4 + type 1 T cells are involved (see Section 6.2.3), CD8 + type 1 T cells are the mediators in the diseases listed under that heading in

TABLE 6.2.1.1. *Known and possible associations among type of immune response, HLA genotype, viral infection, and susceptibility to or occurrence of autoimmune diseases*

Autoimmune disease	Pathogenic mechanism	HLA association	Known or possible infection	Autoantigen
Autoimmune he-molytic anemia	Antibody			RH blood group
Autoimmune thrombocyto-penia purpura	Antibody			Platelet integrin
Pemphigus vul-garis	Antibody	DR3		Adherin
Rheumatic fever	Antibody		Streptococcus	Cardiac muscle
SLE	Antibody	DR3	C-type retroviruses	
Insulin-dependent diabetes mellitus	CMI	DR3, DR4	Coxsackievirus	Pancreatic B-cell antigens*
EAE	CMI			Myelin basic pro-teins†
Multiple sclerosis	CMI	Dw2		
Rheumatoid ar-thritis	CMI	DR4	Epstein-Barr virus	Synovial joint anti-gens
Hashimoto's thy-roiditis	CMI	DR5	Mumps virus	Thyroid hormone
Autoimmune neu-ritis	CMI			

CMI, cell-mediated immunity; EAE, experimental autoimmune encephalomyelitis; HLA, human leukocyte antigen; SLE, systemic lupus erythematosus.

*Glutamic acid decarboxylase, insulin, carboxypeptidase.

†Proteolipid protein, myelin, oligodendrocyte glycoprotein.

Data from references 790 through 792 and from Drs. A. Gautam and D. Willenborg, John Curtin School of Medical Research, Australian National University, Canberra.

TABLE 6.2.1.2. *Autoimmune syndromes occurring in HIV-infected persons*

Mechanism of syndrome	Types of syndromes
Antibody-mediated	Thrombocytopenic purpura, anti-phospholipid, gastropathy with hypochlorhydria, hemolytic anemia, neutropenia, pruritic papulovesicular eruption; a variety of other autoantibodies but without symptoms are also found
T-cell mediated	Sjögren's-like syndrome, lymphocytic interstitial pneumonitis, polymyositis, cardiac myositis, chronic active hepatitis
Demyelinating	Guillain-Barré, chronic inflammatory demyelinating polyneurop-athy
Immune complex-mediated	Polyarteritis nodosa-like arteritis, hypersensitivity vasculitis

Data from Gala S, Fulcher DA. (1996) Managing HIV. 3.4. How HIV leads to autoimmune disorders. Med J Aust 164:224–226.

Table 6.2.1.2. A mechanism for the participation of these cells has been proposed,[793] but one probable reason for their involvement is the very high and continuing production of CTLs during this early phase of HIV infection, to the extent that they continually spill over into the circulation in most infected persons. There is a clear correlation between continuing CTL production and delayed appearance of immunodeficiency in HIV-infected persons.[794]

6.2.2. Immunotherapy

There are two main approaches to immunotherapy, one based on the use of specific antibodies and the other based on manipulation of the CMI response. In the former case, specific antibodies conjugated with a toxin such as ricin can be used, and although this has had some success, it does suffer from the disadvantages discussed in Section 6.1.3. Much work has been directed to investigating examples in which CMI responses were experimentally shown to be the major mechanism involved in the immunopathology.

6.2.2.1. Pathogenic T Cells

EAE has become the favorite model for investigating mechanisms involved in the induction of an autoimmune disease, and many studies have shown that in rats and mice autoantigen-specific T cells have played a crucial role in the induction of disease.[790] Myelin basic protein (MBP)–specific T-cell lines and clones administered to naive animals can cause EAE. Similarly, administration of specific T-cell clones to naive animals has induced a range of other autoimmune diseases (Table 6.2.2.1), indicating the generality of this approach.

In contrast, administration of very low doses of the T-cell clone or larger doses of cells inactivated by irradiation rendered rats resistant to attempts to induce the disease. This form of therapy has become known as T-cell vaccination[802] and was successfully applied to several experimental autoimmune diseases.[790] It was found that the T cells had to be activated, because precursor cells of the appropriate specificity had no effect. It has been established that the active T cells are type 1 CD4 + ,

TABLE 6.2.2.1. *Autoimmune diseases induced in experimental animals by administration of specific T-cell clones*

Disease	Reference
Adjuvant arthritis	795
Autoimmune thyroiditis	796
Autoimmune neuritis	797
Autoimmune uveitis	798
Collagen arthritis	799
Insulin-dependent diabetes mellitus	800
Systemic lupus erythematosus	801

that the cytokines secreted by these cells (eg, IL-2, IFNγ, TNFα) contribute to the immunopathology,[803,804] and that shifting to a type 2 response can protect against disease.[805]

An extension of this approach has been to immunize with peptides isolated from the T-cell receptor (TCR) of the activated T cell. EAE was prevented in experimental animals after immunization with peptides from the CDR2 or CDR3 of the β chain of the TCR.[806,807] The rationale of this approach is not clear, because naive T cells, which have TCRs of the same structure, are inactive. Such peptides can associate with the TCR of CD4 + class II MHC-restricted T cells.

6.2.2.2. Immunization With Autoantigens

Identification of the autoantigen is a major step toward developing a vaccination approach to prevent or control autoimmune diseases. In the case of an intact antigen, advantage can be taken of the oral route of administration, whereby in the appropriate conditions a partial tolerance or anergy may be achieved (see Section 2.3.2.9). This approach has been effective in preventing several autoimmune diseases, including EAE, uveitis, and myasthenia, collagen- and adjuvant-induced arthritis, and diabetes in the non-obese diabetic (NOD) mouse.[808] Anergy or suppression of formation of the pathogenic cells may occur, depending on the dose of autoantigen used.[809] Alternatively, the APCs in the gut-associated lymphoid tissue (GALT) may have directed the response to induce the activation of cells with a particular cytokine secretion pattern, including transforming growth factor-β (TGFβ),[809] which would constitute a form of vaccination. In the case of oral administration of MPB to suppress EAE in the Lewis rat model, it is antigen-specific CD8 + T cells that secrete the TGFβ (reviewed elsewhere[810]).

Other routes of immunization with autoantigens, including intravenous injection[810] or neonatal administration of MBP in EAE, have also led to the prevention or treatment of autoimmune diseases.[811]

6.2.2.3. Induction of Antigen-Specific Unresponsiveness With Synthetic Peptides (reviewed elsewhere[812])

Dresser[813] showed that intravenous injection of a soluble protein could induce specific tolerance, and Weigle[814] demonstrated that, at low antigen concentrations particularly, this was mainly an effect at the T-cell level.[813] Much later, it was shown that this T-cell tolerance could be induced with soluble peptides (ie, T-cell determinants) and that dominant peptide determinants were the most effective.[815,816] This led to the "escape from tolerance" concept,[816] which proposed that T cells specific for less dominant peptides could more easily escape tolerance in vivo.

This concept has been put to the test in the case of MBP and EAE. For mice of the H-2[u] haplotype, the dominant peptide in MPB is aa1-9.[817] Injection of CD4 T cells specific for this determinant induces EAE in these mice.[818] Residues 3 and 6 of the peptide interact with the T-cell receptor, and residues 4 and 5 interact with the MHC molecule.[819-821] The wild-type peptide has lysine at position 4 and has relatively low affinity; substitution with more hydrophobic residues, especially tyrosine, greatly increases the affinity for H-2[u] MHC antigen.[822-823] Because of the relatively low affinity of the wild-type peptide determinant, it was proposed that these T cells persist in the periphery and hence are available for recruitment by immunization with adjuvant to induce EAE.[824] The concept was tested by using H-2[u] mice transgenic for the TCR specific for this peptide. Treatment of such mice with a high-affinity peptide made them unresponsive to repeated immunization with the wild-type peptide.[825]

6.2.2.4. Peripheral T Cells Affected by Soluble Peptide

Intravenous administration of high-affinity peptide, compared with the wild-type peptide, can induce almost complete unresponsiveness in the mice, as judged by the subsequent failure to induce disease by immunization with the peptide in Freund's complete antigen (FCA).[826] This tolerance may be profound, involving CD4+ T1 and T2 cells, and may last for more than 1 month.

Mice already sensitized for disease by immunization with peptide in adjuvant can be made refractory by subsequent administration of soluble peptide,[826] although some time is required before tolerance is obtained in this way. Soluble peptides can be administered intranasally, but larger amounts are required if oral administration is used.

In another approach, mice with EAE, already established by administration of a T-cell clone recognizing a determinant (p87–99) of myelin basic protein, were treated with an analog of that determinant.[827] The analog differed at one position (ie, alanine replacing phenylalanine at position 96). This treatment reversed paralysis, and the inflammatory infiltrate in the brain regressed. Antibody to IL-4 reversed this induced tolerance. The altered peptide silenced the pathogenic T cells and signaled for the efflux of other T cells recruited to the site of disease as a result of the production of IL-4 and a reduction of TNFα in the lesion. There is also evidence to suggest that experimental chronic or chronic-relapsing autoimmune conditions may be treated in this way.[828]

The construction of transgenic mice to increase T-cell precursor numbers has enabled a greater understanding of mechanisms involved in the induction of anergy.[829] T cells specific for a given peptide were obtained from transgenic mice and adoptively transferred to normal mice. Their fate could be followed by using a specific MAb. When challenged with specific peptide in FCA, the cells proliferated and then migrated into lymph node follicles (see Section 2.2.5); when challenged with soluble peptide (no FCA), some proliferation occurred, but the cells failed to enter the follicles, and those that could be recovered were found to be anergic.

Administration with adjuvant may have a profound influence on the effect of soluble peptide. This process may involve the uptake of the peptide by APCs and activation of the APC by the adjuvant so that the T cell undergoes the normal activation and proliferation cycles and avoids becoming anergic.

6.2.2.5. Early Human Trials

Advances in understanding the causes of some autoimmune diseases have already led to some clinical trials. A small double-blind trial was conducted with patients who had episodes of relapsing, remitting multiple sclerosis (MS).[830] They were fed bovine myelin or a placebo daily for 1 year. There was a decrease in MBP-reactive T cells in patients receiving the MBP. Although not conclusive, the patients receiving myelin suffered fewer major MS attacks compared with the controls. The treatment was well tolerated.

Similarly, a double-blind trial involving 60 patients with rheumatoid arthritis who received oral collagen showed a decrease in joint swelling and disease index compared with those who received the placebo (reviewed elsewhere[808]). Four patients who received collagen apparently had complete remissions of their arthritis. The treatment was well tolerated, and a multicenter trial is being planned.[808]

6.2.2.6. Comment

Section 2.3.2.9 described conjugation of a protein to the β subunit of cholera toxin (CTB) made by rDNA technology to avoid contamination with intact cholera toxin. Given orally, CTB profoundly enhanced the level of peripheral tolerance to erythrocytes.[325] A single dose of MBP conjugated to CTB, given before or after disease induction, protected rats against EAE. This approach using an intact protein seems to hold promise for use with an outbred population.

Another promising area is the use of peptide determinants as a form of immunotherapy for autoimmune diseases. Presumably, a range of peptides may be required, but it would be of interest if such an approach could be tested initially for a well-studied autoimmune condition in outbred rats or guinea pigs.

CHAPTER 6.3. VACCINATION TO CONTROL FERTILITY

6.3.1. Control of Human Fertility

The world's population is growing at the rate of about 1 billion persons per decade, with most of this increase occurring in developing countries.[831] This population explosion could have disastrous social and environmental consequences, and there is an urgent need for new and improved methods of birth control. Vaccination to regulate fertility is a relatively new approach to this problem, and substantial progress has been made in the development of birth control vaccines by immunization against reproductive antigens.[832] In this section, work in the area of human immunocontraception is outlined, along with the prospects for the widespread use of this approach to fertility control.

6.3.1.1. Natural Infertility Due to Immunologic Factors

Immunologic factors appear to be involved in about 20% of unexplained human infertility cases and in as many as 85% of unexplained, recurrent spontaneous abortions.[833] These natural cases of infertility provide evidence that immunologic causes can impair fertility. Reproduction may be adversely affected by antibody-, cell-, and cytokine-mediated phenomena before or after fertilization or implantation. Male and female reproductive tracts contain populations of immunocytes, particularly T cells, B cells, macrophages, and NK cells, and other factors that normally facilitate reproduction.[834]

Cytokines such as TNFα and IFNτ secreted by local lymphocytes and macrophages have been shown to influence sperm motility. Anti-sperm IgG and IgA antibodies in serum, largely directed against sperm tails, have been found in a high percentage of males and females who are apparently incapable of fertilization. In the male, the testis is normally an immunologically privileged site, but conditions such as vasectomy, aging, and malignancy may lead to a breakdown of the blood-testis barrier and expose the highly antigenic spermatozoa to immune cells. Lymphoid cells are not normally present in the testicular interstitium, but obstruction of the vas deferens may lead to anti-sperm antibody formation and lymphocyte infiltration, with resultant release of factors toxic to sperm.

In females, ovarian immunocytes may inhibit estrogen production and normal follicle development through their secretion of IL-1α, TNFα, and IFNτ. The cytokine IFNδ may inhibit embryo development, implantation, and trophoblast proliferation, and women with unexplained infertility have increased numbers of endometrial T cells capable of secreting this factor. It is also likely that leukocytes in vaginal and cervical tissues produce factors detrimental to sperm viability after exposure to antigens in seminal fluid. Premature ovarian failure may be caused by serum antibodies directed against ovarian antigens, and IgA or IgG antibodies against sperm components are present in the cervicovaginal secretions of infertile women. IgA and IgG antibodies in uterine tissues are present in abundance in uterine secretions, and they are clearly under hormonal regulation, because they occur in greatly increased concentrations before ovulation.

The cytokines secreted by immunocytes within the peritoneal cavity may affect normal reproduction through their influence on adjacent reproductive organs. Greater insight into the involvement of these components of the immune system in cases of natural infertility should help the development of birth control vaccines.

6.3.1.2. Can Fertility Be Controlled by Vaccination?

Vaccines have been designed to protect against pathogens, and the concept of vaccination against self antigens such as those of the reproductive system is relatively new. Prospects of exploiting the immune system for selective reactivity against autoantigens began with a demonstration of the immunogenicity of the β subunit of the pregnancy hormone, human chorionic gonadotropin (hCG).[835] Ideally, a vaccine to regulate fertility should be directed against antigens of gametes or early products of fertilization that are present only transiently and only on the target itself. Unlike oral contraceptives, which interfere with the hypothalamic-pituitary-gonadal axis, vaccination should not disrupt hormone production and function or ovulation. The chosen antigen should elicit immune responses of great specificity and of the desired type, magnitude, and duration in all vaccinated individuals, but unlike conventional vaccines, the effects of contraceptive vaccines should be reversible. The ability to conceive after a period of immunocontraception is an essential requirement of any potential fertility vaccine.

Figure 6.3.1.2 illustrates the major events in the human reproductive cycle. The reproductive process can theoretically be intercepted by vaccination at a number of these stages. The two major processes for which intervention by contraceptive vaccines has been considered have been oocyte fertilization and embryonic implantation.[831] Particular targets have included hormones, hormone receptors, gamete antigens, and embryo-associated antigens. The most advanced of these candidate vaccines under development are based on hCG, although problems have arisen with crossreactivity and the lack of efficacy of antibodies against this hormone. Increased understanding of the molecular processes of sperm-egg fusion has led to the discovery of new target antigens for vaccination. Subsequent sections describe the progress for each of these approaches.

6.3.1.3. Hormones as Targets

6.3.1.3.1. Choice of Hormones

Several hormones have been the targets of human fertility vaccination studies, including hCG, follicle-stimulating hormone (FSH), and gonadotropin-releasing hormone (GnRH), also known as luteinizing hormone–releasing hormone. The most prominent contraceptive vaccine candidates are those based on the placental pregnancy hormone, hCG, which is widely employed as a marker in testing for pregnancy and belongs to the same family as luteinizing hormone (LH), FSH, and thyroid-stimulating hormone.[831] Each of these hormones consists of two noncovalently bonded subunits: the α subunit, which is common to all four members, and the β subunit, which is immunologically distinct. The β chain of hCG and hLH share 85% sequence homology, but the former has a unique 37–amino acid C-terminal peptide.

HCG is known to play a vital role in maintenance of the endometrium for implantation of the embryo and in the continued secretion of progesterone.[836] The successful blocking of hCG by antibody should therefore prevent the establishment of pregnancy by acting between fertilization and implantation. This approach avoids the disadvantages of disruption of the pituitary-ovarian axis and ovulation or of the

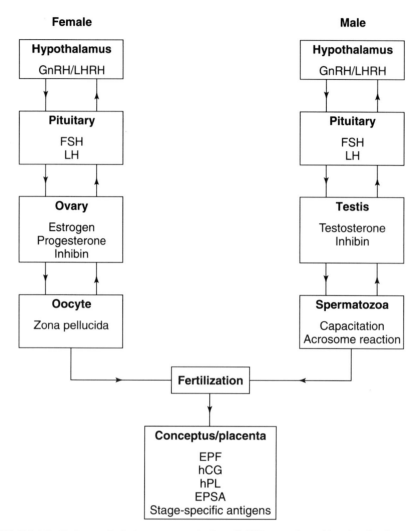

FIG. 6.3.1.2. Early events in human reproduction. GnRH, gonadotrophin-releasing hormone; LHRH, luteinizing hormone–releasing hormone; FSH, follicle-stimulating hormone; LH, luteinizing hormone; EPF, early pregnancy factor; hCG, human chorionic gonadotrophin; hPL, human placental lactogen; EPSA, early pregnancy-specific antigen.

normal production of steroid hormones. Successful immunization against hCG should not interfere with the regularity of the menstrual cycle. In theory, a vaccine against hCG could be used throughout the reproductive life of the female. It was formerly thought that hCG was made only during pregnancy and that an anti-hCG vaccine would therefore be pregnancy specific. However, hCG is made in males and in nonpregnant women.[831] A clearer picture of the physiologic relevance of these findings is required before any widespread use of hCG vaccines to control fertility.

Antibodies elicited by the β chain of hCG have higher avidity for the hCG molecule than those induced by the carboxy-terminal peptide (CTP), and this may be an important factor for the use of the former components for successful vaccination. Receptors on the corpus luteum have very high affinity for hCG, and it follows that specific antibodies should have at least similar binding avidity to achieve neutralization in vivo.[837] A potential disadvantage of this approach is the generation of antibodies crossreactive with LH, although these are apparently of sufficiently low affinity not to interfere with ovulation. Primates vaccinated with the CTP of the hCG β chain generated antibodies reactive to somatostatin-producing cells of the pancreas, striated muscle, and pituitary.[838] A further disadvantage is that there are no T-cell determinants on the CTP, and the low immunogenicity of this peptide means that frequent boosting may be required, seriously undermining the suitability of this candidate as a fertility vaccine.[831] This becomes a minor concern if the peptide is coupled to a foreign protein, such as diphtheria toxoid, which is then the source of T-cell determinants.

FSH is required for spermatogenesis and the maintenance of fertility in males and therefore represents another attractive candidate for immunocontraception.[839] This hormone is produced by the pituitary and binds receptors on the testicular Sertoli cells, which are present throughout life. Although the precise role of FSH in regulating spermatogenesis remains unclear, immunization of primates with ovine FSH results in marked impairment of this process and causes infertility.[839] It also appears that the small numbers of sperm produced after immunization are incapable of fertilizing oocytes. Encouragingly, neutralization of FSH in vivo did not inhibit testosterone production or lead to a loss of libido and was entirely reversible. Data from several studies of the immunogenicity of ovine FSH in nonhuman primates (reviewed elsewhere[839]) have shown that

- Antibodies are generated that are crossreactive with FSH of other species, including human FSH.
- The crossreactive antibodies exhibit the high affinity and antigen-binding capacity of human FSH.
- Neutralizing antibodies are highly specific for FSH; levels of testosterone and LH are unaffected in immunized monkeys.
- Sperm quality (eg, motility, oocyte gel penetration, acrosin activity, viability) was markedly diminished after immunization, as were numbers of spermatozoa per ejaculate.

GnRH plays a major regulatory role in the reproductive systems of vertebrates. This decapeptide is synthesized as part of a 92–amino acid prohormone by the hypothalamus and stimulates the production and release of gonadotropins, particularly FSH and LH, which play key roles in the production of sperm and ova.[840] Neutralization of this factor should result in infertility by impairment of ovulation and spermatogenesis and inhibition of the secretion of sex steroids. Although these effects would be reversible and usually be desirable in a fertility vaccine for animals, many would appear to disadvantageous for human use. Vaccination against

GnRH in females during the postpartum period may increase amenorrhea and potentially increase the interval between offspring; otherwise, the resultant suppression of ovulation would count against its widespread acceptance.[841] Neutralization against GnRH should also control fertility in males, but sex steroids would have to be administered for maintenance of libido and other functions.[841]

Immunization against GnRH has been associated with testicular atrophy in rabbits, a castration-like effect including weight loss in young rams and blockage of ovulation and menstrual cycling in baboons and marmosets, which was reversible over time with declining antibody levels (reviewed elsewhere[841]). Anti-GnRH MAbs blocked estrus and terminated pregnancy when passively administered to mice and caused abortion preceded by a rapid decline in CG levels when given to baboons early in pregnancy.[841] GnRH also stimulates release of hCG from human placental tissue,[844] and it is therefore possible that abortion would also follow GnRH neutralization during the early stages of pregnancy in humans.

6.3.1.3.2. Clinical Trials With Hormone Vaccines

There are at least six formulations using reproductive hormones that are under development as human fertility vaccines. One of these involves FSH, two are directed against GnRH, and three target hCG and represent the most advanced of the six candidates. Three anti-hCG vaccines as conjugates in adjuvant are in trials:

1. The β chain of hCG is covalently linked to tetanus toxoid (TT) as a carrier and adsorbed onto alum as an adjuvant.[835,843]
2. A heterospecies dimer (HSD) consists of the β chain of hCG noncovalently linked to the α subunit of ovine LH and conjugated to TT or diphtheria toxoid (DT) as carriers. The conjugates are used in alternating sequence to avoid the likelihood of hyperimmunization to the carrier. These conjugates are adsorbed on alum and sodium phthalyl derivative of polysaccharide (SPLPS) as an adjuvant.[844]
3. The CTP of the β chain of hCG is conjugated to DT at a ratio of 20 to 30 peptides per carrier molecule. This formulation is given as an oil-in-water emulsion that is made using Squalene and Arlacel-A, with muramyl dipeptide used as an adjuvant.[845]

In phase I clinical trials involving 79 women, the βhCG-TT vaccine (1) gave a reversible anti-hCG antibody response that eventually declined to background levels but did not disturb menstrual regulation.[835] An extended phase I trial carried out in India, Finland, Sweden, Chile, and Brazil gave similar results without notable side effects.[837] Phase I trials have also been conducted using the HSD vaccine (2) or a simple mixture of βhCG and β-ovine LH linked to carriers.[837] Of the two, the HSD vaccine displayed higher immunogenicity and generated antibodies with greater neutralizing capacity. Neither of the vaccines upset menstruation or ovulation; no hematologic abnormalities were found; and there was no evidence for the generation of autoantibodies. A phase I trial of the CTP vaccine (3) in 30 premenstrual females who had previously been surgically sterilized demonstrated anti-hCG antibody responses in all subjects and no evidence of crossreactivity with LH or FSH.[845] However, others have reported that the CTP vaccine, which is supported by the World Health Organization, is of relatively low immunogenicity and fails to elicit antibodies capable of neutralizing hCG.[846]

Doubts have been expressed about the safety of the βhCG-TT, HSD, and CTP vaccines, because several epitopes on the hCG β chain are accessible to antibody binding on receptor-bound hCG.[836] This finding raises the possibility of autoimmune responses against ovarian cells that bear hCG receptors,[831] and it is essential that clinical studies monitor the effects of any autoantibody production.

Phase II clinical trials of the efficacy of the HSD vaccine have been conducted with women of reproductive age, each of whom had two living children, an active sexual life, and normal ovulatory cycles.[844] Subjects were given three intramuscular injections of a mixture of HSD-TT and HSD-DT, the first with SPLPS adjuvant, at intervals of 6 weeks. Pregnancy occurred in only one woman, in whom levels of anti-hCG antibodies that were generated remained above 50 ng/mL. Collectively, 1227 menstrual cycles were recorded during the course of the trial. Preliminary epitope mapping studies revealed that antibodies against a single domain of hCG were present in all subjects and that titers of these antibodies correlated with the neutralization capacity of their sera. It appears that the HSD vaccine, which induces antibodies against hCG, is safe and reversible (phase I trials) and effective above certain antibody titers (phase II trials). The use of this formulation has demonstrated the feasibility of vaccination for fertility control, notwithstanding the need for ongoing monitoring of autoimmune reactions.

6.3.1.4. Gamete Proteins as Antigens

Gamete-specific antigens offer an alternative to hormones as targets for birth control vaccination. Immunologic disruption of processes such as sperm activation, adhesion between sperm and egg molecules, and sperm-egg fusion should prevent fertilization with few or no side effects. This approach may have certain advantages over those that target postconception events, such as blastocyst implantation (eg, for anti-hCG vaccines), given the social considerations that will influence the acceptance of fertility vaccines in some parts of the world. Several sperm and ova antigens are the subject of research as targets for fertility control.

6.3.1.4.1. Candidate Sperm Antigens

Spermatozoa may elicit anti–sperm antibodies in females and males (present in up to 70% of men after vasectomy), and about 30% of infertility may result from such antibodies in one or both partners of an infertile couple.[847] Sperm can act as autoantigens and isoantigens, and anti-sperm antibodies are capable of inhibiting fertilization when present in the genital tract. Only sperm-specific antigens should be considered as targets for an anti-sperm vaccine to fulfill the criteria for birth control vaccination described in Section 6.3.1.2. Several such antigens have been isolated and characterized, and the cDNA that encodes them has been cloned and sequenced.[847] Those that appear to have potential as target antigens are described here.

Lactate dehydrogenase (LDH)-C4 is a sperm enzyme that has been isolated from the testes and is apparently specific to the acrosome.[848] LDH appears to be reactive across each of the species from which it has been isolated. PH-20 is a glycosyl phosphatidylinositol-anchored membrane hyaluronidase present on the plasma membrane and acrosomal membrane. Originally isolated in guinea pigs,[849] it has also been cloned from monkeys and humans[850] but does not appear to be crossreactive. Sperm protein-10 (SP-10) is a polymorphic acrosomal antigen isolated from human spermatozoa, and MAbs against this protein cause sperm agglutination and impairment of motility.[851] HSA-63 is a sperm glycoprotein isolated from rabbits and mice that shows significant sequence homology with SP-10.[852] MAbs and polyclonal antisera against HSA-63 inhibit in vitro fertilization in mice and impair sperm penetration in humans. Other proteins isolated from the sperm of rabbits are called rabbit sperm autoantigens (RSA)-1, -2, and -3.[853] These low-molecular-weight, lectin-like molecules appear to function in binding of spermatozoa to oocytes. Monoclonal antibodies against RSA appear to crossreact with human sperm and inhibit their penetration into zona-free hamster oocytes.

Fertilization antigen-1 (FA-1) is a glycoprotein that has been isolated from human and murine sperm and is present during the later stages of spermatogenesis.[854] It is also present in rabbits, bulls, and monkeys and may perform a similar function in each of these species. MAbs to FA-1 completely block in vitro fertilization in animals and impair sperm motility in humans.[847] Antibodies against FA-1 are found in infertile individuals and after vasectomy and may be a prime causative agent of infertility.[855] The immunogenicity of FA-1 in humans, together with molecular analyses showing that its expression is limited to testes,[847] indicate that this antigen is a promising target for immunocontraception.

FA-2 is an antigen identified using the sperm-specific MAb, Vic-1.[856] This antibody blocks sperm penetration of the ovum in vitro and inhibits the acrosome reaction and release of acrosin from human sperm.[857] FA-2 appears to be a component of the signal transduction pathway leading to the acrosome reaction and may be involved in the binding of sperm to the ovum zona pellucida (ZP) antigen, ZP-3, as with FA-1.[847] Further characterization awaits cloning and sequencing of the relevant human cDNA.

A surface antigen that appears to provide the signal required for the first cleavage of the fertilized oocyte has been identified on sperm of several mammals, including humans and mice.[857] Antibodies to this molecule, termed cleavage signal protein 1 (CS-1), are also found in infertile individuals and act by inhibiting early stage zygote cleavage. The potential of this antigen as a target for fertility vaccination awaits further study.

6.3.1.4.2. Candidate Ova Antigens

The ZP is a translucent extracellular matrix that surrounds the mammalian oocyte from the onset of growth until shortly before implantation and is expressed only in the ovary.[858] Spermatozoa must bind specific receptor sites and penetrate the ZP before fertilization can occur. Sperm penetration of the ZP appears to be relatively species specific. Binding is followed by release of sperm acrosomal contents, leading to fusion of the fertilizing spermatozoon with the oocyte and changes in the ZP that inhibit penetration by other sperm. Disruption of any of these processes should prevent successful fertilization, making the ZP an attractive target for fertility control. Moreover, relatively low levels of antibodies against ZP antigens may be sufficient to inhibit fertilization, because few mature ova are likely to be present at any one time.[831]

The ZP consists of three glycoproteins—ZP1, ZP2, and ZP3—that have been well characterized, especially in the pig (reviewed elsewhere[859]). In particular, porcine ZP3 and its homologs in other mammals, including humans and mice, appear to constitute the primary receptor for acrosome binding. It also appears that O-linked oligosaccharide components of the ZP glycoproteins are essential for the interaction between sperm and ova, but the delineation of antibody epitopes on these sugar chains to target for vaccination awaits further studies of their conformation.[858]

6.3.1.4.3. Studies of Candidate Gamete Antigens

Several studies of the potential of gamete-specific antigens for fertility control have been conducted. A potential problem for vaccination against sperm antigens may be the requirement for extremely large quantities of antibodies in the female reproductive tract because of the huge mass of sperm delivered in a single ejaculate. This may be overcome by vaccination against antigens exposed only during particular stages of the reproductive process, such as during the sperm acrosome reaction. Systemic immunization with the acrosomal isoenzyme LDH-C4 stimulated local immunity in the reproductive tracts of female baboons, rabbits, and mice, which led to a 50% reduction in fertility.[848] A synthetic peptide representing the immunodominant epitope of human LDH-C4 was used to immunize female baboons, but up to 30% of individuals failed to mount an immune response.[860] It appears that LDH-C4 is a relatively poor immunogen; however, Goldberg and colleagues[860] are attempting to increase the immunogenicity of this enzyme by expression in recombinant vaccinia virus vectors.

At this stage, LDH-C4 is the only sperm antigen shown to significantly reduce fertility in primates. However, female baboons given recombinant human SP-10, another acrosome antigen, developed high titers of antibodies against the cognate protein, but only a few baboons displayed a partial reduction in fertility.[848] Immunization of male and female guinea pigs with PH-20, which is essential for sperm-egg fusion, induced total and reversible contraception,[849] and studies in primates are doubtless underway now that the human and monkey homologs of this sperm protein have been cloned.[850]

Immunization studies with HSA-63 or any of the RSA family have not been reported, and it is unknown whether infertile individuals have antibodies to these antigens in their sera. However, active immunization of female rabbits with purified FA-1 protein had effects ranging from a significant reduction to complete blockade of fertility.[847] FA-1 antibodies have been found in infertile and vasectomized men,[855] and active immunization trials, using a synthetic decapeptide epitope that is recognized by anti-FA-1 MAbs, are planned in nonhuman primates.[847] It may be that the sperm-specific antigens known to be present in infertile individuals (ie, FA-1 and CS-1) will be the most useful candidates for fertility control vaccines. These immunogens could be used singly or as components of multivalent preparations of antigens involved at various stages of the interaction between sperm and ovum.

The ZP of the ovum is the major unique antigen that has been identified in the ovary and represents a logical target for birth control vaccination. Sustained high levels of local anti-ZP antibodies may not be needed to block fertility because, unlike the antigenic mass of sperm deposited in the reproductive tract, there are few mature oocytes present at any given time. Anti-ZP antibodies generated in several species after immunization with ZP antigens inhibit sperm attachment and penetration and block fertility. For example, immunization with porcine ZP induced infertility in rabbits, dogs, horses, deer, and several nonhuman primates that was entirely reversible.[858]

Fertility trials using recombinant ZP antigens from rabbits and mice are planned. Synthetic peptides representing epitopes of ZP3 are also being tested as immunocontraceptive antigens. A 16–amino acid peptide of murine ZP3, incorporating a linear B-cell epitope and conjugated to keyhole limpet hemocyanin (KLH), elicited antibodies that induced reversible infertility in 75% of immunized female mice.[861] A 15–amino acid peptide representing the human homolog of the murine sequence and also coupled to KLH was given to two macaques and prevented conception for five or six ovulatory cycles.[858] In neither experiment was ovarian function otherwise impaired. However, other investigators have reported the development of oophoritis and loss of immature oocytes in animals immunized with proteins or synthetic peptides of ZP3, and these reactions appear to have an autoimmune basis (reviewed elsewhere[858]). There is evidence that a CD4 + T-cell response to ZP3 is the primary mechanism for such autoimmune reactions.[862] It may be possible to overcome T-cell–mediated autoimmune phenomena by presenting B-cell epitopes of the ZP along with selected foreign T helper epitopes as components of synthetic immunogens.[858] However, the development of fertility vaccines based on ZP antigens will depend on further analyses of the pathogenesis of ovarian disease in immunized animals.

6.3.1.5. How Best to Immunize for Fertility Control

Many of the fertility control vaccines under development are designed to disrupt processes occurring in the reproductive tract, especially those against gamete antigens, and they require the generation and maintenance of effective local immune responses. The important features of the mucosal immune system have been outlined in Chapter 2.3, but it is appropriate here to review options available to vaccinate for mucosal responses to control fertility. Elements of humoral and cellular immunity are present in the reproductive tracts of males and females and normally mediate protective responses without compromising reproduction. However, as described in Section 6.3.1.1, many cases of natural infertility can be ascribed to immunologic factors.

Relatively little is known of the immunobiology of the male genital tract, although these tissues contain significant numbers of APCs, B cells, and T cells and have epithelia capable of synthesizing secretory component (SC).[294] CD4 + and CD8 + T cells bearing the integrin $\alpha_E\beta_7$, which is found exclusively on mucosal lymphocytes, are found in the human urethra but not usually in healthy testis. Macrophages are abundant in most tissues of the tract. The urethra also contains numerous IgA-staining plasma cells in the submucosa and epithelia capable of synthesizing SC, and sIgA, IgG, and IgM antibodies have been found in prostatic and preejaculatory fluid. Specific sIgA antibodies against a range of local pathogens have also been detected in the semen of infected individuals.[863] All of the elements required for local production of secretory antibodies are therefore present in various regions of the male reproductive tract. It has been suggested that these may be activated only during overt local infection.[863]

Far more is known about the immunology of the female reproductive tract. Components of mucosal and systemic immunity are found throughout the tract from the vagina to the ovaries,[864,865] but there is little evidence for organized lymphoid structures, except for the presence of nodules in the vagina.[863] The T-cell population of the tract varies with location, being relatively sparse in the vagina and ectocervix, but CD4 + and CD8 + T cells are present in reasonable numbers in the endometrium during the secretory phase and at high numbers in the transformation zone of the cervix.[863,866] Potent APCs, including Langerhans cells, are also found in the lower parts of the tract, especially in the cervix and vulva.[866] Local plasma cells are found in their greatest concentrations beneath the epithelia of the vagina, cervix, and fallopian tubes, but they are rarely seen in the ovaries or endometrium. Most of these cells secrete antibodies of the IgA isotype, although IgG- and IgM-producing cells are also found in reasonable numbers. SC is also expressed by epithelial cells of the fallopian tubes and cervical glands and has been found in vaginal secretions; thus elements for local production of secretory antibodies are present throughout large portions of the tract. Cervical secretions contain high concentrations of antibodies, with IgA and IgG present in a ratio of about 1:2. Although most IgA is associated with SC, indicative of local production, the close correlation between the levels of albumin and IgG in these secretions suggest that the latter is derived from serum.

Several studies have been made of the nature of mucosal and systemic responses after immunization by different routes (reviewed elsewhere[863]). Overall, it appears that challenge of the cervix or vagina in female humans and primates leads to local production of specific antibodies that are largely of the IgA isotype, although IgG predominates in the uterus and is derived largely from serum. Titers of vaginal and cervical IgA antibodies generated after local immunization have ranged from high to very low in these studies, but does appear that injection of antigen into the pelvic presacral space can markedly improve local antibody levels. Antibodies may also be found in the reproductive tract after intraperitoneal immunization, possibly resulting from injected antigen gaining direct access to draining lymph nodes or stimulation of the peritoneal B1 cell population.[307] There is some evidence that rectal, rather than vaginal, immunization is more efficient for the generation of vaginal IgA responses,[867] probably because of lymphoid nodules in the rectum and the shared lymph nodes draining these tissues.[863] The lower genital tract and rectum also share draining lymph nodes in males.

A combination of oral priming and vaginal boosting with a subunit vaccine against simian immunodeficiency virus was used to induce vaginal sIgA and IgG, serum IgG and IgA, and T cells in lymph nodes draining the genital tract, all of which were specific for the immunogen.[868] This and similar approaches, such as oral priming and rectal boosting,[869] may be extremely useful for the generation of effective local responses in male and female reproductive tracts. The effectiveness of such regimes probably results from activation and migration of lymphoid cells in the gut after oral immunization, and the local boost may provide an antigen-specific homing or proliferative signal.[863] It is possible that the traffic of sensitized immunocytes from GALT to the genital tract as part of the common mucosal immune system[282,283] may be exploited to generate effective local responses. The B-cell population of the reproductive tract may arise primarily in GALT.[847]

An oral birth control vaccine would be an attractive option, particularly in terms of expense and ease of administration. It should be remembered, however, that immunization by the oral route generally requires substantial amounts of antigen to achieve effective mucosal responses and often generates systemic tolerance to protein antigens (see Section 2.3.2.8), which would not be a desirable feature for immunocontraception. Successful oral immunization requires survival of antigen in the gut environment, effective delivery for presentation of antigen to GALT, and development of appropriate protective immune responses. Much effort is being directed toward meeting these requirements (reviewed elsewhere[863]). Biodegradable microspheres, immune-stimulating complexes, liposomes, and live bacterial and viral vectors are being studied, with some success, for their ability to deliver a range of immunogens for the generation of mucosal responses largely by the oral route. Adjuvants such as cholera toxin as well as tetanus and diphtheria toxoids, some cytokines (particularly type 2 factors such as IL-5 and IL-6), and hybrids of delivery systems and adjuvants have also been used to enhance the development of vaccine-induced mucosal immunity (see Chapter 2.3), and some of these approaches are being applied to the goal of immunocontraception. The feasibility of oral immunization for birth control remains to be established, although strategies involving oral priming and local boosting have been successful for the generation of significant specific B- and T-cell responses in the reproductive tract.

These findings suggest a number of strategies for fertility control that are worthy of further study.[863] Strong secretory antibody responses may be mounted in the lower reproductive tract of the female, especially in the cervix and, to a lesser extent, in the vagina, so that a vaccine that targets mucosal responses against processes such as sperm migration may have a reasonable chance of success. In contrast, the uterus does not appear to mount sIgA responses, but significant levels of serum IgG are able to permeate these tissues. Immunocontraception in the uterus may be best achieved by systemic vaccination strategies. Although more information on the generation of mucosal immune responses in the male reproductive tract is essential, it appears that oral vaccination followed by local boosting (perhaps provided by natural reproductive processes) holds promise for achieving effective mucosal responses in both sexes. Research in the areas of mucosal antigen delivery systems and adjuvants should provide new options for immunocontraception.

6.3.1.6. Comment

Perhaps the greatest problem facing the world today is the population explosion and many believe that this must be brought under control if a habitable earth it is to survive. One obvious way to tackle this problem is to be able to regulate human fertility in an acceptable way. Five types of family planning methods currently can be offered to couples: steroidal preparations, intrauterine devices, barrier methods, surgical sterilization, and the so-called natural methods.[870] Immunization offers an additional option that has several advantages over the others. Optimally, it would provide 12 to 18 months protection against unplanned pregnancy after a single administration; it would not produce the bleeding irregularities and the other side effects associated with hormonal methods; it would be easy to administer and not require constant attention (as with taking a daily pill); and it would be relatively inexpensive. There are several potential disadvantages,[870] such as the apparent low efficacy of this approach relative to established contraceptive methods, the variability in response by different persons in an outbred population, and the possible need to monitor recipients at intervals to check blood antibody levels. It may be possible in time to overcome these difficulties. However, when millions instead of hundreds of women are immunized, will a very small proportion suffer serious side effects? These vaccines will be given to otherwise healthy persons who may have alternative interventions to choose from, and consequently, safety is of prime importance.

The relative simplicity of this approach makes it attractive as an instrument of policy for different groups to serve particular ends. The history of family planning shows that sterilization and contraception have been forced on vulnerable groups for ethnic, cultural, religious, or economic reasons. "The consequences for the individuals involved and for the cause of informed and voluntary family planning have been detrimental and tragic."[871] The many areas of violent conflict in the world offer the potential for misuse of fertility control vaccines for human use.

6.3.2. Control of Fertility in Animals

6.3.2.1. General Principles

Fertility vaccines are an attractive approach for human fertility control and for the control of animal reproduction. From the data summarized in Section 6.3.1, it is clear that infertility can be induced in experimental animals by the use of immunocontraceptive techniques. Most of the approaches taken toward birth control vaccination in humans have relevance for the regulation of breeding patterns in domestic animals and for the control of animal pests. The major difference is that long-term or permanent effects are generally desirable in animals. Nevertheless, in the case of pests, target animal species may vary from those causing devastation, such as rabbits and foxes in Australia (see Section 6.3.2.1), to those that are only locally or temporarily over abundant, such as elephants in Zimbabwe, white tail deer and urban skunks in North America, kangaroos in Australia, and the Assateague horses of Virginia.

In the case of widespread pests, control by immunosterilization requires consideration of the cost of the vaccine and of the risks of affecting domestic herds in certain situations (eg, feral pigs). In cases of temporary overpopulation, there may be a requirement for reversible sterility agents that could be precisely targeted to individual animals for which relatively high costs of delivery would be acceptable. Attempts to control the numbers of wild horses on Assateague Island represent a notable example of the latter approach.[872] Overpopulation of these horses has caused great environmental damage, and a trial is underway involving the vaccination of mares with porcine ZP glycoprotein delivered by dart gun, with the aim of maintaining stock at the carrying capacity of the island. The success of such trials may eventually allow the abandonment of crude methods such as shooting and poisoning for more effective means of control in urban and natural habitats.

6.3.2.2. Fertility Control of Vertebrate Pests in Australia

An Australian initiative has been the establishment of a government-funded Cooperative Research Centre (CRC) for Biological Control of Vertebrate Pest Populations.[873] It aims to control feral rabbits, foxes, and mice, which cause massive environmental damage throughout the continent, as illustrated in Figure 6.3.2.2. The chief aim of the CRC is "to achieve sterilization by inducing immunologic responses in the target species to proteins involved in gamete-gamete interaction at

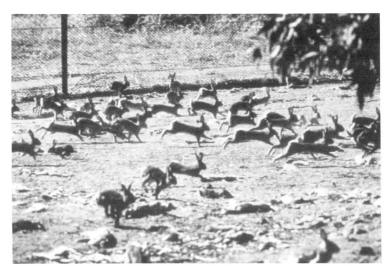

FIG. 6.3.2.2. The rabbit pest demonstrated by a scene in the Australian countryside. After the myxoma virus was introduced into Australia in 1950, the rabbit population decreased dramatically, but it has since "stabilized" at 10% to 15% of the original numbers, with myxoma virus infections, usually nonlethal, endemic in the population. (Photograph courtesy of the Cooperative Research Centre for Biological Control of Vertebrate Pest Populations, Australia.)

fertilization or embryo implantation. These proteins will be administered directly in baits or indirectly by infection of the target species with genetically modified viruses or bacteria that express the genes encoding these proteins. The infectious agents may be nontransmissible or may be species specific contagious agents that spread naturally through the target population."[874] The CRC has three major interrelated components—reproductive immunology, molecular virology, and ecology and social behavior—and is primarily addressing the following issues:

- The proportion of a wild population that must be sterilized to induce a negative growth rate
- The development of delivery systems that can reach the required proportion of the population
- The development of an immunocontraceptive that is species specific, long acting, and effective after a single dose.

The first issue is being addressed in rabbits by the establishment of large scale, 3-year field experiments in different parts of Australia.[873] These involve surgical sterilization of different proportions (0% to 80%) of the adult population, a process repeated annually in each area. Similar experiments are being planned for foxes. A crucial issue is whether dominant members of the population, when sterilized, maintain the prime habitat and continue to inhibit successful reproduction by subordinate members. Initial results for sterilizing rabbits and foxes are encouraging.

Overall, these studies should reveal whether fertility control is feasible in a wild population and will also be important in determining the requirements for an effective delivery system.

Systems for the delivery of immunocontraceptive agents under investigation by CRC scientists include poxviruses such as myxoma, vaccinia, and ectromelia; the herpesvirus murine cytomegalovirus (MCMV); *Salmonella*; nucleic acid vaccines (NAV); and microspheres.[874] Myxoma virus has been circulating in Australian rabbit populations since its release in 1950 and is apparently specific for this species,[875] as is MCMV for mice. The rate of spread of recombinant strains of myxoma in competition with existing strains in the wild will be an important determination of this work. A fox-specific vector has not been identified, but the potential of NAV, *Salmonella*, vaccinia, and microspheres for oral immunization to elicit immune responses in the reproductive tract is being studied in all three species.

Research is also being directed toward isolating genes encoding gamete proteins with immunocontraceptive potential for expression in recombinant vectors or baits.[874] Several rabbit sperm genes (*PH-20*, *PH-30a* and *b*, *acrosin*, *LDH-C4*), a rabbit zona gene (*rec 55*), fox sperm genes (*PH-20*, *LDH-C4*), fox ova genes (*ZP2*, *ZP3*), and corresponding murine genes are ready for insertion into the previously described vector systems, and in some cases, laboratory trials of their ability to elicit appropriate immune responses are underway. Effective immunocontraception will probably require the persistence of high levels of specific anti–gamete antibody. The ability of cytokine genes to enhance mucosal and systemic immune responses when coexpressed in recombinant vectors is another important aspect of this work. The need for a sustained immune response is particularly important in the case of rabbits, for which there is only one small window of opportunity for the immunocontraceptive recombinant myxoma virus to compete successfully with circulating field strains in the new litter. The delivery vector, the reproductive antigen, and even the adjuvant cytokine chosen have the capacity to confer species specificity on the immunocontraceptive agent.

The CRC has been established to tackle the immense problem of fertility control of feral pests. Because it is a novel concept that involves the release of genetically modified organisms, there should be ongoing and informed public discussion of all foreseeable consequences at each major step of the work.[873] At the very least, this effort should supply valuable knowledge concerning fertility control. At best, it may lead to an effective means of controlling the populations of many problem animal species, including those that are devastating the Australian environment.

BIBLIOGRAPHY

Ada GL, ed. (1994) Strategies in vaccine design. RG Landes, Austin, TX, pp. 1–217.

Andre F, Cholat J, Furminger I, eds. (1994) Proceedings of the Second European Conference on Vaccinology. Biologicals 22:297–391.

Brown F, ed. (1994) Recombinant vectors in vaccine development. Dev Biol Standard 82:3–268.

Colten HR, Ravetch JV, eds. (1995) Innate immunity. Curr Opin Immunol. 6:1–64.

Cutts FT, Smith PG, eds. (1994) Vaccination and world health. John Wiley & Sons, Chichester, pp. 1–294.

Division of Microbiology and Infectious Diseases, NIAID. (1995) The Jordan report: accelerated development of vaccines. Division of Microbiology and Infectious Diseases. NIAID, NIH, Washington, DC, pp. 1–82.

Ibelgaufts H. (1994) Dictionary of cytokines. VCH, Weinheim, Germany.

Janeway CA Jr, Travers P, eds. (1994) Immunobiology: the immune system in health and disease. Curr Biol 1.1–12.47.

Janeway CA Jr, Marrack P, Kelly, Natvig JB. (1995) Immunology highlights: proceedings reports from the Sixth International Congress of Immunology. Immunologist 3:165–274.

McFadden G, ed. (1995) Viroceptors, virokines and related immune modulators encoded by DNA viruses. RG Landes, Austin, TX, pp. 1–218.

Möller G, ed. (1995) Tumor immunology. Immunol Rev 145:1–250.

Möller G, ed. (1996) Immunological memory. Immunol Rev 150:1–167.

Paul WE, ed. (1993) Fundamental immunology. Raven Press, New York, pp. 1–1490.

Plotkin SA, Mortimer EA. (1994) Vaccines. WB Saunders, Philadelphia, pp. 1–996.

Seder R, Paul WE. (1994) Acquisition of lymphokine-producing phenotype by CD4 + T cells. Ann Rev Immunol 12:635–673.

Stratton KR, Howe CJ, Johnston RB, eds. (1994) Adverse events associated with childhood vaccines: evidence bearing on causality. Institute of Medicine, National Academy Press, Washington, DC, pp. 1–464.

Talwar GP, Raghupathy R, eds. (1995) Birth control vaccines. RG Landes, Austin, TX, pp. 1–177.

Wick G, ed. (1995) Aspects of vaccination. Int Arch Allergy Immunol 108:303–359.

World Health Organization. (1994) World Health Organization meeting on nucleic acid vaccines. Vaccine 12:16.

Wraith DC. (1995) Induction of antigen-specific unresponsiveness with synthetic peptides: specific immunotherapy for treatment of allergic and autoimmune conditions. Int Arch Allergy Immunol 108:355–359.

REFERENCES

1. Fenner F, Henderson DA, Arita I, Jezek Z, Ladnyi ID. (1988) Smallpox and its Eradication. World Health Organization, Geneva, p. 1–1460.
2. Koch R. (1888) The aetiology of anthrax based on the ontogeny of the anthrax bacillus. Beitr Biol Pflanz 2:277 [Reprinted in Med Classics 1937;2:787].
3. Davain C. (1961) Researches into infusoria of the blood in the disease known as sang de rati. In: London NJ, ed. Louis Pasteur: a master of scientific enquiry. Hutchison, London.
4. Pasteur L, Chamberland CE, Roux E. (1881) Sur la vaccination charbonneux. C R Acad Sci Paris 92:1378.
5. Salmon DE, Smith T. (1886) On a new method of producing immunity from contagious diseases. Am Vet Res 10:63.
6. Roux E, Yersin A. (1888) Contribution a l'etude de la diphtherie. Ann Inst Pasteur 2:629.
7. Von Behring E, Kitasao S. (1890) Uber das Zustandekommen der Diphtherie-Immunitat und der Tetanus-Immunitat bei Thieren. Dtsch Med Wochenschr 16:1113–1114.

8. Plotkin SL, Plotkin SA. (1994) A short history of vaccination. In: Plotkin SA, Mortimer EA, eds. Vaccines, 2nd ed. WB Saunders, Philadelphia, pp. 1–12.
9. Metchnikoff E. (1893) Lectures on the comparative pathology of inflammation. Keegan, Paul, Trench, Trubner, London [Reprinted by Dover, New York, 1968].
10. Ehrlich P. (1897) Die Wertbemessung desdiphtherieheilserums. Klin Jahrb 60:299.
11. Burnet FM. (1957) A modification of Jerne's theory of antibody production using the concept of clonal selection. Aust J Sci 20:67–70.
12. Marrack JR. (1934) The Chemistry of Antigens and Antibodies. Special report Ser. Med Res Council. London, no. 194. pp. 135.
13. Landsteiner K. (1947) The specificity of serological reactions. Harvard University Press, Boston, pp. 1–310.
14. Glenny AT, Hopkins BE. (1923) Diphtheria toxoid as an immunising agent. Br J Exp Pathol 4:283.
15. Landsteiner K, Chase MW. (1942) Experiments on transfer of cutaneous sensitivity to simple compounds. Proc Soc Exp Biol Med 49:688–690.
16. Miller JFAP, Mitchell GM. (1968) Cell to cell interaction in the immune response. II. The source of hemolysin-forming cells in irradiated mice given bone marrow and thymus or thoracic duct lymphocytes. J Exp Med 128:821–837.
17. Bloom BR, Bennett B. (1968) Migration inhibitory factor associated with delayed type hypersensitivity. Fed Proc 27:13–15.
18. Brunner K, Mauel J, Cerotinn J-C, Chapuis B. (1968) Quantitative assay of the lytic action of immune lymphoid cells on ^{51}Cr-labelled allogeneic cells in vitro: inhibition by isoantibody and by drugs. Immunology 14:181–196.
19. Zinkernagel RM, Doherty PC. (1974) Restriction of in vitro cell-mediated cytotoxicity in lymphocytic choriomeningitis with a syngeneic or semi-allogeneic system. Nature 248:701–702.
20. Doherty PC, Zinkernagel RM. (1975) A biological role for the major histocompatibility antigens. Lancet 1:1406–1409.
21. Ada GL. (1994) Twenty years into the saga of MHC restriction. Immunol Cell Biol 72:447–454.
22. Miller JFAP, Vadas MA, Whitelaw A, Gamble J. (1975) H-2 gene complex restricts transfer of delayed-type hypersensitivity in mice. Proc Natl Acad Sci USA 72:5095–5098.
23. Ada G. (1996) The immunological principles of vaccination. In: Plotkin SA, Fantini B, eds. Vaccinia, Vaccination, Vaccinology. Jenner, Pasteur and their successors. Elsevier, Paris, pp. 25–32.
24. Hooper B, Whittingham S, Matthews DJ, Mackay IR, Curnow DH. (1972) Autoimmunity in a rural community. Clin Exp Immunol 12:79–87.
25. Wilson GS. (1967) The hazards of immunization. Athlone Press, London.
26. Storke JR, Connelly KK. (1994) Bacille Calmette-Guerin (BCG) vaccine. In: Plotkin SA, Mortimer EA, eds. Vaccines, 2nd ed. WB Saunders, Philadelphia, pp. 439–474.
27. De Cock KM, Soro B, Koulibaly IM, Lucas SB. (1992) Tuberculosis and HIV infection in sub-Saharan Africa. JAMA 268:1581–1587.
28. Robbins FC. (1994) Polio-historical. In: Plotkin SA, Mortimer EA, eds. Vaccines, 2nd ed. WB Saunders, Philadelphia, pp. 137–154.
29. McIntosh K, Chanock RM. (1985) Respiratory syncytial viruses. In: Fields BN, et al, eds. Viruses. Raven Press, New York, pp. 1285–1304.
30. Merz DC, Scheid A, Choppin PW. (1980) Importance of antibodies to the fusion glycoprotein of paramyxoviruses in the prevention of infection. J Exp Med 151:275–288.
31. Leung K-N, Ada GL. (1982) Different functions and immunopathological effects of subsets of effector T cells in murine influenza virus infection. Cell Immunol 67:312–324.
32. Parkman PD, Hardegree MC. (1994) Regulation and testing of vaccines. In: Plotkin SA, Mortimer EA, eds. Vaccines, 2nd ed. WB Saunders, Philadelphia, pp. 889–902.
33. Salk J, Drucker J, Malvey D. (1994) Non-infectious polio virus vaccines. In: Plotkin SA, Mortimer EA, eds. Vaccines, 2nd ed. WB Saunders, Philadelphia, pp. 205–228.
34. Prince AM, Moor-Jankowski J, Eichberg JW, et al. (1988) Chimpanzees and AIDS research. Nature 333:513.
35. Ballou WR, Sherwood JA, Hoffman SL, et al. (1987) Safety and efficacy of a recombinant DNA *Plasmodium falciparum* sporozoite vaccine. Lancet 1:1277–1281.
36. Herrington DA, Clyde DF, Losonsky G, et al. (1987) Safety and immunogenicity in man of a synthetic peptide malaria vaccine against *Plasmodium falciparum* sporozoites. Nature 328:257.
37. World Health Organization, Advisory Committee on Health Research. Report of a Subcommittee on Enhancement of Transfer of Technology to Developing Countries with Special Reference to Health. (WHO/RPD/ACHR/TT/87. Annex 3). World Health Organization, Geneva.

38. Fenner FJ. (1970) The effects of changing social organization on the infectious diseases of man. In: Boyden SW, ed. The impact of civilization on the biology of man. University of Toronto Press, Toronto, p. 48–68.

39. Willem JS, Sanders CR. (1981) Cost-effectiveness and cost-benefit analysis of vaccines. J Infect Dis 144:486–493.

40. White DO, Fenner FJ. (1994) Medical virology, 4th ed. Academic Press, New York, pp. 1–603.

41. Freestone DS. (1994) Yellow fever vaccine. In: Plotkin SA, Mortimer EA, eds. Vaccines, 2nd ed. WB Saunders, Philadelphia, pp. 741–780.

42. Melnick JL. (1994) Live, attenuated polio vaccines. In: Plotkin SA, Mortimer EA, eds. Vaccines, 2nd ed. WB Saunders, Philadelphia, pp. 155–204.

43. Stanway G, Hughes PJ, Mountford RC, et al. (1984) Comparison of the complete nucleotide sequence of the genomes of the neurovirulent poliovirus P3/Leon/37 and its attenuated Sabin vaccine derivative P3/Leon/12a$_1$b. Proc Natl Acad Sci USA 81:1539–1543.

44. Burke KL, Dunn G, Ferguson M, et al. (1988) Antigen chimeras of poliovirus as potential new vaccines. Nature 332:81–82.

45. Evans DMA, Dunn G, Minor PD, et al. (1985) Increased neurovirulence associated with a single nucleotide change in a non-coding region of the sabin type 3 polio vaccine genome. Nature 314:548–550.

46. Rubin BA, Rorke LB. (1994) Adenovirus vaccines. In: Plotkin SA, Mortimer EA, eds. Vaccines. WB Saunders, Philadelphia, pp. 475–502.

47. Fuenzalida E, Palacios R, Borgono JM. (1964) Anti-rabies antibody response in man to vaccine made from infected suckling mouse brains. Bull WHO 30:431–436.

48. Wiktor TJ, Plotkin SA, Grella DW. (1973) Human cell culture rabies vaccine. JAMA 224:1170–1171.

49. Maassab HF, Shaw MW, Heilman CA. (1994) Live influenza virus vaccine. In: Plotkin SA, Mortimer EA, eds. Vaccines, 2nd ed. WB Saunders, Philadelphia, pp. 781–802.

50. Govaert T ME, Thijs CT, Masurel N, et al. (1994) The efficacy of influenza vaccination in elderly individuals. JAMA 272:1661–1664.

51. Patriarca PA. (1994) A randomized controlled trial of influenza vaccine in the elderly. Scientific scrutiny and ethical responsibility. JAMA 272:1700–1701.

52. Krugman S. (1994) Hepatitis B vaccine. In: Plotkin SA, Mortimer EA, eds. Vaccines, 2nd ed. WB Saunders, Philadelphia, p. 419–438.

53. Chanock RM, Murphy BR, Collins PL, et al. (1988) Live viral vaccines for respiratory and enteric tract diseases. Vaccine 6:129–133.

54. Wright PF, Johnson PR, Karzon D. (1986) Clinical experience with live attenuated vaccines in children. In: Kendal AP, Patriarca P, eds. Options for the control of influenza. Alan R Liss, New York, pp. 243–253.

55. Plotkin SA. (1994) Cytomegalovirus vaccines. In: Plotkin SA, Mortimer EA, eds. Vaccines, 2nd ed. WB Saunders, Philadelphia, p. 803–808.

56. Starr SE, Glazer JP, Friedman HM, Plotkin SA. (1981) Specific cellular and humoral immunity after immunization with live Towne strain cytomegalovirus vaccine. J Infect Dis 143:585–589.

57. Brandt WE. (1990) Development of dengue and Japanese encephalitis vaccines. J Infect Dis 162:577–583.

58. Wilson G, Dick HM. (1983) Topley and Wilson's principles of bacteriology, virology and immunity, vol 1, 7th ed. Williams & Wilkins, Baltimore.

59. Storke JR, Connelly KK. (1994) Bacillus Calmette-Guerin vaccine. In: Plotkin SA, Mortimer EA, eds. Vaccines, 2nd ed. WB Saunders, Philadelphia, pp. 439–474.

60. Levine MM. (1994) Typhoid fever vaccines. In: Plotkin SA, Mortimer EA, eds. Vaccines, 2nd ed. WB Saunders, Philadelphia, pp. 597–634.

61. Austrian R. (1985) Polysaccharide vaccines. Ann Inst Pasteur Microbiol 136B:295–307.

62. Holmgren J, Svennerholm AM, Clemens JD, et al. (1987) An oral B subunit whole cell against cholera: from concept to successful field trial. Adv Exp Med Biol 216B:1649–1660.

63. Tropical Disease Research. (1995) Twelfth Programme Report. UNDP/World Bank WHO Special Programme for Research and Training in Tropical Diseases, Geneva, p. 110.

64. Leishmaniasis dog vaccine trials in Brazil. (1994) TDR News 46:4.

65. Mortimer EA. (1994) Pertussis vaccine. In: Plotkin SA, Mortimer EA, eds. Vaccines, 2nd ed. WB Saunders, Philadelphia, pp. 91–136.

66. Galaska AM, Lauer BA, Henderson RH, Keja J. (1984) Indications and contraindications for vaccines used in the Expanded Programme of Immunization. Bull World Health Organ 62:357–366.

67. Garenne M, Leroy O, Beau JP, et al. (1991) Child mortality after high titer measles; prospective study in Senegal. Lancet 388:903–907.
68. Stratton KR, Howe CJ, Johnston RB, eds, for the Vaccine Safety Committee, Division of Health Promotion and Disease Prevention. Institute of Medicine. (1994) Adverse events associated with childhood vaccines. Evidence bearing on causality. National Academy Press, Washington, DC, pp. 1–464.
69. De Quadros CA, Andrus JK, Olive JM, et al. (1991) Eradication of poliomyelitis. Progress in the Americas. Pediatr Infect Dis J 10:222–229.
70. De Quadros CA. (1994) Strategies for disease control/eradication in the Americas. In: Cutts FT, Smith PG, eds. Vaccination and world health. John Wiley & Sons, Chichester, pp. 17–34.
71. Measles elimination by the year 2000! Expanded Program of Immunization in the Americas. (1994) EPI Newsletter 16:1–2.
72. Peltola H, Heinonen OP, Valle M, et al. (1994) The elimination of indigenous measles, mumps and rubella from Finland by a 12-year, two dose vaccination program. N Engl J Med 331:1397–1402.
73. Henderson DA. (1995) Vaccination policies and practices. Aust J Pub Health 19:634–638.
74. Begg N, Cutts FT. (1994) The role of epidemiology in the development of a vaccination programme. In: Cutts FT, Smith PG, eds. Vaccination and world health. John Wiley & Sons, Chichester, pp. 123–137.
75. Adams WG, Deaver KA, Cochi S, et al. (1993) Decline of childhood *Haemophilus influenzae* type b (Hib) disease in the Hib vaccine era. JAMA 269:221–226.
76. Bloom BR, Murray CJ. (1992) Tuberculosis: commentary on a re-emergent killer. Science 257:1055–1064.
77. Plotkin SA, Koprowski H. (1994) Rabies vaccine. In: Plotkin SA, Mortimer EA, eds. Vaccines, 2nd ed. WB Saunders, Philadelphia, pp. 649–670.
78. Convit J, Aranzazu N, Ulrich M, et al. (1982) Immunotherapy with a mixture of *Mycobacterium leprae* and BCG in different forms of leprosy and Mitsuda-negative contacts. Int J Lepr 50:413–426.
79. Convit J, Catellanos PI, Rondon A, et al. (1987) Immunotherapy versus chemotherapy in localized cutaneous leishmaniasis. Lancet 1:401–403.
80. Salk J. (1987) Prospects for the control of AIDS by immunizing seropositive individuals. Nature 327:473–476.
81. Zagury D, Bernard J, Cheynier R, et al. (1988) A group-specific anamnestic reaction against HIV-1 induced by a candidate vaccine against AIDS. Nature 332:344–346.
82. Redfield RR, Birx DL, Ketter N, et al. (1991) A phase I evaluation of the safety and immunogenicity of vaccination with recombinant gp160 in patients with early human immunodeficiency virus infection. N Engl J Med 324:1677–1684.
83. Wain-Hobson S. (1995) Virological mayhem. Nature 373:102.
84. Ho DD, Neumann AU, Perelson AS, et al. (1995) Rapid turnover of plasma virions and CD4 lymphocytes in HIV-1 infection. Nature 373:123–126.
85. Wei X, Ghosh SK, Taylor ME, et al. (1995) Viral dynamics in human immunodeficiency virus type 1 infection. Nature 373:117–122.
86. Ukwu HN, Graham BS, Lambert JS, et al. (1992) Perinatal transmission of human immunodeficiency virus-1 infection and maternal immunization strategies for prevention. Obstet Gynecol 80:458–68.
87. Snydman DR. (1990) Cytomegalovirus immunoglobulins in the prevention and treatment of cytomegalovirus disease. Rev Infect Dis 12:S839–S848.
88. Zaia JA, Levin MJ, Preblud SR, et al. (1983) Evaluation of varicella-zoster immune globulin: protection of immunosuppressed children after household exposure to varicella. J Infect Dis 147:737–743.
89. Plotkin SA, Mortimer EA, eds. (1994) Vaccines, 2nd ed. WB Saunders, Philadelphia, App. 2.
90. Insel RA, Amstey M, Pichichero M. (1985) Postimmunization antibody to *H. influenzae* type b capsule in breast milk. J Infect Dis 152:407–408.
91. Riddell SR, Watanabe KS, Goodrich JM, et al. (1992) Restoration of viral immunity in immunodeficient humans by the adoptive transfer of T cell clones. Science 257:238–240.
92. Kuzushima K, Yamamoto M, Kimura H, et al. (1996) Establishment of Epstein-Barr virus (EBV) cellular immunity by adoptive transfer of virus specific cytotoxic T lymphocytes from an HLA matched sibling to a patient with severe chronic active EBV infection. Clin Exp Immunol 103:192–198.

93. Boulianne GL, Hozumi ZN, Schulman MJ. (1984) Production of functional chimeric mouse/human antibody region domains. Nature 312:643–646.
94. Jones PT, Dear PH, Foote J. (1986) Replacing the complementarity-determining regions in a human antibody with those from a mouse. Nature 321:522–525.
95. Burton DR, Barbas CF III. (1994) Human antibodies from combinatorial libraries. Adv Immunol 57:191–280.
96. Fenner FJ, Gibbs EPJ, Murphy FA, Rott R, Studdert MJ, White DO. (1993) Veterinary virology, 2nd ed. Academic Press, New York, pp. 1–666.
97. Shahid NS, Steinhoff MC, Hoque SS, et al. (1995) Serum, breast milk and infant antibody after maternal immunisation with pneumococcal vaccine. Lancet 346:1252–1257.
98. Henderson RH. (1994) Vaccination: successes and challenges. In: Cutts FT, Smith PG, eds. Vaccination and world health. John Wiley & Sons, Chichester, pp. 3–16.
99. Recommended childhood immunization schedule—United States, January-June, 1966. Morb Mortal Wkly Rep 51/52:940–943.
100. Declaration of New York, September 10, (1990) New York, NY.
101. Ramachandran S, Russell PK. (1994) A new technological synthesis. The Children's Vaccine Initiative. Int J Tech Assess Health Care 10:193–196.
102. Scientific Advisory Group of Experts (SAGE). (1994) Global programme for vaccines and immunization. WHO/GPV/GEN/94.1. World Health Organization, Geneva.
103. Nowak R. (1994) U.S. national program going nowhere fast. Science 265:1375–1376.
104. Salisbury D. (1994) Do vaccines reach those who need them most? In: Cutts FT, Smith PG, eds. Vaccination and world health. John Wiley & Sons, Chichester, pp. 238–242.
105. Global Programme for Vaccines and Immunization. (1995) Immunization policy. World Health Organization Expanded Programme of Immunization/95.3. World Health Organization, Geneva, p. 15.
106. Lane JM, Ruben L, Neff JM, Miller JD. (1969) Complications of smallpox vaccination, 1968. National surveillance in the United States. N Engl J Med 281:1201–1205.
107. Institute of Medicine. (1985) New vaccine development: establishing priorities, vol I. Diseases of importance in the United States. National Academy Press, Washington, DC.
108. Institute of Medicine. (1986) New vaccine development: establishing priorities, vol II. Diseases of importance in developing countries. National Academy Press, Washington, DC.
109. Bloom B. (1986) Learning from leprosy: a perspective on immunology and the third world. J Immunol 137:i–x.
110. US Department of Health and Human Services. (1992) Report of the Task Force on Microbiology and Infectious Diseases. Public Health Service, National Institutes of Health, Bethesda, MD.
111. Morse SS, ed. (1993) Emerging viruses. Oxford University Press, New York, p. 1–317.
112. Murphy FA. (1994) New, emerging and re-emerging infectious diseases. Adv Virus Res 43:2–52.
113. Ada GL. (1994) The development of new vaccines. In: Cutts FC, Smith PG, eds. Vaccination and world health. John Wiley & Sons, Chichester, pp. 67–79.
114. Plotkin SA. (1994) Discussion. In: Cutts FC, Smith PG, eds. Vaccination and world health. John Wiley & Sons, Chichester, pp. 80–88.
115. Root RK. (1996) Host responses to infection: fever, hyperthermia and hypothermia. In: Root RK, Stamm W, Waldvogel F, Corey L, eds. Clinical infectious diseases: a practical approach. Oxford University Press, Oxford (in press).
116. Styrt B, Sugarman B. (1990) Antipyresis and fever. Arch Intern Med 150:1589–1596.
117. Brown E, Atkinson JP, Fearon DT. (1994) Innate immunity: 50 ways to kill a microbe. Curr Opin Immunol 6:73–74.
118. Ashman RB, Mullbacher A. (1984) Infectious disease, fever and the immune response. Immunol Today 5:268–271.
119. Mullbacher A. (1984) Hyperthermia and the generation and activity of murine influenza-immune cytotoxic T cells in vitro. J Virol 52:928–931.
120. Sweet C, Smith H. (1980) Pathogenicity of influenza viruses. Microbiol Rev 44:303–330.
121. Hussein RH, Sweet C, Collie MH, Smith H. (1982) Elevation of nasal viral levels by suppression of fever in ferrets infected with influenza viruses of differing virulence. J Infect Dis 145:520–524.
122. Mak NK, Schiltnecht E, Ada GL. (1983) Protection of mice against influenza virus infection: enhancement of non-specific cellular responses by *Corynebacterium parvum*. Cell Immunol 78:314–325.
123. Haller O. (1981) Inborn resistance of mice to influenza viruses. Curr Top Microbiol Immunol 92:25–52.

124. Dale DC. (1994) Physiology, function and role of the neutrophil in host defense. Amgen, Kew, Victoria, pp. 1–32.
125. Denson P, Mandell GL. (1990) Granulocyte phagocytes. In: Mandell GL, Douglas RG Jr, Bennett JL, eds. Principles and practice of infectious disease, 3rd ed. Churchill Livingstone, New York, pp. 81–101.
126. Yokoyama WM, Seaman WE. (1993) The Ly-49 and NKR-P1 gene families encoding lectin-like receptors on natural killer cells. Annu Rev Immunol 1:613–635.
127. Farrar MA, Schreiber RD. (1993) The molecular cell biology of interferon-γ and its receptor. Annu Rev Immunol 11:571–611.
128. Liebson PJ. (1995) MHC-recognizing receptors: they're not just for T cells anymore. Immunity 3:5–8.
129. Taterka J, Cebra JJ, Rubin DH. (1995) Characterization of cytotoxic cells from reovirus-infected SCID mice: activated cells express natural killer- and lymphokine-activated killer-like activity but fail to clear infection. J Virol 69:3910–3914.
130. Bancroft GJ, Schreiber RD, Unanue ER. (1992) Natural immunity: a T cell-independent pathway of macrophage activation, defined in the SCID mouse. Immunol Rev 124:5–24.
131. Mond JJ, Carman J, Ohara SC, Finkelman FD. (1986) Interferon gamma suppresses B cell stimulation factor (BSF-1) induction of class II MHC determinants on B cells. J Immunol 137:3534–3537.
132. Pujol-Borrell R, Todd I, Doshi M, et al. (1987) HLA class II induction in human islet cells by interferon gamma plus tumor necrosis factor or lymphotoxin. Nature 326:304–306.
133. Adams DO, Hamilton TA. (1984) The cell biology of macrophage activation. Annu Rev Immunol 2:283–318.
134. Mantovani A, Dejana E. (1989) Cytokines as communication signals between leukocytes and endothelial cells. Immunol Today 10:370–375.
135. Buchmeier NA, Schreiber RD. (1985) Requirement of endogenous interferon gamma for resolution of *Listeria monocytogenes* infection. Proc Natl Acad Sci USA 82:7404–7408.
136. Susuki Y, Orellana MA, Schreiber RD, Remington JS. (1988) Interferon gamma: the major mediator of resistance against *Toxoplasma gondii*. Science 240:516–518.
137. Green SJ, Crawford RM, Hockmeyer JT, Meltzer MS, Nacy CA. (1990) *Leishmana major* amastigotes initiate L-arginine-dependent killing mechanism in IFN-gamma-stimulated macrophages by induction of tumor necrosis factor-alpha. J Immunol 145:4290–4297.
138. Karupiah G, Xie Q-W, Buller ML, et al. (1993) Inhibition of viral replication by interferon-γ-induced nitric oxide synthase. Science 261:1445–1448.
139. Welsh RM. (1978) Cytotoxic cells induced during lymphocytic choriomeningitis virus infection of mice. 1. Characterization of NK cell induction. J Exp Med 148:163–174.
140. Hirsch RL. (1982) The complement system: its importance in the host response to viral infection. Microbiol Rev 46:71–85.
141. Aaskov JG, Hadding U, Bitter-Suermann D. (1985) Interaction of Ross River virus with the complement system. J Gen Virol 66:121–129.
142. Jokiranta TS, Jokiph L, Meri S. (1995) Complement resistance of parasites. Scand J Immunol 42:9–20.
143. Doukas J, Pober JS. (1990) IFN-gamma enhances endothelial activation induced by tumor necrosis factor but not IL-1. J Immunol 145:1727–1733.
144. Munro JM, Pober JS, Cotran RS. (1989) Tumor necrosis factor and interferon gamma induce distinct patterns of endothelial activation and associated leukocyte accumulation in skin of *Papio anubis*. Am J Pathol 135:121–131.
145. Erbe DV, Collis JE, Shen L, Graziano RF, Fanger MW. (1990) The effect of cytokines on the expression and function of Fc receptors for IgG on human myeloid cells. Mol Immunol 27:57–67.
146. Strunk R, Cole FS, Perlmutter DH, Colten HR. (1985) Gamma interferon increases expression of class III complement genes C2 and factor B in human monocytes and in murine fibroblasts transfected with human C2 and factor B genes. J Biol Chem 260:15280–15285.
147. Aversa G, Punnonen J, De Vries JE. (1993) The 26 kD transmembrane form of tumor necrosis factor alpha on activated CD4 + T cell clones provides a costimulatory signal for human B cell activation. J Exp Med 177:1575–1585.
148. Snapper CM, Yamagguchi H, Moorman MA, et al. (1993) Natural killer cells induce activated murine B cells to secrete Ig. J Immunol 151:5251–5280.

149. Fearon DT, Carter RH. (1995) The CD19/CR2/TAPA-1 complex of B lymphocytes; linking natural to acquired immunity. Annu Rev Immunol 13:127–140.

150. Kincade PW, Gimble JM. (1993) B lymphocytes. In: Paul WE, ed. Fundamental immunology, 3rd ed. Raven Press, New York, pp. 43–74.

151. Sprent J. (1993) T lymphocytes and the thymus. In: Paul WE, ed. Fundamental immunology, 3rd ed. Raven Press, New York, pp. 75–110.

152. Williams AF, Barclay AN. (1988) The immunoglobulin superfamily—domains for cell surface recognition. Annu Rev Immunol 6:381–405.

153. Roes J, Rajewsky K. (1993) Immunoglobulin D (IgD)-deficient mice reveal an auxiliary receptor function for IgD in antigen-mediated recruitment of B cells. J Exp Med 177:45–55.

154. Van Oss CJ. (1992) Antigen:antibody reactions. In: Van Regenmortel MHV, ed. Structure of antigens. CRC Press, Boca Raton, FL, pp. 99–126.

155. Van Regenmortel MHV. (1992) Molecular dissection of protein antigens. In: Van Regenmortel MHV, ed. Structure of antigens. CRC Press, Boca Raton, FL, pp. 1–27.

156. Nara PL, Smit L, Dunlop N, et al. (1990) Emergence of viruses resistant to neutralization by V3 specific antibodies in experimental human immunodeficiency virus type IIIB infection of chimpanzees. J Virol 64:3779–3791.

157. Parry N, Fox G, Rowlands D, et al. (1990) Structural and serological evidence for a novel method of antigenic variation in foot and mouth disease virus. Nature 347:569–572.

158. Stern LJ, Brown JH, Jardetzky TS, et al. (1994) Crystal structure of the human class II MHC protein HLA-DR1 complexed with an influenza virus peptide. Nature 368:215–221.

159. Bjorkman PJ, Saper MA, Samraoui B, et al. (1987) Structure of the human class I histocompatibility antigen. Nature 329:506–511.

160. Unanue ER. (1993) Macrophages, antigen-presenting cells and the phenomena of antigen handling and presentation. In: Paul WE, ed. Fundamental immunology, 3rd ed. Raven Press, New York, pp. 111–144.

161. Lafferty KJ, Warren HS, Woolnough JA, Talmage DW. (1978) Immunological induction of T lymphocytes. Role of antigen and the lymphocyte costimulator. Blood Cells 4:395–404.

162. Welch PA, Namen AE, Goodwin RG, Armitage R, Cooper MD. (1989) Human IL-7: a novel T cell growth factor. J Immunol 143:3562–3566.

163. Alderson MR, Sassenfeld HM, Widmer MB. (1990) Interleukin-7 enhances cytolytic T lymphocyte generation and induces lymphokine-activated killer cells from human peripheral blood. J Exp Med 172:577.

164. Kos FJ, Mullbacher A. (1992) Induction of primary anti-viral cytotoxic T cells by in vitro stimulation with short synthetic peptide and interleukin-7. Eur J Immunol 22:3183–3185.

165. Kos FJ, Mullbacher A. (1993) IL-2-independent activity of IL-7 in the generation of secondary antigen-specific cytotoxic T cell responses in vitro. J Immunol 150:387–393.

166. Yssel H, Schneider PV, Lanier LL. (1993) Interleukin-7 specifically induces the B7/BB1 antigen on human cord blood and peripheral blood T cells and T cell clones. Int Immunol 5:753–759.

167. Elliott T, Smith M, Driscoll P, McMichael A. (1993) Peptide selection by class I molecules of the major histocompatibility complex. Curr Biol 3:854–866.

168. Arnoldi J, Kaufmann SHE. (1994) The contribution of CD8+ cytolytic T cells to the control of bacterial and parasitic infections. In: Ada GL, ed. Strategies in vaccine design. RG Landes, Austin, TX, pp. 83–112.

169. Mossmann TR, Coffman RL. (1987) Two types of mouse helper T cell clones—implications for immune regulation. Immunol Today 8:223–227.

170. Mossmann TR, Schumacher JH, Street NF, et al. (1991) Diversity of cytokine synthesis and function of mouse CD4+ T cells. Immunol Rev 123:209–229.

171. Firestein S, Roeder WD, Laxer JA, et al. (1989) A new murine CD4+ T cell subset with an unrestricted cytokine profile. J Immunol 143:518–525.

172. Street NE, Schumacher JH, Fong TAT, et al. (1990) Heterogeneity of mouse helper T cells: evidence from bulk cultures and limit dilution cloning for precursors of TH1 and TH2 cells. J Immunol 144:1629–1639.

173. Heinzel FP, Sadick MD, Holaday BJ, Coffman RL, Locksley RM. (1989) Reciprocal expression of interferon gamma or IL-4 during the resolution or progression of murine leishmaniasis. Evidence for expansion of distinct helper T cell subsets. J Exp Med 169:59–72.

174. Henzel FP, Sadick MD, Mutha SS, Locksley RM. (1991) Production of IFN-γ, IL-2, IL-4 and IL-10 by CD4+ lymphocytes during healing and progressive murine leishmaniasis. Proc Natl Acad Sci USA 88:7011–7015.

175. Sadick MD, Heinzel FP, Holaday BJ, et al. (1990) Cure of murine leishmaniasis with anti-interleukin 4 monoclonal antibody. Evidence for a T cell-dependent, interferon gamma-independent mechanism. J Exp Med 171:115–122.

176. Scott P, Pearce E, Cheever AW, Coffmann RL, Sher A. (1989) Role of cytokines and CD4+ T cell subsets in the regulation of parasite immunity and disease. Immunol Rev 112:161–182.

177. Hsieh C-S, Macatonia SE, Tripp CS, et al. (1993) Development of TH1 CD4+ T cells through IL-12 produced by *Leishmania*-induced macrophages. Science 260:547–549.

178. Heinzel FP, Schoenhaut DS, Rerko RM, Rosser LE, Gately MK. (1993) Recombinant interleukin 12 cures mice infected with *Leishmania major*. J Exp Med 177:1505–1510.

179. Scott P. (1993) IL-12: initiation cytokine for cell-mediated immunity. Science 260:496–497.

180. Orange JS, Wolf SF, Biron CA. (1994) Effects of IL-12 on the response and susceptibility to experimental viral infections. J Immunol 152:1253–1265.

181. Trinchieri G, Scott P, eds. (1995) Interleukin-12: a proinflammatory cytokine with immunoregulatory functions. Res Immunol 146:423–651.

182. Bretscher PA. (1992) Establishment of stable cell-mediated immunity that makes "susceptible" mice resistant to *Leishmania major*. Science 257:539–542.

183. Bretscher PA. (1994) Requirements and basis for efficacious vaccination by a low antigen dose regimen against intracellular pathogens uniquely susceptible to a cell-mediated attack. In: Ada GL, ed. Strategies for vaccine design. RG Landes, Austin, TX, pp. 99–112.

184. Del Prete CF, De Carli M, Mastromauro C, et al. (1991) Purified protein derivative (PPD) of *Mycobacterium tuberculosis* and excretory-secretory antigen(s) (TES) of *Toxocara canis* select human T cell clones with stable and opposite (TH1 or TH2) profiles of cytokine production. J Clin Invest 88:346–350.

185. Romagnani S. (1994) Lymphokine production by human T cells in disease states. Annu Rev Immunol 12:227–257.

186. Clerici M, Shearer G. (1993) A TH1 to TH2 switch is a critical step in the etiology of HIV infection. Immunol Today 14:107–111.

187. Montaner LJ, Shearer GM, Virelizier JL. (1994) Cytokine HIV regulation in macrophages and lymphocytes and in AIDS pathogenesis: from in vitro to in vivo. The 60th forum in immunology. Res Immunol 145:575–725.

188. Keene JA, Forman J. (1982) Helper activity is required for the in vivo generation of cytotoxic T cells. J Exp Med 155:768–782.

189. Buller RM, Holmes KJ, Hugin A, et al. (1987) Induction of cytotoxic T cell responses in vivo in the absence of CD4+ helper cells. Nature 328:77–79.

190. Wu Y, Liu Y. (1994) Viral induction of co-stimulatory activity on antigen-presenting cells bypasses the need for CD4+ T-cell help in CD8+ T-cell responses. Curr Biol 4:500–505.

191. Mullbacher A, Ada GL. (1987) How do cytotoxic T cells work in vivo? Microb Pathog 3:315–318.

192. Kyburz D, Speiser DE, Battegay M, Hengartner H, Zinkernagel RM. (1993) Lysis of infected cells in vivo by anti-viral cytotoxic T cells demonstrated by release of cell internal viral proteins. Eur J Immunol 23:1540–1545.

193. Tschopp J, Nabholz M. (1990) Perforin-mediated target cell lysis by cytolytic T lymphocytes. Annu Rev Immunol 8:279–302.

194. Kagi D, Ledermann B, Burki K, et al. (1994) Cytotoxicity mediated by T cells and natural killer cells is greatly impaired in perforin-deficient mice. Nature 369:31–36.

195. Harty JT, Bevan MJ. (1995) Specific immunity to Listeria monocytogenes in the absence of IFN-γ. Immunity 3:109–117.

196. Kagi D, Ledermann B, Burki K, et al. (1994) CD8+ T cell-mediated protection against an intracellular bacterium by perforin-dependent cytotoxicity. Eur J Immunol 24:3068–3072.

197. Ramshaw I, Ruby J, Ramsay A, Ada GL, Karupiah G. (1992) Expression of cytokines by recombinant vaccinia viruses. A model for studying cytokines in viral infections in vivo. Immunol Rev 127:157–182.

198. Lin Y-L, Askonas BA. (1981) Biological properties of an influenza virus-specific killer cell clone. J Exp Med 154:225–234.

199. Ruby J, Ramshaw IA. (1991) The anti-viral activity of immune CD8+ T cells is dependent upon interferon-γ. Lymph Cytol Res 10:353–358.

200. Zinkernagel RM. (1996) Immunology taught by viruses. Science 271:173–178.
201. Huang S, Hendriks W, Althage A, et al. (1993) Immune response in mice that lack the interferon-γ receptor. Science 259:1742–1745.
202. Misko IS, Pope JS, Hutter R, et al. (1984) HLA-DR antigen-associated restriction of EBV-specific cytotoxic T cell clones. Int J Cancer 33:239–243.
203. Lukacher AE, Morrison LA, Braciale VA, et al. (1985) Expression of specific cytolytic activity by H-2 I-region-restricted influenza-specific T lymphocyte clones. J Exp Med 162:171–187.
204. Orentas RJ, Hildreth JF, Obeh E, et al. (1990) Induction of human CD4 cytotoxic T cells specific for HIV-infected cells by a gp160 subunit vaccine. Science 248:1234–1237.
205. Muller D, Koller BH, Whitton JL, et al. (1992) LCMV-specific class II-restricted cytotoxic T cells in B_2-microglobulin deficient mice. Science 255:1576–1577.
206. Spriggs MK, Koller BH, Sato T, et al. (1992) $β_2$-Microglobulin-CD8+ T cell-deficient mice survive inoculation with high doses of vaccinia virus and exhibit altered IgG responses. Proc Natl Acad Sci USA 89:6070–6074.
207. Rothstein TL, Wang JKM, Panka DJ, et al. (1995) Protection against Fas-dependent TH1–mediated apoptosis by antigen receptor engagement in B cells. Nature 374:163–165.
208. Doherty PC. (1995) Cytotoxic T cell effector and memory function in viral immunity. In: Chisari FV, Oldstone MBA, eds. Transgenic models of human viral and immunological disease. Springer, Berlin, pp. 1–14.
209. Seder RA, Boulay JL, Finkelman F, et al. (1992) CD8+ T cells can be primed in vitro to produce IL-4. J Immunol 148:1652–1656.
210. Erard F, Wild MT, Garcia-Sanz JA, Le Gros GG. (1993) Switch of CD8+ T cells to non-cytolytic CD8– CD4– cells that make TH2 cytokines and help B cells. Science 260:1802–1805.
211. Croft M, Carter L, Swain SL, Dutton RW. (1994) Generation of polarized antigen-specific CD8+ effector populations: reciprocal action of IL-4 and IL-12 in promoting type 2 versus type 1 cytokine profiles. J Exp Med 180:1715–1728.
212. Maggi E, Giudizi MG, Biagiotti R, et al. (1994) TH2–like CD8+ T cells showing B helper function and reduced cytolytic activity in human immunodeficiency virus type 1 infection. J Exp Med 180:489–495.
213. Paganelli R, Scala E, Ansotegui IJ, et al. (1994) CD8+ T lymphocytes provide helper activity for IgE synthesis in human immunodeficiency virus-infected patients with hyper IgE. J Exp Med 181:423–428.
214. Ada GL, Blanden RV. (1994) CTL immunity and cytokine regulation in viral infection. Res Immunol 145:625–629.
215. Seder RA, Le Gros GG. (1995) The functional role of CD8+ T helper type 2 cells. J Exp Med 181:5–7.
216. McMichael AJ, Ting A, Zweerink HJ, Askonas BA. (1977) HLA restriction of cell mediated lysis of influenza-infected human cells. Nature 270:524–526.
217. McMichael AJ, Michie CA, Gotch FM, Moss B. (1986) Recognition of influenza virus nucleoprotein by human cytotoxic T lymphocytes. J Gen Virol 67:719–726.
218. Kuwano K, Scott M, Young JF, Ennis FA. (1988) HA2 subunit of influenza A H1 and H2 subtype viruses induces a prototype cross-reactive cytotoxic T lymphocyte response. J Immunol 140:1264–1268.
219. Hill AB, Lobigs M, Blanden RV, Kulkarni A, Mullbacher A. (1993) The cellular immune response to flaviviruses. In: Thomas DB, ed. Viruses and the cellular immune response. Marcel Dekker, New York, pp. 363–388.
220. Livingstone PG, Kurane I, Dai L-C, et al. (1995) Dengue virus specific HLA-B35–restricted, human CD8+ cytotoxic T cell clones. J Immunol 154:1287–1295.
221. Demkowicz WE, Ennis FA. (1993) Vaccinia virus-specific CD8+ cytotoxic T lymphocytes in humans. J Virol 67:1538–1544.
222. Rickinson AB, Moss DJ, Wallace LE, et al. (1981) Long-term cell-mediated immunity to Epstein-Barr virus. Cancer Res 41:4216–21.
223. Levy JA. (1993) Pathogenesis of human immunodeficiency virus infection. Microbiol Rev 57:183–289.
224. Modlin RL, Melancon-Kaplan J, Young SSM, et al. (1988) Learning from lesions: patterns of tissue inflammation in leprosy. Proc Natl Acad Sci USA 85:1213–1217.
225. Rossi GA, Balbi M, Manca F. (1987) Evidence for the selective presence of PPD-specific T lymphocytes at site of inflammation in the early stage of infection. Am Rev Respir Dis 136:575–579.

226. Sinigaglia F, Matile H, Pink JRL. (1987) *Plasmodium falciparum*-specific human T cell clones: evidence for helper and cytotoxic activities. Eur J Immunol 17:187–192.

227. Romero P, Maryanski L, Corradin G, et al. (1989) Cloned cytotoxic T cells recognize an epitope in the circumsporozoite protein and protect against malaria. Nature 341:323–325.

228. Malik A, Egan E, Houghten RA, et al. (1991) Human cytotoxic T lymphocytes against the *Plasmodium falciparum* circumsporozoite protein. Proc Natl Acad Sci USA 88:3300–3303.

229. Doolan DL, Houghten RA, Good MF. (1991) Location of human cytotoxic T cell epitopes within a polymorphic domain of the *Plasmodium falciparum* circumsporozoite protein. Int Immunol 3:511–518.

230. Hill AVS, Elvin J, Willis AC, et al. (1992) Molecular analysis of the association of HLA-B53 and resistance to severe malaria. Nature 360:434–438.

231. Hodgkin PD, Basten A. (1995) B cell activation, tolerance and antigen presenting function. Curr Opin Immunol 7:114–122.

232. Blanchard D, Gaillard C, Hermann P, Banchereau J. (1994) Role of CD40 antigen and inter-leukin-2 in T cell-dependent human B lymphocyte growth. Eur J Immunol 24:330–335.

233. Van den Eartwegh AJ, Noelle RJ, Roy M, et al. (1993) In vivo CD40-gp39 interactions are essential for thymus-dependent humoral immunity. 1. In vivo expression of CD40 ligand, cytokines, and antibody production delineates sites of cognate T-B cell interactions. J Exp Med 178:1555–1565.

234. Nemazee D, Burki K. (1989) Clonal deletion of B lymphocytes in a transgenic mouse bearing anti-MHC class antibody genes. Nature 337:562–566.

235. Hartley SB, Cooke MP, Fulcher DA, et al. (1993) Elimination of self-reactive B lymphocytes proceeds in two stages: arrested development and cell death. Cell 72:325–335.

236. Goodnow CC, Crosbie J, Adelstein S, et al. (1988) Altered immunoglobulin expression and functional silencing of self-reactive B lymphocytes in transgenic mice. Nature 334:676–682.

237. Goodnow CC, Crosbie J, Jorgensen H, Brink RA, Basten A. (1989) Induction of self tolerance in mature peripheral B lymphocytes. Nature 342:385–391.

238. Kennedy MK, Mohler KM, Shanebeeck KD, et al. (1994) Induction of B cell costimulatory function by recombinant murine CD40 ligand. Eur J Immunol 24:116–123.

239. Eris JM, Basten A, Brink R, Doherty K, Kehry MR, Hodgkin PD. (1994) Anergic, self-reacting B cells present self antigen and respond normally to CD40-dependent T cell signals but are defective in antigen-receptor-mediated functions. Proc Natl Acad Sci USA 91:4392–4396.

240. Nossal GJV. (1994) Negative selection of lymphocytes. Cell 76:229–239.

241. Von Boehmer H. (1994) Positive selection of lymphocytes. Cell 76:219–228.

242. Picker LJ, Siegelman MH. (1993) Lymphoid tissues and organs. In: Paul WE, ed. Fundamental immunology, 3rd ed. Raven Press, New York, pp. 145–198.

243. Rowley D, Turner KJ. (1966) Number of molecules of antibody required to phagocytose one bacterium. Nature 210:496–499.

244. Gray D, Skarvall H. (1988) B cell memory is short-lived in the absence of antigen. Nature 336:70–72.

245. Burton GF, Kapasi ZF, Szakal AK, Tew JG. (1994) The generation of antibody and B cell memory: the role of retained antigen and follicular dendritic cells. In: Ada GL, ed. Strategies for vaccine design. RG Landes, Austin, TX, pp. 35–50.

246. Wang D, Wells SM, Stall AM, Kabat EA. (1994) Reaction of germinal centers in the T cell-independent response to the bacterial polysaccharide $\alpha(1-6)$ dextran. Proc Natl Acad Sci USA 91:2502–2506.

247. Kosko-Vilbois MH, ed. (1995) An antigen depository of the immune system: follicular dendritic cells. Curr Top Microbiol Immunol 201:1–209.

248. Kapasi ZF, Burton GF, Schultz LD, Tew J, Szakal AK. (1993) Induction of functional follicular dendritic cell development in severe combined immunodeficiency mice. J Immunol 150:2648–2658.

249. Mandel TE, Phipps RP, Abbot A, Tew JG. (1980) The follicular dendritic cell: long term antigen retention during immunity. Immunol Rev 53:29–59.

250. Tenner-Racz K, Racz P. (1995) Follicular dendritic cells initiate and maintain infection of the germinal centers by human immunodeficiency virus. Curr Top Microbiol Immunol 201:141–160.

251. Heath SL, Tew J Grant, Tew JG, Szakal AK, Burton GF. (1995) Follicular dendritic cells and human immunodeficiency virus infectivity. Nature 377:740–744.

252. Ada GL. (1991) Vaccination and the immune response. Curr Biol 1:221–222.

253. Nossal GJV, Ada GL. (1971) Antigens, lymphoid cells and the immune response. Academic Press, New York, pp. 1–324.

254. Gray D. (1993) Immunological memory. Annu Rev Immunol 11:49–77.
255. Bruce J, Symington FW, McKearn J, Sprent J. (1981) A monoclonal discriminating between subsets of T and B cells. J Immunol 127:2446–2451.
256. Linton P-J, Klinman NR. (1992) The generation of memory B cells. Semin Immunol 4:3–9.
257. Linton P-J, Decker D, Klinman NR. (1989) Primary antibody forming cells and secondary B cells are generated from separate precursor populations. Cell 59:1949–1959.
258. Linton P-J, Lo D, Lai L, Thorbecke JG, Klinman NR. (1992) Among naive precursor cell subpopulations, only progenitors of memory B cells originate germinal centers. Eur J Immunol 22:1293–1297.
259. Johnson JG, Jemmerson R. (1991) Relative frequencies of secondary B cells activated by cognate vs other mechanisms. Eur J Immunol 21:951–958.
260. Terry LA, Brown MH, Beverly PC. (1988) The monoclonal antibody, UCHL-1, recognises a 180,000 MW component of the human leucocyte-common antigen, CD45. Immunology 64:331–336.
261. Dianzani U, Lugman M, Rojo J, et al. (1990) Molecular associations on the T cell surface correlate with immunological memory. Eur J Immunol 20:2249–2257.
262. Powrie F, Mason DW. (1990) Subsets of rats CD4 + T cells defined by their differential expression of variants of the CD45 antigen: developmental relationships and in vitro and in vivo functions. Curr Top Microbiol Immunol 159:79–96.
263. Byrne JA, Butler JL, Cooper MD. (1988) Differential activation requirements for virgin and memory T cells. J Immunol 141:3249–3257.
264. Mullbacher A, Flynn K. (1996) Aspects of cytotoxic T cell memory. Immunol Rev 150:113–128.
265. Ashman RB. (1982) Persistence of cell mediated immunity to influenza A virus in mice. Immunology 47:165–168.
266. Eichelberger MC, Wang M, Allan W, et al. (1991) Influenza virus RNA in the lung and lymphoid tissue of immunologically intact and CD4-depleted mice. J Gen Virol 72:1695–1698.
267. Demkowicz WE, Littaua RA, Wang J, Ennis FA. (1996) Human cytotoxic T cell memory: long-lived responses to vaccinia virus. J Virol 70:2627–2631.
268. Gray D, Matzinger P. (1991) T cell memory is short-lived in the absence of antigen. Nature 336:969–974.
269. Mullbacher A. (1994) The long-term maintenance of cytotoxic T cell memory does not require persistence of antigen. J Exp Med 179:317–321.
270. Hou S, Hyland L, Ryan KW, Portner A, Doherty PC. (1994) Virus-specific CD8 + T-cell memory is determined by clonal burst size. Nature 369:652–654.
271. Lau LL, Jamieson BD, Somasundaram T, Ahmed R. (1994) Cytotoxic T cell memory without antigen. Nature 369:648–651.
272. Mak N-K, Sweet C, Ada GL, Tannock GA. (1984) The sensitization of mice with wild-type and cold-adapted variant of influenza A virus. II. Secondary cytotoxic T cell responses. Immunology 51:407–416.
273. Jones PD, Ada GL. (1987) Persistence of influenza virus-specific antibody-secreting cells and B cell memory after primary murine influenza virus infection. Cell Immunol 109:53–64.
274. Schittek B, Rajewsky K. (1990) Maintenance of B cell memory by long-lived cells generated from proliferating precursors. Nature 346:749–751.
275. Haas W, Pereira P, Tonegawa S. (1993) Gamma/delta cells. Annu Rev Immunol 11:637–686.
276. Sim G-K. (1995) Intraepithelial lymphocytes and the immune system. Adv Immunol 58:297–334.
277. Besredka A. (1919) De la vaccination contre les etats typhoides par voie buccale. Ann Inst Pasteur 33:882–903.
278. Chodirker WB, Tomasi TB Jr. (1963) Gamma globulins: quantitative relationships in human serum and nonvascular fluids. Science 142:1080–1081.
279. Halpern MS, Koshland ME. (1970) Novel subunit in secretory IgA. Nature 223:1276–1279.
280. Brandtzaeg P. (1989) Overview of the mucosal immune system. Curr Top Microbiol Immunol 146:13–25.
281. Czerkinsky C, Holmgren J. (1995) The mucosal immune system and prospects for anti-infectious and anti-inflammatory vaccines. Immunologist 3:97–103.
282. Rudzik O, Clancy RL, Perey DYE, Day RP, Bienenstock J. (1975) Repopulation with IgA-containing cells of bronchial and intestinal lamina propria after transfer of homologous Peyer's patches and bronchial lymphocytes. J Immunol 114:1599–1604.
283. Mestecky J. (1987) The common mucosal immune system and current strategies for induction of immune responses in external secretions. J Clin Immunol 7:265–276.

284. Owen RL, Jones AL. (1974) Epithelial cell specialization within human Peyer's patches: an ultra-structural study of intestinal lymphoid follicles. Gastroenterology 66:189–203.
285. Lebman DA, Griffin PM, Cebra JJ. (1987) Relationship between expression of IgA by Peyer's patch cells and functional IgA memory cells. J Exp Med 166:1405–1418.
286. Craig SW, Cebra JJ. (1971) Peyer's patches: an enriched source of precursors for IgA-producing immunocytes in the rabbit. J Exp Med 134:188–200.
287. Bienenstock J, Johnston N, Perey DYE. (1973) Bronchial lymphoid tissue. I. Morphological characteristics. Lab Invest 28:686–692.
288. Pabst R. (1992) Is BALT a major component of the human lung immune system? Immunol Today 13:119–121.
289. Picker LJ. (1994) Control of lymphocyte homing. Curr Opin Immunol 6:390–406.
290. Cepek KL, Shaw SK, Parker CM, et al. (1994) Adhesion between epithelial cells and T lymphocytes mediated by E-cadherin and the $\alpha E\beta 7$ integrin. Nature 372:190–193.
291. Guy-Grand D, Malassis-Seris M, Briottet C, Vassalli P. (1991) Cytotoxic differentiation of mouse gut thymodependent and independent intraepithelial T lymphocytes is induced locally. Correlation between functional assays, presence of perforin and granzyme transcripts, and cytotoxic granules. J Exp Med 173:1549–1552.
292. Weiner HL. (1994) Oral tolerance. Proc Natl Acad Sci USA 91:10762–10765.
293. Blumberg RS, Balk SP. (1994) Recognition of intestinal epithelial cell ligands by T cells. Mucos Immunol Update 2:3–5.
294. Miller CJ, McGhee JR, Gardner MB. (1992) Mucosal immunity, HIV transmission and AIDS. Lab Invest 68:129–145.
295. Kawanishi H, Saltzman L, Strober W. (1983) Mechanisms regulating IgA class-specific immunoglobulin production in murine gut-associated lymphoid tissue. I. T cells derived from Peyer's patches that switch sIgM cells to sIgA cells in vitro. J Exp Med 157:433–450.
296. Ramsay AJ. (1995) Genetic approaches to the study of cytokine regulation of mucosal immunity. Immunol Cell Biol 73:484–488.
297. Defrance T, Vanbervliet B, Briere F, et al. (1992) Interleukin-10 and transforming growth factor beta co-operate to induce anti-CD40–activated naive human B cells to secrete immunoglobulin A. J Exp Med 175:671–682.
298. Taguchi T, McGhee JR, Coffman RL, et al. (1990) Analysis of Th1 and Th2 cells in murine gut-associated tissues. Frequencies of CD4[+] and CD8[+] T cells that secrete IFNγ and IL-5. J Immunol 145:68–77.
299. Xu-Amano J, Kiyono H, Jackson R, et al. (1992) Helper T cell subsets for immunoglobulin A responses: oral immunisation with tetanus toxoid and cholera toxin as adjuvant selectively induces Th2 cells in mucosa-associated lymphoid tissues. J Exp Med 172:921–929.
300. Lin Y, Shockett P, Stavnezer J. (1991) Regulation of the antibody class switch to IgA. Immunol Res 10:376–380.
301. Vajdy M, Kosco-Vilbois MH, Kopf M, et el. (1995) Impaired mucosal immune responses in interleukin 4-targeted mice. J Exp Med 181:41–53.
302. Ehrhardt RO, Strober W, Harriman GR. (1992) Effects of transforming growth factor (TGF)-$\beta 1$ on IgA isotype expression. TGF-$\beta 1$ induces a small increase in sIgA[+] cells regardless of the method of B cell activation. J Immunol 148:3830–3836.
303. Islam KB, Nilsson L, Sideras P, et al. (1991) TGF-beta-1 induces germline transcripts of both IgA subclasses in human B lymphocytes. Int Immunol 3:1099–1106.
304. Kopf M, Brombacher F, Hodgkin PD, et al. (1996) IL-5–deficient mice have a developmental defect in CD5[+] B-1 cells and lack eosinophilia but have normal antibody and cytotoxic T cell responses. Immunity 4:15–24.
305. Ramsay AJ, Husband AJ, Ramshaw IA, et al. (1994) The role of interleukin-6 in mucosal IgA responses in vivo. Science 264:561–563.
306. Beagley KW, Bao S, Ramsay AJ, et al. (1995) IgA production by peritoneal cavity B cells is IL-6-independent: implications for intestinal IgA responses. Eur J Immunol 25:2123–2126.
307. Pecquet SS, Ehrat C, Ernst PB. (1992) Enhancement of mucosal antibody responses to *Salmonella typhimurium* and the microbial hapten phosphorylcholine in mice with X-linked immunodeficiency by B-cell precursors from the peritoneal cavity. Infect Immun 60:503–509.
308. Kroese GFM, Butcher GC, Stall AM, et al. (1998) Many of the IgA-producing plasma cells in the murine gut are derived from self-replenishing precursors in the peritoneal cavity. Int Immunol 1:75–84.

309. Brandtzaeg P. (1995) Basic mechanisms of mucosal immunity. Immunologist 3:89–96.
310. Mazanec MB, Nedrud JG, Kaetzel CS, Lamm ME. (1993) A three-tiered view of the role of IgA in mucosal defense. Immunol Today 14:430–435.
311. Dimmock NJ, Taylor JP, Carver AS. (1993) Interaction of neutralised influenza virus with avian and mammalian cells. In: Compans RW, Bishop DWL, eds. Segmented negative strand viruses. Raven Press, New York, pp. 355–365.
312. Wold AE, Mestecky J, Tomana M. (1990) Secretory immunoglobulin A carries oligosaccharide receptors for *Escherichia coli* type 1 fimbrial lectin. Infect Immun 58:3073–3077.
313. Kilian M, Mestecky J, Russell MW. (1988) Defense mechanisms involving Fc-dependent functions of immunoglobulin A and their subversion by immunoglobulin A proteases. Microbiol Rev 52:296–303.
314. Tagliabue A. (1989) Immune response to oral *Salmonella* vaccines. Curr Top Microbiol Immunol 146:225–231.
315. Davies MDJ, Parrott DMW. (1981) Cytotoxic T cells in small intestine epithelium, lamina propria and lung lymphocytes. Immunology 44:367–371.
316. Klein JR, Kagnoff MF. (1987) Spontaneous in vitro evolution of lytic specificity of cytotoxic T lymphocyte clones isolated from murine intestinal epithelium. J Immunol 138:58–62.
317. Issekutz TB. (1984) The response of gut-associated T lymphocytes to intestinal viral immunisation. J Immunol 133:2955–2960.
318. Offit PA, Dudzik KI. (1989) Rotavirus-specific cytotoxic T lymphocytes appear at the intestinal mucosal surface after rotavirus infection. J Virol 63:3507–3512.
319. Lohman BL, Miller CJ, McChesney MB. (1995) Anti-viral cytotoxic T lymphocytes in the vaginal mucosa of simian immunodeficiency virus-infected rhesus macaques. J Immunol 155:5855–5861.
320. Wells H. (1911) Studies on the chemistry of anaphylaxis. III. Experiments with isolated proteins, especially those of hen's egg. J Infect Dis 9:147–171.
321. Chase MW. (1946) Inhibition of experimental drug allergy by prior feeding of the sensitizing agent. Proc Soc Exp Biol 61:257–259.
322. Mowat AM. (1987) The regulation of immune responses to dietary protein antigens. Immunol Today 8:93–98.
323. Whitacre C, Gienapp C, Orosz IE, Bitar D. (1991) Oral tolerance in experimental immune encephalomyelitis. III. Evidence for clonal anergy. J Immunol 147:2155–2163.
324. Chen Y, Kuhroo VK, Inobe JI, Hafler DA, Weiner HL. (1994) Regulatory T cell clones induced by oral tolerance: suppression of autoimmune encephalomyelitis. Science 265:1237–1240.
325. Sun JB, Holmgren J, Czerkinsky C. (1994) Cholera toxin B subunit: an efficient transmucosal delivery system for induction of peripheral tolerance. Proc Natl Acad Sci USA 91:10795–10799.
326. Elson CO, Ealding W. (1984) Cholera toxin did not induce oral tolerance in mice and abrogated oral tolerance to an unrelated antigen. J Immunol 133:2892–2897.
327. Burnet FM, Fenner F. (1949) The production of antibodies, 2nd ed. Macmillan, Melbourne, pp. 1–142.
328. Medawar PB. (1945) A second study of the behaviour and fate of skin homografts in rabbits. J Anat 79:157–176.
329. Lawton AR. (1994) Immunization of the neonate. Int J Technol Assess Health Care 10:154–160.
330. Solvason N, Kearney JF. (1992) The human fetal omentum. A site of B cell generation. J Exp Med 175:397–404.
331. Gathings WE, Lawton AR, Cooper MD. (1977) Immunofluorescent studies on the development of pre-B cells, B lymphocytes and immunoglobulin isotype diversity. Eur J Immunol 7:804–810.
332. Cancro MP, Wylie DE, Gerhard W, et al. (1979) Patterned acquisition of the antibody repertoire: diversity of the hemagglutinin-specific B cell repertoire in neonatal Balb/c mice. Proc Natl Acad Sci USA 76:6577–6581.
333. Sigal NH, Pickard AR, Metcalf ES, et al. (1977) Expression of phosphoryl choline-specific B cells during murine development. J Exp Med 146:933–948.
334. Gathings WE, Lawton AR, Cooper MD. (1977) Immunofluorescent studies on the development of pre-B cells, B lymphocytes and immunoglobulin isotype diversity. Eur J Immunol 7:804–810.
335. Gandini M, Kubagawa H, Gathings WE, et al. (1981) Expression of three immunoglobulin isotypes by individual B cells during development: implications for heavy chain switching. Am J Reprod Immunol 1:161–163.
336. Splawski JB, Lipsky PE. (1991) Cytokine regulation of immunoglobulin secretion by neonatal lymphocytes. J Clin Invest 88:967–977.

337. Clement LT, Vink PE, Bradley GE. (1990) Novel immunoregulatory functions of phenotypically distinct subpopulations of CD4 + cells in the human neonate. J Immunol 145:102–198.
338. Sidiropoulos D, Hermann U, Morell A, et al. (1986) Transplacental passage of intravenous immunoglobulin in the last trimester of pregnancy. J Pediatr 109:505–508.
339. de Almeida MFB, Schoettler JJ, Kornbrot BB, et al. (1988) IgG subclass levels in maternal and cord sera of appropriate and small-for-gestational age preterm and full-term newborn infants. J Allergy Clin Immunol 81:289–295.
340. Black FL. (1989) Measles active and passive immunity in a worldwide perspective. Prog Med Virol 36:1–33.
341. Insel RA, Amstey M, Woodin K, Pichichero M. (1994) Maternal immunization to prevent infectious diseases in the neonate and infant. Int J Technol Assess Health Care 10:143–153.
342. Weisz-Carrington P, Roux ME, McWilliams M, et al. (1979) Organ and isotype distribution of plasma cells producing specific antibody after oral administration. Evidence for a generalized secretory immune system. J Immunol 123:1705–1708.
343. Slade H, Schwartz S. (1987) Mucosal immunity: the immunology of breast milk. J Allergy Clin Immunol 80:348–358.
344. Gill TJ, Repetti CF, Metlay LA, et al. (1983) Transplacental immunization of the human fetus to tetanus by immunization of the mother. J Clin Invest 72:987–996.
345. McCormick J, Gusmao H, Nakamura S, et al. (1980) Antibody response to serogroup A and C meningococcal polysaccharide vaccine in infants born of mothers vaccinated during pregnancy. J Clin Invest 65:1141–1144.
346. Amstey MS, Insel RA, Munoz J, et al. (1985) Fetal-neonatal passive immunization against *Haemophilus influenzae*, type b. Am J Obstet Gynaecol 63:105–108.
347. Vanderbeeken Y, Sarfati M, Bose R, et al. (1985) In utero immunization of the fetus to tetanus by maternal immunization during pregnancy. Am J Reprod Immunol Microbiol 8:39–42.
348. Eloi-Santos SM, Novato-Silva E, Maselli VM, et al. (1989) Idiotypic sensitization in utero of children born to mothers with schistosomiasis or Chagas' disease. J Clin Invest 84:1028–1931.
349. Hahn-Zoric M, Carlsson B, Bjorkander J, et al. (1992) Presence of non-maternal antibodies in newborn of mothers with antibody deficiencies. Pediatr Res 32:150–154.
350. Ada GL, Jones PD. (1986) The immune response to influenza infection. Curr Top Microbiol Immunol 128:1–54.
351. Sharma DP, Ramsay AJ, Maguire DJ, Rolph MS, Ramshaw IA. (1996) Interleukin-4 mediates down regulation of antiviral cytokine expression and cytotoxic T-lymphocyte responses and exacerbates vaccinia virus infection in vivo. J Virol. 70 (in press).
352. Kent SJ, Clancy RL, Ada GL. (1995) Prospects for a prophylactic HIV vaccine. Med J Aust. 165 (in press).
353. Koup RA, Safrit JT, Cao Y, et al. (1994) Temporal association of cellular immune responses and initial control of viremia in HIV-1 infection. J Virol 68:4650–4655.
354. Borrow P, Lewicki H, Hahn BH, Shaw GM, Oldstone MAB. (1994) Virus-specific CD8 + cytotoxic T lymphocyte activity associated with control of viremia in primary human immunodeficiency virus type 1 infection. J Virol 68:6103–6110.
355. Nestorowizc A, Laver G, Jackson DC. (1985) Antigenic determinants of influenza virus hemagglutinin. X. A comparison of the physical and antigenic properties of monomeric and trimeric forms. J Gen Virol 65:1687–1695.
356. Rossman MG, Arnold E, Erickson JW, et al. (1985) Structure of a human common cold virus and functional relationships to other picornaviruses. Nature 317:145–153.
357. Minor PD, Ferguson M, Evans DMA, et al. (1986) Antigenic structure of polioviruses of serotypes 1, 2 and 3. J Gen Virol 67:1283–1291.
358. Almond JW, Burke KL. (1990) Polio as a vector for the presentation of foreign antigens. Semin Virol 1:11–20.
359. Acharya R, Fry E, Stuart D, et al. (1989) The three dimensional structure of foot and mouth disease virus at 2.9 A resolution. Nature 337:709–716.
360. LaRosa GJ, Davide JP, Weinhold K, et al. (1990) Conserved sequences and structural elements in the HIV-1 principal neutralizing determinant. Science 249:932–935.
361. Caldwell HD, Berry IJ. (1982) Neutralization of *Chlamydia trachomatis* infectivity with antibodies to the major outer membrane protein. Infect Immun 38:745–754.
362. Stephens RS, Sanchez-Pescador R, Wagar EA, et al. (1987) Diversity of *Chlamydia trachomatis* major outer membrane protein genes. J Bacteriol 169:3879–3885.

363. Zhang YX, Stewart S, Joseph T, Taylor HR, Caldwell HT. (1987) Protective monoclonal antibodies recognize epitopes located on the major outer membrane protein of *Chlamydia trachomatis*. J Immunol 138:575–581.
364. Mandel B. (1976) Neutralization of poliovirus: a hypothesis to explain the mechanism and the one-hit character of the neutralization reaction. Virology 69:500–510.
365. Wetz K, Willingman P, Zucchardt H, Harbermehl KV. (1986) Neutralization of poliovirus by polyclonal antibodies requires binding of a single IgG molecule per virion. Arch Virol 91:207–220.
366. Colman PM, Air GM, Webster RG, et al. (1987) How antibodies recognize viral proteins. Immunol Today 8:323–326.
367. Stein BS, Gowda SD, Lifson JD, et al. (1987) pH-independent entry into CD4-positive T cells via virus envelope fusion to the plasma membrane. Cell 49:659–668.
368. Possee RD, Schild DC, Dimmock NJ. (1982) Studies on the mechanism of neutralization by antibody: evidence that neutralizing antibody (anti-hemagglutinin) inactivates influenza virus in vivo by inhibiting virion transcriptase activity. J Gen Virol 58:373–386.
369. Taylor HP, Dimmock NJ. (1985) Mechanisms of neutralization of influenza virus by secretory IgA is different from that of monomeric IgA or IgG. J Exp Med 161:198–209.
370. Taylor HP, Dimmock NJ. (1985) Mechanism of neutralization of influenza virus by IgM. J Gen Virol 66:903–907.
371. Watson DL. (1987) Serological response of sheep to live and killed *Staphylococcus aureus* vaccines. Vaccine 5:275–278.
372. Shellam GR, Grundy JE, Harnett GB, Allen JE. (1986) Natural killer cells. Prog Immunol 6:209–217.
373. Bukowski JF, Woder BA, Welch RM. (1984) Pathogenesis of murine cytomegalovirus infection in natural killer cell-depleted mice. J Virol 52:119–128.
374. Rosenberg ZF, Fauci AS. (1993) Immunology of HIV infection. In: Paul WE, ed. Fundamental immunology. Raven Press, New York, pp. 1375–1398.
375. Liszewski MK, Atkinson JP. (1993) The complement system. In: Paul WE, ed. Fundamental immunology. Raven Press, New York, pp. 917–940.
376. Butterworth AE. (1984) Cell-mediated damage to helminths. Adv Parasitol 23:143–235.
377. Capron A, Dessaint JP, Capron M, Ouma JH, Butterworth AE. (1987) Immunity to schistosomes: progress towards vaccine. Science 238:1065–1072.
378. Hagan P, Blumenthal UJ, Dunn D, et al. (1991) Human, IgE, IgG4 and resistance to reinfection with *Schistosoma haematobium*. Nature 349:243–245.
379. Rihet P, Demeure CE, Burgois A, et al. (1991) Evidence for an association between human resistance to *Schistosoma mansoni* and high anti-larval IgE levels. Eur J Immunol 21:2679–2686.
380. Scott PA, Sher A. (1993) Immunoparasitology. In: Paul WE, ed. Fundamental vaccinology, 3rd ed. Raven Press, New York, pp. 1179–1210.
381. Ada GL. (1996) Overview of vaccines. In: Robinson A, Wiblin C, Farrar G, eds. Vaccine protocols. Humana Press, Totowa, New Jersey.
382. Shvartsman YS, Zykov MP. (1976) Secretory influenza immunity. Adv Immunol 22:291–330.
383. Maiztegui JI, Fernandez JI, de Damilano AJ. (1979) Efficacy of immune plasma in treatment of Argentine haemorrhagic fever and association between treatment and late neurological syndrome. Lancet 2:1216–1217.
384. Yap KL, Ada GL. (1979) The effect of specific antibody on the generation of cytotoxic T lymphocytes and the recovery of mice from influenza virus infection. Scand J Immunol 10:325–332.
385. Askonas BA, McMichael AJ, Webster RG. (1982) The immune response to influenza virus and the problem of protection against infection. In: Beare H, ed. Basic and applied influenza research. CRC Press, Boca Raton, FL, pp. 159–188.
386. Kris RM, Asofsky R, Evans CB, Small PA. (1985) Protection and recovery in influenza virus-infected mice immunosuppressed with anti-IgM. J Immunol 132:1230–1235.
387. Scherle PA, Palladino G, Gerhard W. (1992) Mice can recover from pulmonary influenza virus infection in the absence of class I restricted cytotoxic T cells. J Immunol 148:212–217.
388. Taylor G. (1994) The role of antibody in controlling and/or clearing virus infections. In: Ada GL, ed. Strategies in vaccine design. RG Landes, Austin, TX, pp. 17–34.
389. Griffin DE, Levine B, Tyor WB, Irani DN. (1992) The immune response in viral encephalitis. Semin Immunol 4:111–119.
390. Tishon AS, Eddelston M, de la Torre JC, Oldstone MBA. (1993) Cytotoxic T lymphocytes cleanse viral gene products from individually infected neurones and lymphocytes in mice persistently infected with lymphocytic choriomeningitis virus. Virology 187:463–467.

391. Blanden RV. (1974) Mechanisms of cell-mediated immunity in viral infection. In: Brent L, Holborow J, eds. Progress in immunology, vol 4. II: Clinical Aspects. North Holland, Amsterdam, pp. 117–125.
392. Zinkernagel RM, Welsh RM. (1976) H-2 compatibility requirements for virus-specific T cell-mediated effector functions in vivo. 1. Specificity of T cells conferring antiviral protection against lymphocytic choriomeningitis virus is associated with H-2K and H-2D. J Immunol 117:1495–1502.
393. Yap KL, Ada GL, McKenzie IFC. (1978) Transfer of specific cytotoxic T lymphocytes protects mice inoculated with influenza virus. Nature 273:238–239.
394. Nash AA, Phelan J, Wildy P. (1981) Cell-mediated immunity in herpes simplex virus infected mice: H-2 mapping of the delayed-type hypersensitivity response and the anti-viral T cell response. J Immunol 126:1260–1262.
395. Melief CJM, Kast WM. (1993) T-cell- and natural killer cell-mediated immunity to Sendai virus. In: Thomas DG, ed. Viruses and the cellular immune response. Marcel Dekker, New York, pp. 271–278.
396. Randall RE. (1993) Paramyxoviruses: the role of CD8+ T cells in protective immunity and the development of solid matrix-antibody-antigen complexes as vaccines. In: Thomas DG, ed. Viruses and the cellular immune response. Marcel Dekker, New York, pp. 293–313.
397. Cannon MJ, Stott EJ, Taylor G, Askonas BA. (1987) Clearance of persistent respiratory virus infections in immunodeficient mice following transfer of primed cells. Immunology 62:133–138.
398. Koszinowski UH, Reddehase MJ. (1993) The role of T lymphocyte subsets in the control of cytomegalovirus infection. In: Thomas DG, ed. Viruses and the cellular immune response. Marcel Dekker, New York, pp. 429–445.
399. Niewiesk S, Brinkmann U, Bankamp B, et al. (1993) Susceptibility to measles virus-induced encephalitis in mice correlates with impaired antigen presentation to cytotoxic T lymphocytes. J Virol 67:75–81.
400. Rodriguez M, Dunkel AJ, Thiemann RI, et al. (1993) Abrogation of resistance to Theiler's virus-induced demyelination in H-2$_b$ mice deficient in β_2-microglobulin. J Immunol 151:266–276.
401. Jackson DC, Ada GL, Tha Hla R. (1976) Cytotoxic T cells recognize very early minor changes in ectromelia virus-infected target cells. Aust J Exp Biol Med Sci 54:349–363.
402. Zinkernagel RM, Althage A. (1977) Anti-viral protection by virus-immune cytotoxic T cells: infected target cells are lysed before infectious virus progeny is assembled. J Exp Med 145:644–651.
403. Geisow M. (1991) Unravelling the mysteries of molecular audit: MHC class I restriction. Tibtech 9:403–404.
404. Gotch F, Rowland-Jones S, Nixon D. (1992) Longitudinal study of HIV-gag specific cytotoxic T lymphocytes responses over time in several patients. In: Racz P, Letvin NL, Gluckman JC, eds. Cytotoxic T cells in HIV and other retroviral infections. Karger, Basel, pp. 60–65.
405. Baier M, Werner A, Bannert M, et al. (1995) HIV suppression by interleukin-16. Nature 378:563.
406. Cocchi F, DeVic AL, Garzino-Demo A, et al. (1995) Identification of RANTES, MIP-1a, and MIP-1b as the major HIV-suppressive factors produced by CD8+ T cells. Science 270:1811–1813.
407. Cheynier R, Langlade-Demoyen P, Marescot M, et al. (1992) CTL responses in the PBMC of children born to HIV-1 infected mothers. Eur J Immunol 22:2211–2217.
408. Rowland-Jones SL, Sutton J, Ariyoshi K, et al. (1993) HIV-specific CTL activity in an HIV-exposed but uninfected infant. Lancet 341:860–861.
409. Langlade-Demoyen P, Ngo-Giang-Huong N, Ferchat F, Oksenhendler E. (1994) Human immunodeficiency virus (HIV) nef-specific cytotoxic T lymphocytes in noninfected heterosexual contact of HIV-infected patients. J Clin Invest 93:1293–1297.
410. Rowland-Jones S, Sutton J, Ariyoshi K, et al. (1995) HIV-specific cytotoxic T-cells in HIV-exposed but uninfected Gambian women. Nat Med 1:59–64.
411. Pinto LA, Sullivan J, Berzofsky JA. (1995) Env-specific cytotoxic T lymphocytes in HIV seronegative health care workers occupationally exposed to HIV-contaminated body fluids. J Clin Invest 96:867–876.
412. Yamamura M, Uyemura K, Deans RJ, et al. (1991) Defining protective responses to pathogens: cytokine profiles in leprosy lesions. Science 254:277–279.
413. Salgami P, Abrams JS, Clayberger C, et al. (1991) Differing lymphokine profiles of functional subsets of human CD4 and CD8 T cell clones. Science 254:279–282.
414. Modlin RL, Mehra VB, Wong L, et al. (1986) Suppressor T lymphocytes from lepromatous leprosy skin lesions. J Immunol 137:2831–2834.

415. Vandenberg J, Nussenzweig R, Most H. (1969) Protective immunity produced by injection of X-irradiated sporozoites of *P. berghei*. Mil Med 134:1183–1190.

416. Egan JE, Hoffman SL, Haynes JD, et al. (1993) Humoral immune responses in volunteers immunized with irradiated *Plasmodium falciparum* sporozoites. Am J Trop Med Hyg 49:166–173.

417. Kumar S, Miller LH, Quakyi IA, et al. (1988) Cytotoxic T cells specific for the circumsporozoite protein of *Plasmodium falciparum*. Nature 334:258–260.

418. Doolan DL, Houghton RA, Good MP. (1991) Location of human cytotoxic T cell epitopes within a polymorphic domain of the *Plasmodium falciparum* circumsporozoite protein. Int Immunol 3:511–516.

419. Doolan DL, Kamboonruang C, Beck H-P, et al. (1993) Cytotoxic T lymphocyte (CTL) low-responsiveness to the *Plasmodium falciparum* circumsporozoite protein in naturally exposed endemic populations: analysis of human CTL response to most known variants. Int Immunol 5:37–46.

420. Sedegah M, Kim Lee Sim B, Mason C, et al. (1992) Naturally acquired CD8+ cytotoxic T lymphocytes against the *Plasmodium falciparum* circumsporozoite protein. J Immunol 149:966–971.

421. Blum-Tirouvanziam U, Servis C, Habluetzel A, et al. (1995) Localization of HLA-A2.1-restricted T cell epitopes in the circumsporozoite protein of *Plasmodium falciparum*. J Immunol 154:3922–3931.

422. Aidoo M, Lavlani A, Allsopp CEM, et al. (1995) Identification of conserved antigenic components for a cytotoxic T lymphocyte-inducing vaccine against malaria. Lancet 345:1003–1007.

423. Good MF. (1995) Harnessing cytotoxic T lymphocytes for vaccine design. Lancet 345:999–1000.

424. Wizel B, Houghten RA, Parker KC, et al. (1995) Irradiated sporozoite vaccine induces HLA-B8-restricted cytotoxic T lymphocyte responses against two overlapping epitopes of the *Plasmodium falciparum* sporozoite surface protein 2. J Exp Med 182:1435–1445.

425. Weiss WR, Sedegah M, Berzofsky JA, Hoffman SL. (1993) The role of CD4+ T cells in immunity to malaria sporozoites. J Immunol 151:2690–2698.

426. Tarleton RL. (1990) Depletion of CD8+ T cells increases susceptibility and reverses vaccine-induced immunity in mice infected with *Trypanosoma cruzi*. J Immunol 144:717–724.

427. Rotzschke O, Falk K, Deres K, et al. (1990) Isolation and analysis of naturally processed viral peptides as recognized by cytotoxic T cells. Nature 348:252–254.

428. Townsend A, Ohlen C, Bastin J, et al. (1989) Association of class I major histocompatibility heavy and light chains induced by viral peptides. Nature 340:443–448.

429. Rammensee H-G, Friede T, Stevanovic S. (1995) MHC ligands and peptide motifs. Immunogenetics 41:178–228.

430. Nixon DF, Broliden K, Ogg G, Broliden P-A. (1992) Cellular and human cellular epitopes in HIV and SIV. Immunology 76:515–534.

431. Shearer GM, Clerici M. (1994) CD4+ functional T cell subsets: their roles in infection and vaccine development. In: Ada GL, ed. Strategies in vaccine design. RG Landes, Austin, TX, pp. 113–124.

432. Fauci AS. (1993) Multifactorial nature of human immunodeficiency virus disease. Science 262:1101–1108.

433. Hilleman MR. (1992) The dilemmas of HIV vaccine and therapy. Possible clues from comparative pathogenesis with measles. AIDS Res Hum Retroviruses 8:1743–1747.

434. Mackaness GB. (1962) Cellular resistance to infection. J Exp Med 116:381–406.

435. Mielke MEA, Ehlers S, Hahn H. (1988) T-cell subsets in delayed type hypersensitivity, protection and granuloma formation in primary and secondary Listeria infection in mice: superior role of Lyt-2+ cells in acquired immunity. Infect Immun 56:1920–1925.

436. Harty JT, Bevan MJ. (1992) CD8+ T cells specific for a single nonamer epitope of *Listeria monocytogenes* are protective in vivo. J Exp Med 175:1531–1538.

437. Pedrazzini T, Hug K, Louis JA. (1987) Importance of L3T4+ and LYt-2+ cells in the immunologic control of infection with *Mycobacterium bovis* strain bacillus Calmette-Guerin in mice. J Immunol 139:2032–2037.

438. Leveton C, Barnass S, Champion B, et al. (1989) T cell-mediated protection of mice against virulent *Mycobacterium tuberculosis*. Infect Immun 57:390–395.

439. Roberts AD, Ordway DJ, Orme IM. (1993) *Listeria monocytogenes* infection in β-2 microglobulin deficient mice. Infect Immun 61:1113.

440. Flynn JL, Goldstein MM, Triebold KJ, Koller B, Bloom BR. (1993) Major histocompatibility class I-restricted T cells are required for resistance to *Mycobacterium tuberculosis* infection. Proc Natl Acad Sci USA 89:12013–12017.

441. Manickan M, Francotte M, Kuklin N, et al. (1995) Vaccination with recombinant vaccinia viruses expressing ICP27 induces protective immunity against herpes simplex virus through CD4 + Th1 T cells. J Virol 69:4711–4716.
442. Simmons A, Nash AA. (1984) Zosteriform spread of herpes simplex virus as a model of recrudescence and its use to investigate the role of immune cells in prevention of recurrent disease. J Virol 52:816–821.
443. Simmons A, Tscharke DC. (1992) Anti-CD8 impairs clearance of herpes simplex virus from the nervous system: implications for the fate of virally infected neurones. J Exp Med 175:1337–1344.
444. Fu Y-X, Roark CE, Kelly K, et al. (1994) Immune protection and control of inflammatory tissue necrosis by γ,δ T cells. J Immunol 153:3101–3105.
445. Rosal J-P, MacDonald HR, Louis JA. (1993) A role for γ,δ T cells during experimental infection of mice with *Leishmania major*. J Immunol 150:550–555.
446. Askenase PW, Szczepanik M, Ptak M, et al. (1995) γ,δ T cells in normal spleen assist immunized α,β T cells in the adoptive transfer of contact sensitivity. J Immunol 154:3644–3653.
447. Kaufman SHE. (1995) Immunity to intracellular bacteria and protozoa. Immunologist 3:221–225.
448. Marrack P, Kappler J. (1994) Subversion of the immune system by pathogens. Cell 76:323–332.
449. Smith GL. (1994) Virus strategies for evasion of the host response to infection. Trends Microbiol 2:81–88.
450. Dawkins R. (1976) The selfish gene. Oxford University Press, Oxford.
451. Marasco WA, Phan S, Krutzch H, et al. (1984) Purification and identification of met-leu-phe as the major peptide neutrophil chemotactic factor produced by *Escherichia coli*. J Biol Chem 259:5430–5439.
452. Hartshorn KL, Liou LS, White MR, et al. (1995) Neutrophil deactivation by influenza A virus. J Immunol 154:3952–3960.
453. Franke-Ullmann G, Pfortner C, Walter P, et al. (1995) Alteration of pulmonary macrophage function by respiratory syncytial virus infection in vitro. J Immunol 154:268–280.
454. Turner PC, Musy PY, Moyer RW. (1995) Poxvirus serpins. In: McFadden G, ed. Viroceptors, virokines and related immune modulators encoded by DNA viruses. RG Landes, Austin, TX, pp. 67–88.
455. Alcami A, Smith GL. (1995) Interleukin-1 receptors encoded by poxviruses. In: McFadden G, ed. Viroceptors, virokines and related immune modulators encoded by DNA viruses. RG Landes, Austin, TX, pp. 17–28.
456. Smith CA, Goodwin RG. (1995) Tumor necrosis factor receptors in the poxvirus family. Biological and genetic implications. In: McFadden G, ed. Viroceptors, virokines and related immune modulators encoded by DNA viruses. RG Landes, Austin, TX, pp. 29–40.
457. Mossman K, Barry M, McFadden G. (1995) Interferon-γ receptors encoded by poxviruses. In: McFadden G, ed. Viroceptors, virokines and related immune modulators encoded by DNA viruses. RG Landes, Austin, TX, pp. 41–54.
458. Symons JA, Alcami A, Smith GL. (1995) Vaccinia virus encodes a soluble type 1 interferon receptor of novel structure and broad species specificity. Cell 81:551–560.
459. Schall TJ, Stein B, Gorgone G, Bacon KB. (1995) Cytomegalovirus encodes a functional receptor for C-C chemokines. Cell 81:201–214.
460. Wold WSM, Tollefson AE, Hermiston TW. (1995) Strategies of immune modulation by adenoviruses. In: McFadden G, ed. Viroceptors, virokines and related immune modulators encoded by DNA viruses. RG Landes, Austin, TX, pp. 147–186.
461. Swaminathan S, Kieff E. (1995) The role of BCRF1/vIL-10 in the life cycle of Epstein-Barr virus. In: McFadden G, ed. Viroceptors, virokines and related immune modulators encoded by DNA viruses. RG Landes, Austin, TX, pp. 111–126.
462. Isaacs SN, Moss B. (1995) Inhibition of complement activation by vaccinia virus. In: McFadden G, ed. Viroceptors, virokines and related immune modulators encoded by DNA viruses. RG Landes, Austin, TX, pp. 55–66.
463. Albrecht JC, Fleckenstein B. (1995) Complement regulatory proteins of Herpesvirus Saimiri. In: McFadden G, ed. Viroceptors, virokines and related immune modulators encoded by DNA viruses. RG Landes, Austin, TX, pp. 127–146.
464. Holland J, Spindler K, Horodyski F, et al. (1982) Rapid evolution of RNA genomes. Science 215:1577–1585.
465. LaRosa GJ, Davide JP, Weinhold K, et al. (1990) Conserved sequence and structural elements in the HIV-1 principal neutralizing determinant. Science 249:932–935.

466. Karzon DT. (1994) Preventive vaccines In: Broder S, Merigan TC, Bolognesi D, eds. Textbook of AIDS medicine. Williams & Wilkins, Baltimore, pp. 667–692.
467. Murphy BR, Webster RG. (1990) Orthomyxoviruses. In: Fields BN, Knipe DM, eds. Virology, 2nd ed. Raven Press, New York, pp. 1091–1154.
468. Norrby E, Oxman MN. (1990) Measles virus. In: Fields BN, Knipe DM, eds. Virology, 2nd ed. Raven Press, New York, pp. 1013–1044.
469. Temin HW. (1993) The high rate of retrovirus variation results in rapid evolution. In: Morse SS, ed. Emerging viruses. Oxford University Press, New York, pp. 219–225.
470. Holland J. (1993) Replication error, quasispecies populations and extreme evolution rates of RNA viruses. In: Morse SS, ed. Emerging viruses. Oxford University Press, New York, pp. 203–218.
471. Vanhamme L, Pays E. (1995) Control of gene expression in trypanosomes. Microbiol Rev 59:223–240.
472. Mulks MA, Plaut AG. (1978) IgA protease production as a characteristic, distinguishing pathogenic from harmless Neisseriaceae. N Engl J Med 299:973–976.
473. Lawton AR, Asofsky R, Mage RG. (1970) Synthesis of secretory IgA in the rabbit. III. Interaction of colostral IgA fragments with T chain. J Immunol 104:397–408.
474. Haigwood NL, Nara PL, Brooks E, et al. (1992) Native but not denatured recombinant human immunodeficiency virus type 1 gp120 generates broad spectrum neutralizing antibodies in baboons. J Virol 66:172–182.
475. Pruksakorn S, Currie B, Brandt E, et al. (1994) Towards a vaccine for rheumatic fever: identification of a conserved target epitope on M protein of group A streptococci. Lancet 344:639–642.
476. Natali A, Oxford JS, Schild GC. (1981) Frequency of naturally occurring antibody to influenza virus antigenic variants selected in vitro with monoclonal antibody. J Hyg 87:185–190.
477. Halstead SB. (1990) Dengue and dengue hemorrhagic fever. Curr Opin Infect Dis 3:434–436.
478. Robinson WE, Kawamura T, Lake D, et al. (1990) Antibodies to the primary immunodominant domain of human immunodeficiency virus type 1 glycoprotein 41 enhance HIV-1 infection in vivo. J Virol 64:5301–5305.
479. Fujinani RS, Norrby E, Oldstone MBA. (1984) Antigenic modulation induced by monoclonal antibodies: antibodies to measles virus hemagglutinin alter expression of other viral polypeptides in infected cells. J Immunol 132:2618–2628.
480. Levitskaya J, Coram M, Levitsky V, et al. (1995) Inhibition of antigen processing by the internal repeat region of the Epstein-Barr virus nuclear antigen-1. Nature 375:685–687.
481. Ada GL. (1988) Prospects for HIV vaccines. J Acquir Immune Defic Syndr 1:295–303.
482. Blanden RV, Deak BD, McDevitt HO. (1989) Strategies in virus-host interactions. In: Blanden RV, ed. Immunology of viral diseases: proceedings of the first Frank and Bobbie Fenner Conference on Medical Research. Brolga Press, Canberra, pp. 125–138.
483. Patterson S, Gross J, English N, et al. (1995) CD4 expression on dendritic cells and their infection by human immunodeficiency virus. J Gen Virol 76:1155–1163.
484. Gardner ID, Bowern NA, Blanden RV. (1975) Cell-mediated cytotoxicity against ectromelia virus-infected target cells. III. Role of the H2 gene complex. Eur J Immunol 5:122–127.
485. Grundy JE, McKeating JA, Griffiths PD. (1982) Cytomegalovirus strain AD169 binds β_2 microglobulin in vitro after release from cells. J Gen Virol 68:777–784.
486. Paabo S, Severinsson L, Andersonn M, et al. (1989) Adenovirus proteins and MHC expression. Adv Cancer Res 52:151–163.
487. Fruh K, Ahn K, Djaballah K, et al. (1995) A viral inhibitor of peptide transporters for antigen presentation. Nature 375:415–418.
488. Hill A, Jugovic P, York I, et al. (1995) Herpes simplex virus turns off the TAP to evade host immunity. Nature 375:411–414.
489. Pircher H, Moskophidis D, Rohrer U, et al. (1990) Viral escape by selection of cytotoxic T cell resistant virus variant in vivo. Nature 346:629–633.
490. Phillips RE, Rowland-Jones S, Nixon DF, et al. (1991) Human immunodeficiency virus genetic variation that can escape cytotoxic T cell recognition. Nature 354:453–458.
491. Niewiesk S, Daenke S, Parker CE, et al. (1995) Naturally occurring variants of human T-cell leukemia virus type 1 tax protein impair its recognition by cytotoxic T lymphocytes and the transactivation function of tax. J Virol 69:2649–2653.
492. Myerhans A, Dadaglio G, Vartanian J-P, et al. (1991) In vivo persistence of a HIV-1-encoded HLA-B27-restricted cytotoxic T lymphocyte epitope despite specific in vitro reactivity. Eur J Immunol 21:2637–2640.

493. Chen ZW, Shen L, Miller MD, et al. (1992) Cytotoxic T lymphocytes do not appear to select for mutations in an immunodominant epitope of simian immunodeficiency virus gag. J Immunol 149:4060–4066.

494. Klenerman P, Rowland-Jones S, McAdam S, et al. (1994) Cytotoxic T cell activity antagonized by naturally occurring HIV-1 gag variants. Nature 369:403–407.

495. Bertoletti A, Sette A, Chisari FV, et al. (1994) Natural variants of cytotoxic epitopes are T cell receptor antagonists for anti-viral cytotoxic T cells. Nature 369:407–410.

496. Allen PM, Zinkernagel RM. (1994) Promethean viruses. Nature 369:355–356.

497. Nowak MA, May RM, Phillips RE, et al. (1995) Antigenic oscillations and shifting immunodominance in HIV-1 infections. Nature 375:606–609.

498. Whitton JL, Sheng N, Oldstone MBA, McKee TA. (1993) A "string-of-beads" vaccine, comprising linked minigenes, confers protection from a lethal dose virus challenge. J Virol 67:348–352.

499. Berendt AR, McDowell A, Craig AG, et al. (1992) The binding site on ICAM-1 for *Plasmodium falciparum*-infected erythrocytes overlaps but is distinct from the LFA binding site. Cell 68:71–81.

500. Ockenhouse CF, Betageri R, Springer TA, Staunton DA. (1992) *Plasmodium falciparum*-infected erythrocytes bind ICAM-1 at a site distinct from LFA-1, Mac-1 and human rhinovirus. Cell 68:63–69.

501. Hill AB, Mullbacher A, Blanden RV. (1993) Ir genes, peripheral cross-tolerance and immunodominance in MHC class I-restricted T-cell responses: an old quagmire revisited. Immunol Rev 133:75–92.

502. Eichelberger MC, Wang M, Allan W, et al. (1991) Influenza virus RNA in the lung and lymphoid tissue of immunologically intact and CD4 depleted mice. J Gen Virol 72:1695–1698.

503. Francis T Jr. (1955) The current status of the control of influenza. Ann Intern Med 43:534–543.

504. Cooney EL, Collier AC, Greenberg PD, et al. (1991) Safety and immunological response to a recombinant vaccinia virus vaccine expressing HIV-1 glycoprotein. Lancet 337:567–572.

505. Allen JE, Dixon JE, Doherty PC. (1987) Nature of the inflammatory process in the central nervous system of mice infected with lymphocytic choriomeningitis virus. Curr Top Microbiol Immunol 134:131–143.

506. Zinkernagel RM, Hengartner H. (1994) T cell-mediated immunopathology versus direct cytolysis by virus: implications for HIV and AIDS. Immunol Today 15:262–268.

507. Cannon MJ, Openshaw PJM, Askonas BA. (1988) Cytotoxic T cells clear virus but augment pathology in mice infected with respiratory syncytial virus. J Exp Med 168:1163–1168.

508. Peters M, Vierling J, Gershwin ME, et al. (1991) Immunology and the liver. Hepatology 13:977–994.

509. Kohler P, Trembath J, Merril DA, et al. (1974) Immunotherapy with antibody, lymphocytes and transfer factor in chronic hepatitis B. Clin Immunol Immunopathol 2:465–471.

510. Mak NK, Zhang Y-H, Ada GL, Tannock GA. (1982) The humoral and cellular response of mice to infection with a cold-adapted influenza A virus variant. Infect Immun 38:218–225.

511. Yap KL, Ada GL. (1978) The recovery of mice from influenza A virus infection: adoptive transfer of immunity with influenza virus-specific cytotoxic T lymphocytes recognizing a common virion antigen. Scand J Immunol 8:413–420.

512. Ada GL. (1996) Vaccines. In: Nathanson N, ed. Viral pathogenesis. Lippincott-Raven Publishers, Philadelphia (in press).

513. Flynn K, Mullbacher A. (1996) Memory alloreactive cytotoxic T cells do not require costimulation for activation in vitro. Immunol Cell Biol 79 (in press).

514. Davis LE, Hjelle BL, Miller VE, et al. (1992) Early viral brain invasion in iatrogenic human immunodeficiency viral infection. Neurology 42:1736–1739.

515. Allison AC, Byars NE. (1986) An adjuvant formulation that selectively elicits the formation of antibodies of protective isotypes and cell-mediated immunity. J Immunol Methods 95:157–168.

516. Glenny AT, Pope GC, Waddington H, Wallace U. (1926) Immunological notes. XIII. The antigenic value of toxoid precipitated by potassium alum. J Pathol Bacteriol 29:38–39.

517. Freund J, Casals J, Hosmer EP. (1937) Sensitization and antibody formation after injection of tubercle bacilli and paraffin oil. Proc Soc Exp Biol Med 37:509–514.

518. Uhr JW, Salvin SB, Pappenheimer AM. (1957) Delayed hypersensitivity II. Induction of hypersensitivity in guinea pigs by means of antigen:antibody complexes. J Exp Med 105:11–21.

519. Myers KR, Gustafson GL. (1991) Adjuvants for human vaccine usage: a rational design. In: Cryz SJ Jr, ed. Vaccines and immunotherapy. Pergamon Press, New York, pp. 404–411.

520. Cooper PD. (1994) The selective induction of different immune responses by vaccine adjuvants. In: Ada GL, ed. Strategies in vaccine design. RG Landes, Austin, TX, pp. 125–158.

521. Gupta RK, Relyveld EH, Lindblad EB, et al. (1993) Adjuvants—a balance between toxicity and adjuvanticity. Vaccine 11:293–306.
522. Stieneker F, Kersten G, van Bloois L, et al. (1995) Comparison of 24 different adjuvants for inactivated HIV-2 split whole virus as antigen in mice. Induction of titers of binding antibodies and toxicity of the formulations. Vaccine 13:45–53.
523. Chedid L. (1985) Adjuvants of immunity. Ann Immunol Institut Pasteur 136D:283–291.
524. White RG, Coons AH, Connolly JM. (1955) Studies on antibody production. III. The alum granuloma. J Exp Med 102:73.
525. Bomford R. (1984) Relative adjuvant efficacy of Al(OH)$_3$ and saponin is related to the immunogenicity of the antigen. Int Arch Allergy Appl Immunol 75:280–281.
526. Cooper PD, Steele EJ. (1988) The adjuvanticity of gamma inulin. Immunol Cell Biol 66:345–352.
527. Freund J. (1956) The mode of action of immunological adjuvants. Adv Tuberc Res 7:130.
528. Hunter RL, Bennett B. (1986) The adjuvant activity of nonionic block polymer surfactants. Scand J Immunol 23:287–293.
529. Morris W, Steinhoff MC, Russell PK. (1994) Potential of polymer microencapsulation technology for vaccine innovation. Vaccine 12:5–11.
530. O'Hagan DT. (1994) Microparticles as oral vaccines. In: O'Hagan DT, ed. Novel delivery systems for oral vaccines. CRC Press, Boca Raton, FL, pp. 175–205.
531. Gengoux C, Leclerc C. (1995) In vivo induction of CD4 + T cell responses by antigens covalently linked to synthetic microspheres does not require adjuvant. Int Immunol 7:45–53.
532. Nakaoka R, Tabata Y, Ikada Y. (1995) Potentiality of gelatin microspheres as immunological adjuvants. Vaccine 13:653–661.
533. O'Hagan DT, Rahman D, McGee JP, et al. (1991) Biodegradable microparticles as controlled release antigen delivery systems. Immunology 73:239–242.
534. Men Y, Thomasin C, Merkle HP, et al. (1995) A single administration of tetanus toxoid in biodegradable microspheres elicits T cell and antibody responses similar or superior to those obtained with aluminium hydroxide. Vaccine 13:683–689.
535. Eldridge JH, Staas JK, Meulbroek JA, et al. (1991) Biodegradable and biocompatible poly (DL-lactide-co-glycolide) microspheres as an adjuvant for staphylococcal enterotoxin B toxoid which enhances the level of toxin neutralizing antibodies. Infect Immun 59:2978–2986.
536. Stevens VC. (1993) Vaccine delivery systems: potential methods for use in antifertility vaccines. Am J Reprod Immunol 29:176–188.
537. Eldridge JH, Hammond CJ, Meulbroeck JA, et al. (1990) Controlled vaccine release in the gut-associated lymphoid tissues. 1. Orally administered biodegradable microspheres target the Peyer's patches. J Control Rel 11:205–215.
538. Eldridge JH, Staas JK, Meulbroeck JA, et al. (1991) Biodegradable microspheres as a vaccine delivery system. Mol Immunol 28:287–294.
539. Moldoveanu Z, Novak M, Huang W-Q, et al. (1993) Oral immunization with influenza virus in biodegradable microspheres. J Infect Dis 167:84–90.
540. Marx PA, Compans RW, Gettie A, et al. (1993) Protection against vaginal SIV transmission with microencapsulated vaccine. Science 260:1323–1325.
541. Kawamura H, Berzofsky JA. (1986) Enhancement of antigenic potency in vitro and immunogenicity in vivo by coupling the antigen to immunoglobulin. J Immunol 136:58–65.
542. Carayanniotis C, Barber BB. (1987) Adjuvant-free IgG responses induced with antigen coupled to antibodies against class II MHC. Nature 327:59–61.
543. de Aizpurua HJ, Russell-Jones GJ. (1988) Oral vaccination: identification of classes of proteins which provoke an immune response upon oral feeding. J Exp Med 167:440–451.
544. Elson CO, Ealding W. (1984) Generalized systemic and mucosal immunity in mice after mucosal stimulation with cholera toxin. J Immunol 132:2736–2741.
545. Hornquist E, Lycke N. (1993) Cholera toxin adjuvant greatly promotes antigen priming of T cells. Eur J Immunol 23:2136–2143.
546. Dempsey PW, Allison MED, Akkaraju S, Goodnow CC, Fearon DT. (1996) C3d of complement as a molecular adjuvant: bridging innate and acquired immunity. Science 271:348–350.
547. Verma JN, Rao M, Amselem S, et al. (1992) Adjuvant effects of liposomes containing lipid A: enhancement of liposomal antigen presentation and recruitment of macrophages. Infect Immun 60:2438–2444.
548. Warren HS, Vogel FR, Chedid LA. (1986) Current status of immunological adjuvants. Annu Rev Immunol 4:369–388.

549. Ribi E. (1984) Beneficial modification of the endotoxin molecule. J Biol Response Modif 3:1–9.
550. Schultz N, Oratz R, Chen D, et al. (1995) Effect of DETOX as an adjuvant for melanoma vaccine. Vaccine 13:503–508.
551. Cabral GA, Marciano-Cabral F, Funk GA, et al. (1978) Cellular and humoral immunity in guinea pigs to two major polypeptides derived from hepatitis B surface antigen. J Gen Virol 38:339–350.
552. Moriarty AM, McGee JS, Winslow BJ, et al. (1990) Expression of HIV gag and env B cell epitopes on the surface of HBV core particles and analysis of the immune responses generated to those epitopes. In: Brown F, Chanock RM, Ginsberg HS, Lerner RA, eds. Vaccines '90. Cold Spring Harbor Laboratory, Cold Spring Harbor, NY, pp. 225–229.
553. Moore JP. (1995) Back to primary school. Nature 376:115.
554. Harding CV, Unanue ER. (1990) Quantitation of antigen-presenting cell MHC class II/peptide complexes necessary for T-cell stimulation. Nature 346:574–576.
555. Dmotz S, Grey HM, Sette A. (1990) The minimal number of class II MHC-antigen complexes needed for T cell activation. Science 249:1028–1030.
556. Morein B, Lovgren K, Hoglund S, Sundquist B. (1987) The ISCOM: an immunostimulating complex. Immunol Today 8:333–338.
557. Jones PD, Tha Hla R, Morein B, Lovgren K, Ada GL. (1988) Cellular immune responses in the murine lung to local immunization with influenza A glycoproteins in micelles and immunostimulatory complexes (ISCOMS). Scand J Immunol 27:645–652.
558. Takahashi H, Takashita T, Morein B, Putney SD, Germain RN, Berzofsky JA. (1990) Induction of CD8+ cytotoxic T cells by immunization with purified HIV-1 envelope protein in ISCOMS. Nature 344:873–875.
559. Griffiths JC, Berrie EL, Holdsworth LN, et al. (1991) Induction of high titer neutralizing antibodies, using hybrid human immunodeficiency virus V3-Ty virus-like particles in a clinically relevant adjuvant. J Virol 65:450–456.
560. Schlienger K, Mancini M, Riviere Y, et al. (1992) Human immunodeficiency type 1 major neutralizing determinant exposed on hepatitis B surface antigen particles is highly immunogenic in primates. J Virol 66:2570–2576.
561. Evans DJ, McKeating J, Meredith JM, et al. (1989) An engineered polio virus chimaera elicits broadly reactive HIV-1 neutralizing antibodies. Nature 339:385–388.
562. Parish CR. (1972) The relationship between humoral and cell-mediated immunity. Transplant Rev 13:35–66.
563. Salvin SP. (1958) Occurrence of delayed hypersensitivity during the development of Arthus type hypersensitivity. J Exp Med 107:109–118.
564. Parish CR, Liew FY. (1972) The immune response to chemically-modified flagellin. III. Enhanced cell mediated immunity during high and low zone antibody tolerance to flagellin. J Exp Med 135:298–311.
565. Braciale TJ, Yap KL. (1978) Role of viral infectivity in the induction of influenza virus-specific cytotoxic T cells. J Exp Med 147:1236–1252.
566. Fitch FW, Lancki DW, Gajewski TF. (1993) T-cell mediated immune regulation. In: Paul WE, ed. Fundamental immunology, 3rd ed. Raven Press, New York, pp. 733–761.
567. Pike BL. (1992) Cytokines acting on B lymphocytes. In: Roitt IM, Delves PJ, eds. Encyclopedia of immunology. Academic Press, New York, pp. 440–441.
568. Bao S, Goldstone S, Husband AJ. (1993) Localization of IFNγ and IL-6 mRNA in mucosal intestine by in vitro hybridization. Immunology 80:666–670.
569. Moore MW, Carbone FR, Bevan MJ. (1988) Introduction of soluble protein into the class I pathway of antigen processing and presentation. Cell 54:777–786.
570. Harding CW. (1992) Electrophoration of exogenous antigen into the cytosol for antigen processing and class I major histocompatibility complex (MHC) presentation: weak base amines and hypothermia (18°C) inhibit the class I MHC processing pathway. Eur J Immunol 22:1865–1870.
571. Yong K, Ying L, Kapp JA. (1995) Ovalbumin injected with complete Freund's adjuvant stimulates cytolytic responses. Eur J Immunol 25:549–553.
572. Hancock GE, Speelman DJ, Frenchick PJ, et al. (1995) Formulation of the purified fusion protein of respiratory syncytial virus with the saponin QS21 induces protective immune responses in Balb/c mice that are similar to those generated by experimental infection. Vaccine 13:391–400.
573. Bevan MJ. (1987) Class discrimination in the world of immunology. Nature 325:192–194.
574. Bevan MJ. (1995) Antigen presentation to cytotoxic T lymphocytes in vivo. J Exp Med 182:639–641.

575. Zhou F, Rouse BT, Huang L. (1992) Induction of cytotoxic T lymphocytes in vivo with protein entrapped in membranous vehicles. J Immunol 149:1599–1604.
576. Kovacsovics-Bankowski M, Clark K, Benacerraf B, Rock KL. (1993) Efficient major histocompatibility complex class 1 presentation of exogenous antigen upon phagocytosis by macrophages Proc Natl Acad Sci USA 90:4942–4946.
577. Bachmann MF, Kundig TM, Freer G, et al. (1994) Induction of protective cytotoxic T cells with viral proteins. Eur J Immunol 24:2228–2236.
578. Nair S, Buiting AMJ, Rouse RJD, et al. (1995) Role of macrophages and dendritic cells in primary cytotoxic T lymphocyte responses. Int Immunol 7:679–688.
579. Reis e Sousa C, Stahl PE, Austyn JM. (1993) Phagocytosis of antigens by Langerhans cells in vitro. J Exp Med 178:509–519.
580. Srivistava PK, Old LJ. (1988) Individually distinct transplantation antigens of chemically induced mouse tumors. Immunol Today 9:78–83.
581. Udono H, Srivastava PK. (1993) Heat-shock protein-70 associated peptides elicit specific cancer immunity. J Exp Med 178:1391–1396.
582. Srivastava PK, Udono H, Blachere NE, Li ZH. (1994) Heat-shock proteins transfer peptides during antigen processing and CTL priming. Immunogenetics 39:93–98.
583. Srivastava PK. (1996) Heat shock protein-peptide complexes: natural immunogens against cancers and infectious diseases. In: Progress in immunology. 9 (in press).
584. Aiuchele P, Hengartner H, Zinkernagel RM, Schulz M. (1990) Antiviral cytotoxic T cell response induced by in vivo priming with a free synthetic peptide. J Exp Med 171:1815–1820.
585. Schulz M, Zinkernagel RM, Hengartner H. (1991) Peptide-induced antiviral protection by cytotoxic T cells. Proc Natl Acad Sci USA 88:991–993.
586. Kast WM, Roux L, Curren J, et al. (1991) Protection against lethal Sendai virus by in vivo priming of virus-specific cytotoxic T lymphocytes with a free synthetic peptide. Proc Natl Acad Sci USA 88:2283–2287.
587. Blum-Tirouvanziam U, Beghdadi-Rais C, Roggero MA, et al. (1994) Elicitation of specific cytotoxic T cells by immunization with malaria soluble synthetic polypeptides. J Immunol 153:4134–4137.
588. Mullbacher A, Tha Hla R. (1993) In vivo administration of major histocompatibility complex class-1 specific peptides from influenza virus induces specific cytotoxic T cell hyporesponsiveness. Eur J Immunol 23:2526–2531.
589. AIchele P, Brduscha-Reim K, Zinkernagel RM, et al. (1995) T cell priming versus T cell tolerance induced by synthetic peptides. J Exp Med 182:261–266.
590. Deres K, Schild H, Weissmuller K-H, et al. (1989) In vivo priming of virus-specific cytotoxic T lymphocytes with synthetic lipopeptide vaccine. Nature 352:561–564.
591. Sauzet JP, Deprez B, Martinon F, et al. (1995). Long-lasting anti-viral cytotoxic T lymphocytes induced in vivo with chimeric-multirestricted lipopeptides. Vaccine 13:1339–1345.
592. Apostolopoulos V, Pietersz GA, McKenzie IFC. (1996) Cell-mediated immune responses to MUC-1 fusion protein coupled to mannan. Vaccine (in press).
593. Blattner WA. (1991) HIV epidemiology: past, present and future. FASEB J 5:2340–2348.
594. Ada GL. (1991) Do cytotoxic T cells clear some HIV/SIV infections? J Med Primatol (in press).
595. Ada GL. (1993) Vaccines. In: Paul WE, ed. Fundamental immunology, 2nd ed. Raven Press, New York, pp. 985–1032.
596. Brown F. (1990) The potential of peptides as vaccines. Semin Virol 1:67–74.
597. Stevens VC. (1993) Vaccine delivery systems: potential methods for use in antifertility vaccines. Am J Reprod Immunol 29:176–188.
598. Gao XM, Liew FY, Tite JP. (1990) A dominant Th epitope in influenza nucleoprotein. Analysis of the fine specificity and functional repertoire of T cells recognizing a single determinant. J Immunol 144:2730–2737.
599. Clarke BE, Newton SE, Carroll AR, et al. (1987) Improved immunogenicity of a peptide epitope after fusion to hepatitis B core protein. Nature 330:381–384.
600. Donnelly JJ, Deck RR, Liu MA. (1990) Immunogenicity of a *Haemophilus influenzae* polysaccharide-*Neisseria meningitidis* outer membrane protein complex conjugate vaccine. J Immunol 145:3071–3079.
601. Tam JP. (1988) Synthetic peptide vaccine design: synthesis and properties of a high density multiple antigenic peptide system. Proc Natl Acad Sci USA 85:5409–5413.
602. Sela M. (1966) Immunological studies with synthetic polypeptides. Adv Immunol 5:29–129.

603. Wang CW, Looney DJ, Li ML, et al. (1991) Long-term high-titer neutralizing activity induced by octameric synthetic HIV antigen. Science 254:285–288.

604. Marguerite M, Bossus M, Mazxingue C, et al. (1992) Analysis of antigenicity and immunogenicity of the different chemically defined constructs of a peptide. Mol Immunol 29:793–800.

605. Nardin EH, Oliviera GA, Calvo-Calle JM, Nussenzweig R. (1995) The use of multiple antigenic peptides in the analysis and induction of protective immune responses against infectious diseases. Adv Immunol. 50:105–150.

606. Palker TJ, Matthews TJ, Langlois A, et al. (1989) Polyvalent immunodeficiency virus synthetic immunogen comprised of envelope gp120 T helper cell sites and B cell neutralization epitopes. J Immunol 142:3612–3619.

607. Haynes NF, Moody MA, Heinley CS, et al. (1995) HIV-1 gp120 V3 region primer-induced antibody suppression is overcome by administration of HIV-1 gp120 envelope C4-V3 peptides as a polyvalent immunogen. AIDS Res Hum Retroviruses 11:211–221.

608. Haynes BF, Arthur LO, Frost P, et al. (1993) Conversion of an immunogenic human immunodeficiency virus (HIV) envelope synthetic peptide to a tolerogen in chimpanzees by the fusogenic domain of HIV gp41 envelope protein. J Exp Med 177:717–727.

609. Parditos C, Stanley C, Steward M. (1992) The effect of orientation of epitopes on the immunogenicity of chimeric synthetic peptides representing measles virus protein sequences. Mol Immunol 29:651–658.

610. Brown LE, White DO, Agius C, et al. (1996) Synthetic peptides representing sequences within gp41 of HIV as immunogens for murine T- and B-cell responses. Arch Virol 140:635–654.

611. Baba E, Nakamura M, Ohkuma K, et al. (1995) A peptide-based human T cell leukemia virus type 1 vaccine containing T and B cell epitopes that induces high titers of neutralizing antibodies. J Immunol 154:399–412.

612. Wang R, Charoenvit Y, Corradin G, et al. (1995) Induction of protective polyclonal antibodies by immunization with a *Plasmodium yoelii* circumsporozoite protein multiple antigen peptide vaccine. J Immunol 154:2784–2793.

613. Laver WG, Air GM, Webster RG, Smith-Gill S. (1990) Epitopes on protein antigens. Misconceptions and realities. Cell 61:553–556.

614. Dyson HJ, Wright P. (1995) Antigenic peptides. FASEB J 9:37–42.

615. Haumaya PTP, Berndt KD, Heidorn DB, et al. (1990) Synthesis and biophysical characterization of engineered topographic, immunogenic determinants with aa topology. Biochemistry 29:13–23.

616. Mutter M, Tuchscherer GG, Miller C, et al. (1992) Template-assembled synthetic proteins with four-helix-bundle topology. Total chemical synthesis and conformational studies. J Am Chem Soc 114:1463–1470.

617. Rose K. (1994) Facile synthesis of homogeneous artificial proteins. J Am Chem Soc 116:30–33.

618. Berzofsky JA. (1995) Designing peptide vaccines to broaden recognition and enhance potency. Ann NY Acad Sci 754:161–168.

619. Berzofsky JA, Pendelton CD, Clerici M, et al. (1991) Construction of peptides encompassing multideterminant clusters of HIV envelope to induce in vitro T-cell responses in mice and humans of multiple MHC types. J Clin Invest 88:876–884.

620. Patarroyo ME, Romero P, Torres ML, et al. (1987) Induction of protective immunity against experimental infection with malaria using synthetic peptides. Nature 328:629–632.

621. Amador R, Moreno A, Murillo MA, et al. (1992) Safety and immunogenicity of the synthetic malaria vaccine SPf66 in a large field trial. J Infect Dis 166:139–144.

622. Valero MV, Amador LR, Galindo C, et al. (1993) Vaccination with SPf66, a chemically synthesized vaccine against *Plasmodium falciparum* in Columbia. Lancet 341:706–710.

623. Alonso PL, Tanner T, Smith T, et al. (1994) A trial of SPf66, a synthetic malaria vaccine, in Kilombero (Tanzania): rationale and design. Vaccine 12:181–186.

624. D'Alessandro U, Leach A, Drakeley CJ, et al. (1995) Efficacy trial of malaria vaccine SPf66 in Gambian infants. Lancet 346:462–467.

625. Morrison RP, Scott Manning D, Caldwell HD. (1992) Immunology of *Chlamydia trachomatis* infections: immunoprotective and immunopathogenic responses. In: Quinn TC, ed. Sexually transmitted diseases. Raven Press, New York, pp. 57–84.

626. Ertl HCJ, Bona CA. (1988) Criteria to define anti-idiotype antibodies carrying the internal image of the antigens. Vaccine 6:80–84.

627. Pan Y, Yuhasz SC, Amzel LM. (1995) Anti-idiotypic antibodies: biological function and structural studies. FASEB J 9:43–49.
628. Roth C, Roca-Serra J, Somme G, et al. (1985) The gene repertoire of the GAT response. Comparison of the VH$_k$ and D regions used by anti-GAT antibodies and monoclonal antibodies produced after idiotypic immunization. Proc Natl Acad Sci USA 82:4788–4792.
629. Bruck C, Co MS, Zlaoui M, et al. (1986) Nucleic acid sequence of an internal image bearing monoclonal and anti-idiotype and its comparison to that of the internal antigen. Proc Natl Acad Sci USA 83:6578–6582.
630. Marwick C. (1986) Possible defense against the common cold: block that cellular receptor site. JAMA 256:967–971.
631. Germanier R, Furer E. (1975) Isolation and characterization of a Gal E mutant Ty21a of *Salmonella typhi*: a candidate strain for a live, oral typhoid vaccine. J Infect Dis 131:553–558.
632. Silva BA, Gonzalez C, Mora GC, Cabello F. (1987) Genetic characteristics of the *Salmonella typhi* strain Ty21a vaccine. J Infect Dis 155:1077–1078.
633. Rappuoli R, Douce G, Dougan G, Pizza M. (1995) Genetic detoxification of bacterial toxins: a new approach to vaccine development. Int Arch Allergy Immunol 108:327–333.
634. Giannini G, Rappuoli R, Ratti G. (1984) The amino acid sequence of two non-toxic mutants of diphtheria toxin, CRM45 and CRM 197. Nucleic Acid Res 12:4063–4069.
635. Pizza M, Covacci A, Bartolini A, et al. (1989) Mutants of pertussis toxin suitable for vaccine development. Science 246:497–500.
636. Pizza M, Fontana MR, Guiliani MM, et al. (1995) A genetically detoxified derivative of heat-labile *E coli* enterotoxin induces neutralizing antibodies against the A subunit. J Exp Med 180:2147–2153.
637. Fontana MR, Manetti R, Gianneli V, et al. (1995) Construction of non-toxic derivatives of cholera toxins and characterization of the immunological response against the A subunit. Infect Immun 63:2356–2360.
638. Curtiss R III, Kelly SM, Tinge SA, et al. (1994) Recombinant *Salmonella* vectors in vaccine development. Dev Biol Stand 82:23–33.
639. Chatfield S, Roberts M, Li J, et al. The use of live attenuated *Salmonella* for oral vaccination. Dev Biol Stand 82:35–42.
640. Levine MM, Kaper JB, Herrington D, et al. (1988) Safety, immunogenicity and efficacy of recombinant live oral cholera vaccines, CVD 103 and CVD 103 HgR. Lancet 2:467–470.
641. Taylor DN, Killeen KP, Hack DC, et al. (1994) Development of a live, oral, attenuated vaccine against El Tor cholera. J Infect Dis 170:1518–1523.
642. Coster TS, Killeen KP, Waldor MK, et al. (1995) Safety, immunogenicity and efficacy of live attenuated *Vibrio cholerae* 0139 vaccine prototype. Lancet 345:949–952.
643. Goebel SJ, Johnson GP, Perkus ME, et al. (1990) The complete DNA sequence of vaccinia virus. Virology 179:247–266.
644. Paoletti E, Tartaglia J, Taylor J. (1994) Safe and effective poxvirus vectors—NYVAC and AL-VAC. Dev Biol Stand 82:65–69.
645. Moss B. Replicating and host-restricted non-replicating vaccinia virus vectors for vaccine development. Dev Biol Stand 82:55–63.
646. Lee SL, Roos JM, McGuigan LC, et al. (1992) Molecular attenuation of vaccinia virus: mutant generation and animal characteristics. J Virol 66:2617–2630.
647. Harris TJR. (1983) Expression of eukaryotic genes in *E. coli*. In: Williamson R, ed. Genetic engineering, vol 4. Academic Press, London, pp. 128–175.
648. Davis AR, Nayak DP, Veda M, et al. (1983) Immune response to human influenza virus hemagglutinin expressed in *E. coli*. Gene 21:273–284.
649. Hilleman MR. (1992) Vaccine perspectives from the vantage of hepatitis B. Vaccine Res 1:1–17.
650. Valenzuela P, Medina A, Rutter WJ, et al. (1982) Synthesis and assembly of hepatitis B surface antigen particles in yeast. Nature 298:347–350.
651. Jilg W, Schmidt M, Zoulek G, et al. (1984) Clinical evaluation of a recombinant hepatitis B vaccine. Lancet 2:1174–1175.
652. Nayak DP, Jabber MA. (1986) Expression of influenza viral hemagglutinin (HA) in yeast. In: Kendal AP, Patriaca PA, eds. *Saccharomyces cerevisiae*. Alan R Liss, New York, pp. 357–373.
653. Wintsch J, Chaignat C-L, Braun DG, et al. (1991) Safety and immunogenicity of a genetically engineered human immunodeficiency virus vaccine. J Infect Dis 163:219–225.

654. Emslie KR, Miller JM, Slade MB, et al. (1995) Expression of the rota virus SA11 protein VP7 in the simple eukaryote *Dictyostelium discoideum*. J Virol 69:1747–1754.
655. Gething MJ, Sambrook J. (1981) Cell-surface expression of influenza hemagglutinin from a cloned DNA copy of the RNA gene. Nature 293:620–625.
656. Sveda MM, Lai CJ. (1981) Functional expression in primate cells of cloned DNA coding for the hemagglutinin glycoprotein of influenza virus. Proc Natl Acad Sci USA 78:5488–5492.
657. WHO Study Group. (1987) Acceptability of cell substrates for production of biologicals. Tech Rep Series 747:3–29.
658. Berman PW, Matthews TJ, Riddle L, et al. (1990) Protection of chimpanzees from infection by HIV-1 after vaccination with recombinant glycoprotein gp120 but not gp160. Nature 345:622–625.
659. Zinder ND, Lederberg J. (1952). Genetic change in Salmonella. J Bacteriol. 64:679–685.
660. Ada GL. (1991) Strategies for exploiting the immune system in the design of vaccines. Mol Immunol 28:225–230.
661. Weir JP, Bazozar G, Moss B. (1982) Mapping the vaccinia virus thymidine gene by marker rescue and by cell-free translation of selected mRNA. Proc Natl Acad Sci USA 79:1210–1214.
662. Nakano E, Panicalli D, Paoletti E. (1982) Molecular genetics of vaccinia virus. Demonstration of marker rescue. Proc Natl Acad Sci USA 79:1593–1596.
663. Smith GL, Mackett M. (1992) The design, construction and use of recombinant poxviruses. In: Binns M, Smith GL, eds. Recombinant poxviruses. CRC Press, Boca Raton, FL, pp. 123–162.
664. Townsend A, Bastin J, Gould K, et al. (1988) Defective presentation to class I restricted cytotoxic T lymphocytes in vaccinia-infected cells is overcome by enhanced degradation of antigen. J Exp Med 168:1211–1244.
665. Wachsman M, Aurelian L, Smith CC, et al. (1989) Regulation of expression of herpes simplex virus (HSV) glycoprotein D in vaccinia recombinants affects their ability to protect from cutaneous HSV-2 disease. J Infect Dis 159:625–634.
666. Fuerst TR, Earl PI, Moss B. (1987) Use of a hybrid vaccinia virus T7 RNA polymerase system for expression of target genes. Mol Cell Biol 7:2538–2544.
667. Binns MM, Smith GL, eds. (1992) Recombinant poxviruses. CRC Press, Boca Raton, FL, pp. 1–343.
668. Brown F, ed. (1993) Recombinant vectors in vaccine development. Dev Biol Standard. 82:1–268.
669. Cox WI, Tartaglia J, Paoletti E. (1992) Pox virus recombinants as live vaccines. In: Binns M, Smith GL, eds. Recombinant poxviruses. CRC Press, Boca Raton, FL, pp. 123–162.
670. Moss B, Smith GL, Gerin JL, Purcell RH. (1984) Live recombinant vaccinia virus protects chimpanzees against hepatitis B. Nature 311:67–71.
671. Collins PL, Purcell RH, London WT, et al. (1990) Evaluation in chimpanzees of vaccinia virus recombinants that express the surface glycoproteins of respiratory syncytial virus. Vaccine 8:164–168.
672. Buller ML, Palumbo GJ. (1992) Safety and attenuation of vaccinia virus. In: Binns M, Smith GL, eds. Recombinant poxviruses. CRC Press, Boca Raton, FL, pp. 235–268.
673. Pastoret P-P, Brochier B, Blanco J, et al. (1992) Development and deliberate release of a vaccinia-rabies recombinant virus for the oral vaccination of foxes against rabies. In: Binns M, Smith GL, eds. Recombinant poxviruses. CRC Press, Boca Raton, FL, pp. 163–206.
674. Yilma T, Hsu D, Jones L, et al. (1988) Protection of cattle against rinderpest with vaccinia virus recombinants expressing the HA or F gene. Science 242:1058–1061.
675. Yilma TD. (1989) Prospects for the total eradication of rinderpest. Vaccine 7:484–485.
676. Johnston MI. (1995) Progress in AIDS vaccine development. Int Arch Allergy Immunol 108:313–317.
677. Cooney EL, Collier AC, Greenberg PD, et al. (1991) Safety and immunological response to a recombinant vaccinia virus vaccine expressing HIV-1 glycoprotein Lancet 337:567–572.
678. Galletti R, Beauverger P, Wild TF, et al. (1995) Passively administered antibody suppresses the induction of measles virus antibodies by vaccinia-measles recombinant viruses. Vaccine 13:197–201.
679. Murphy BR, Olmsted RA, Collins PL, et al. (1988) Passive transfer of respiratory syncytial virus (RSV) antiserum suppresses the immune response to the RSV fusion (F) and large (G) glycoprotein expressed by recombinant vaccinia viruses. J Virol 62:3907–3910.
680. Fenner F. (1984) Viral vectors for vaccines. In: Bell R, Torrigiani G, eds. New approaches for development. Schwabe, Basel, pp. 187–192.
681. Buller ML, Palumbo G. (1992) Safety and attenuation of vaccinia virus. In: Binns M, Smith GL, eds. Recombinant poxviruses. CRC Press, Boca Raton, FL, pp. 235–268.

682. Tartaglia J, Cox WI, Pincus S, Paoletti E. (1994) Safety and immunogenicity of recombinants based on the genetically engineered vaccina strain, NYVAC. Dev Biol Stand 82:125–130.

683. Sutter G, Moss B. (1992) Nonreplicating vaccinia vector efficiently expresses recombinant genes. Proc Natl Acad Sci USA 89:10847–10851.

684. Taylor J, Tartaglia J, Riviere M, et al. (1994) Application of canarypox (ALVAC) vectors in human and veterinary vaccination. Dev Biol Stand 82:131–136.

685. Gonczol E, Berencsi K, Meric C, et al. (1995) Preclinical evaluation of an ALVAC (canarypox)—human cytomegalovirus glycoprotein B vaccine candidate. Vaccine 13:1080–1085.

686. Natuk RJ, Davis AR, Chanda PK, et al. (1994) Adenovirus vectored vaccines. Dev Biol Stand 82:71–78.

687. Imler J-L. (1995) Adenovirus vectors as recombinant viral vaccines. Vaccine 13:1143–1151.

688. Almond JW, Burke KI. (1990) Polio virus as a vector for the presentation of foreign antigens. Semin Virol 1:11–20.

689. Porter DC, Ansardi DC, Choi WS, Morrow DC. (1993) Encapsidation of genetically engineered polio virus minireplicons which express human immunodeficiency virus type 1 gag and pol proteins upon infection. J Virol 67:3712–3719.

690. Glorioso JC, Goins WF, Fink DJ, Deluca NA. (1994) Herpes simplex virus vectors and gene transfer to brain. Dev Biol Stand 82:79–87.

691. Coen DM. (1990) Molecular genetics of animal viruses. In: Fields BN, Knipe DN, et al, eds. Virology. Raven Press, New York, pp. 123–150.

692. Nauciel C. (1990) Role of CD4+ T cells and T-independent mechanisms in acquired resistance to *Salmonella typhimurium* infection. J Immunol 145:265–269.

693. Strugnell RA, Maskell D, Fairweather N, et al. (1990) Stable expression of foreign antigen from the chromosome of *Salmonella typhimurium* vaccine strain. Gene 88:57–63.

694. Parish CR, Wistar R, Ada GL. (1969) Cleavage of bacterial flagellin with cyanogen bromide. Antigenic properties of the protein fragments. Biochem J 113:501–506.

695. Sambrook J, Fritsh EF, Maniatis T. (1989) Site-directed mutagenesis of cloned DNA. In: Molecular cloning: a laboratory manual. Cold Spring Harbor Press, Cold Spring Harbor, NY, pp. 1–15.

696. Stocker BAD. (1990) Aromatic-dependent Salmonella as a live vaccine presenter of foreign epitopes as inserts in flagellin. Res Microbiol 141:787–796.

697. Tite JP, Gao X-M, Hughes-Jenkins CM, et al. (1990) Anti-viral immunity induced by a recombinant nucleoprotein of influenza A virus. Immunology 70:540–546.

698. Poirer TP, Kehoe MA, Beachey EH. (1988) Protective immunity provoked by oral administration of attenuated aroA *Salmonella typhimurium* expressing cloned streptococcal M protein. J Exp Med 168:25–32.

699. Sadoff JC, Ballou WR, Baron LS, et al. (1988) Oral *Salmonella typhimurium* vaccine expressing circumsporozoite protein protects against malaria. Science 240:336–338.

700. Aggarwal A, Kumar S, Jaffe R, et al. (1990) Oral *Salmonella*:malaria circumsporozoite recombinants induce specific CD8+ cytotoxic T cells. J Exp Med 172:1083–1090.

701. Flynn JL, Weiss WR, Norris KA, et al. (1990) Generation of a cytotoxic T lymphocyte response using a *Salmonella* delivery system. Mol Microbiol 4:2111–2118.

702. Schodel F, Kelly SM, Peterson D, et al. (1994) Development of recombinant Salmonellae expressing hybrid hepatitis B core particles as candidate oral vaccines. Dev Biol Stand 82:151–158.

703. Verma NK, Ziegler HK, Stocker BAD, Schoolnik GK. (1995) Induction of a cellular immune response to a defined T-cell epitope as an insert in the flagellin of a live vaccine strain of *Salmonella*. Vaccine 13:235–244.

704. Verma NK, Ziegler HK, Wilson M, et al. (1995) Delivery of class I and class II MHC-restricted T-cell epitopes of listeriolysin of *Listeria monocytogenes* by attenuated *Salmonella*. Vaccine 13:142–150.

705. Hone DM, Lewis GK, Beier M, et al. (1995) Expression of human immunodeficiency virus antigens in an attenuated *Salmonella typhi* vector vaccine. Vaccine 13:159–162.

706. Stover CK, de la Cruz VF, Fuerst TR, et al. (1991) New use of BCG for recombinant vaccines. Nature 351:456–460.

707. Aldovini A, Young RA. (1991) Humoral and cell-mediated responses to live recombinant BCG-HIV vaccines. Nature 351:479–482.

708. Stover CK, Bansal GP, Langerman S, Hanson MS. (1994) Protective immunity elicited by rBCG vaccines. Dev Biol Stand 82:163–170.

709. Yilma T, Anderson K, Brechling K, Moss B. (1987) Expression of an adjuvant gene (interferon-γ) in infectious vaccinia virus recombinants. In: Vaccines '87. Cold Spring Harbor Laboratory, Cold Spring Harbor, NY, pp. 393–396.

710. Ramshaw IA, Andrew ME, Phillips SM, et al. (1987) Recovery of immunodeficient mice from a vaccinia virus/IL-2 recombinant infection. Nature 329:545–546.

711. Flexner H, Hugin A, Moss B. (1987) Prevention of vaccinia virus infection in immunodeficient mice by vector-directed IL-2 expression. Nature 330:259–262.

712. Ruby J, Brinkman C, Jones S, Ramshaw IA. (1990) Response of monkeys to vaccination with recombinant vaccinia virus which coexpress HIV gp160 and human interleukin-2. Immunol Cell Biol 68:113–117.

713. Karupiah G, Ramsay AJ, Ramshaw IA, Blanden RV. (1992) Recombinant vaccine vector-induced protection of athymic, nude mice from influenza A virus infection. Analysis of protective mechanisms. Scand J Immunol 36:99–105.

714. Karupiah G, Coupar BEH, Andrew ME, Boyle DB, Phillips SM, Blanden RV, Ramshaw IA. Elevated natural killer cell responses in mice infected with recombinant vaccinia virus encoding IL-2. J Immunol 144:290–298.

715. Karupiah G, Blanden RV, Ramshaw IA. (1990) Interferon is involved in the recovery of athymic nude mice from recombinant vaccinia/interleukin 2 infection. J Exp Med 172:1495–1503.

716. Kohonen-Corish M, King M, Woodhams C, Ramshaw IA. (1990) Immunodeficient mice recover from infection with vaccinia virus expressing interferon-γ. Eur J Immunol 20:157–161.

717. Sambhi SK, Kohonen-Corish M, Ramshaw IA. (1991) Local production of tumour necrosis factor encoded by recombinant vaccinia virus is effective in controlling viral replication in vivo. Proc Natl Acad Sci USA 88:4025–4029.

718. Ramsay AJ, Kohonen-Corish M. (1993) Interleukin-5 expressed by a recombinant vaccinia virus enhances specific mucosal IgA reactivity in vivo. Eur J Immunol 23:3141–3145.

719. Ramsay AJ. (1995) Vector-encoded IL-5 and IL-6 enhance specific mucosal immunoglobulin IgA reactivity in vivo. Adv Exp Med Biol 371A:35–42.

720. Leong KH, Ramsay AJ, Boyle DB, Ramshaw IA. (1994) Selective induction of immune responses by cytokines co-expressed in recombinant fowlpoxvirus. J Virol 68:8125–8130.

721. Ruby J, Fordham S, Kasprzak A, et al. (1991) The immunobiology of murine interleukin-1a encoded by recombinant vaccinia virus. Cytokine 3:92–97.

722. Xing Z, Braciak T, Jordana M, Croitoru K, Graham FL, Gauldie J. (1994) Adenovirus-mediated cytokine gene transfer at tissue sites. Overexpression of IL-6 induces lymphocytic hyperplasia in the lung. J Immunol 153:4059–4069.

723. Dunstan SJ, Ramsay AJ, Strugnell RA. (1996) Expression of interleukin-6 in recombinant *Salmonella* vaccine vectors. Infect Immun 64:2730–2736.

724. Carrier MJ, Chatfield SN, Dougan G, et al. (1992) Expression of human IL-1β in *Salmonella typhimurium*. A model system for the delivery of recombinant therapeutic proteins in vivo. J Immunol 148:1176–1181.

725. Denich K, Borlin P, O'Hanley PD, et al. (1993) Expression of the murine interleukin-4 gene in an attenuated aroA strain of *Salmonella typhimurium*: Persistence and immune response in BALB/c mice and susceptibility to macrophage killing. Infect Immun 61:4818–4827.

726. Raz E, Watanabe A, Baird SM, Eisenberg RA, Parr TB, Lotz M, Kipps TJ, Carson DA. (1993) Systemic immunological effects of cytokine genes injected into skeletal muscle. Proc Natl Acad Sci USA 90:4523–4527.

727. Arnon R, Levi R. (1995) Synthetic recombinant vaccines against viral antigens. Int Arch Allergy Immunol 108:321–326.

728. Ada GL, Nossal GJV, Pye J, Abbot A. (1964) Antigens in immunity. 1. Preparation and properties of flagellar antigens from *Salmonella adelaide*. Aust J Exp Biol Med Sci 42:267–282.

729. Rowley MJ, Mackay IR. (1969) Measurement of antibody-producing capacity in man. 1. The normal response to flagellin from *Salmonella adelaide*. Clin Exp Immunol 5:407–418.

730. Garcia-Sastre A, Percy N, Barclay W, Palese P. (1994) Introduction of foreign sequences into the genome of influenza A virus. Dev Biol Stand 82:237–246.

731. Rodrigues M, Li S, Murata K, et al. (1994) Influenza and vaccinia viruses expressing malaria CD8+ T and B cell epitopes. J Immunol 153:4636–4648.

732. Kalyan NK, Lee SG, Wilhelm J, et al. (1994) Immunogenicity of recombinant influenza virus hemagglutinin carrying peptides from the envelope protein of human immunodeficiency virus type 1. Vaccine 12:753–760.

733. Val MD, Schlist HJ, Ruppert T, et al. (1991) Efficient processing of an antigenic sequence for presentation by class I MHC molecules depends on its neighboring residues in the protein. Cell 66:1145.
734. World Health Organization. (1994) Proceedings of the WHO meeting on nucleic acid vaccines. Vaccine 12:1491–1568.
735. McDonnell WM, Askari FK. (1995) Molecular medicine. DNA vaccines. N Engl J Med 334:42–45.
736. Pardoll DM, Beckering AM. (1995) Exposing the immunology of naked DNA vaccines. Immunity 3:165–169.
737. Donnelly JJ, Friedman FA, Martinez D, et al. (1995) Preclinical efficacy of a prototype NA vaccine: enhanced protection against antigenic drift in influenza virus. Nat Med 1:583–587.
738. Xiang Z, Ertl HCJ. (1995) Manipulation of the immune response to a plasmid-encoded antigen by coinoculation with plasmids expressing cytokines. Immunity 2:129–135.
739. Hilleman MR. (1995) DNA vectors. Precedents and safety. Ann NY Acad Sci 772:1–14.
740. Moffat AS. (1995) Exploring transgenic plants as a new vaccine source. Science 268:658–660.
741. Haq TA, Mason HS, Clements JD, Arntzen CJ. (1995) Oral immunization with a recombinant bacterial antigen produced in transgenic plants. Science 268:714–716.
742. Ma J K-C, Hiatt A, Hein M, et al. (1995) Generation and assembly of secretory antibodies in plants. Science 268:716–719.
743. McCafferty J, Griffiths AD, Winter G, Chiswell DJ. (1990) Phage antibodies: filamentous phage displaying antibody variable domains. Nature 348:552–554.
744. Winter G, Milstein C. (1991) Man-made antibodies. Nature 349:293–299.
745. Barbas III CF, Kang AS, Lerner RA, Benkovic SJ. (1991) Assembly of combinatorial libraries on phage surfaces: the gene III site. Proc Natl Acad Sci USA 88:7978–7982.
746. Winter G, Griffiths AD, Hawkins RE, Hoogenboom HR. (1994) Making antibodies by phage display technology. Annu Rev Immunol 12:433–455.
747. Griffiths AD. (1993) Production of human antibodies using bacteriophage. Curr Opin Immunol 5:263–267.
748. Chanock RM, Crowe JE, Murphy BR, Burton DR. (1993) Human monoclonal antibody Fab fragments cloned from combinatorial libraries: potential usefulness in prevention and/or treatment of major human viral disease. Infect Agents Dis 2:118–131.
749. Spiegelberg HL, Weigle WO. (1965) The catabolism of homologous and heterologous 7S gamma globulin fragments. J Exp Med 121:323–338.
750. Ada GL. (1944) Combination vaccines: present practices and future possibilities. Biologicals 22:329–332.
751. Conclusions of Workshop III. Vaccination policy: Second European Conference on Vaccinology. Biologicals 22:435–436.
752. Ada GL. (1995) Global aspects of vaccination. Int Arch Allergy Immunol 108:304–308.
753. Graham BS, Matthews TJ, Belshe RB, et al. (1993) Augmentation of human immunodeficiency virus type 1 neutralizing antibody by priming with gp160 recombinant vaccinia and boosting with rgp160 in vaccinia-naive adults. J Infect Dis 167:533–537.
754. Leong KH, Ramsay AJ, Morin MJ, Robinson HL, Boyle DB, Ramshaw IA. (1995) Generation of enhanced immune responses by consecutive immunization with DNA and recombinant fowlpox virus. In: Brown F, Chanock R, Ginsberg H, Norrby E, eds. Vaccines 95. Cold Spring Harbor Laboratory Press, pp. 327–331.
755. Pisetsky DS. (1993) DNA vaccination. A clue to memory. Hum Immunol 38:241–242.
756. Thomas L. (1959). In: Lawrence HS, ed. Cellular and humoral aspects of the hypersensitive state. Hoeber-Harper, New York, p. 529–532.
757. Burnet FM. (1957) Cancer—a biological approach. Br Med J 1:779–786, 841–847.
758. Frazer IH. (1996) The role of vaccines in the control of STDs—HPV vaccines. Genitourin Med (in press).
759. Burrows SR, Gardner J, Khanna A, et al. (1944) Five new cytotoxic T cell epitopes identified within Epstein-Barr virus nuclear antigen 3. J Gen Virol 75:2489–2493.
760. Schirrmacher V. (1995) Tumor vaccine design: concepts, mechanisms and efficacy testing. Int Arch Allergy Immunol 108:340–344.
761. Blanden RV, McKenzie IFC, Kees U, et al. (1977) Cytotoxic T cell response to ectromelia virus-infected cells. Different H2 requirements for triggering precursor cell induction or lysis by effector T cells defined by the BALB/c-h-2^{db} mutation. J Exp Med 146:669–680.
762. Zier K, Gansbacher B, Salvadori S. (1996) Preventing abnormalities in signal transduction of T cells in cancer: the promise of cytokine gene therapy. Immunol Today 17:39–45.

763. Thrush GR, Lark LR, Clinchy BC, Vitetta ES. (1996). Immunotoxins: an update. Annu Rev Immunol 14:49–72.
764. Renner C, Pfreundschuh M. (1995) Tumor therapy by immune recruitment with bispecific antibodies. Immunol Rev 145:179–209.
765. Mazumder A, Rosenberg AS. (1984) Successful immunotherapy of NK-resistant established pulmonary metastases by the intravenous adoptive transfer of syngeneic lymphocytes activated in vitro by interleukin-2. Science 255:1487–1489.
766. Lafreniere R, Rosenberg AS. (1985) Successful immunotherapy of murine experimental metastases with lymphokine-activated killer cells and recombinant interleukin-2. Cancer Res 45:3735–3741.
767. Kawakami Y, Eliyahu S, Jennings C, et al. (1995) Recognition of multiple epitopes in the human melanoma antigen gp100 by tumor-infiltrating T lymphocytes associated with in vivo tumor regression. J Immunol 154:3961–3968.
768. Van Pel A, Van Der Bruggen P, Coule PG, et al. (1995) Genes coding for tumor antigens by cytolytic T lymphocytes. Immunol Rev 145:229–250.
769. Ressing ME, Sette A, Brandt RMP, et al. (1995) Human CTL epitopes encoded by human papillomavirus type 16 E6 and E7 identified through in vivo and in vitro immunogenicity studies of HLA-A0201-binding peptides. J Immunol 154:5934–5943.
770. Feltcamp MCW, Vreugdenil GR, Vierboom MPM, et al. (1995) Cytotoxic T lymphocytes raised against a subdominant epitope offered as a synthetic peptide eradicate human papillomavirus type 16-induced tumors. Eur J Immunol 25:2638–2642.
771. Fin OJ, Jerome KR, Henderson RA, et al. (1995) MUC-1 epithelial tumor mucin-based immunity and cancer vaccines. Immunol Rev 145:61–90.
772. Domenech N, Henderson RA, Fin OJ. (1995) Identification of an HLA-A11-restricted epitope from the tandem repeat domain of the epithelial tumor antigen mucin. J Immunol 155:4766–4774.
773. Apostolopoulos V, Loveland BE, Petersz GA, McKenzie IFC. (1995) CTL in mice immunized with human mucin 1 are MHC-restricted. J Immunol 155:5089–5094.
774. Visseren MJW, van Elsas A, van der Voort EIH, et al. (1995) CTL specific for the tyrosinase autoantigen can be induced from healthy donor blood to lyse melanoma cells. J Immunol 154:3991–3998.
775. Hellstrom KE, Hellstrom I, Chen L. (1995) Can co-stimulated tumor immunity be therapeutically efficacious? Immunol Rev 145:123–146.
776. Gilbert KM, Weigle WO. (1994) Tolerogenicity of resting and activated B cells. J Exp Med 179:249–258.
777. Chen L, Ashe S, Brady WA, et al. (1992) Costimulation of anti-tumor immunity by the B7 counter receptor for the T lymphocyte molecules, CD28 and CTLA-4. Cell 71:1093–1102.
778. Gresser I. (1989) Anti-tumor effects of interferon. Acta Oncol 28:347.
779. Ferrantini M, Proietti E, Santodonato L, et al. (1993) Interferon αl transfer into metastatic Friend leukemia cells abrogated tumorigenicity in immunocompetent mice: anti-tumor therapy by means of interferon producing cells. Cancer Res 53:1107–1116.
780. Dranoff G, Jaffee E, Lazenby A, et al. (1993) Vaccination with irradiated tumor cells, engineered to secrete murine GMCSF, stimulates potent specific and long-lasting anti-tumor immunity. Proc Natl Acad Sci USA 90:3539–3543.
781. Mayordomo JI, Zorina T, Storkus WJ, et al. (1995) Bone marrow-derived dendritic cells pulsed with synthetic tumor peptides elicit protective and therapeutic antitumor immunity. Nat Med 1:1297–1302.
782. Bakker ABH, Marland G, de Boor AJ, et al. (1995) Generation of anti-melanoma cytotoxic T lymphocytes from healthy donors after presentation of melanoma-associated antigen-derived epitopes by dendritic cells in vitro. Cancer Res 55:5330–5334.
783. Mandelboim O, Vadai E, Fridkin M, et al. (1995) Regression of established murine carcinoma metastases following vaccination with tumor associated antigen peptides. Nat Med 1:1179–1183.
784. Apostolopoulos V, Pietersz GA, Loveland B, et al. (1995) Oxidative/reductive conjugation of mannan to antigen selects for T1 or T2 immune responses. Proc Natl Acad Sci USA 92:10128–10132.
785. Zhai H, Yang JC, Kawakami Y, et al. (1996) Antigen-specific tumor vaccines. Development and characterization of recombinant adenoviruses encoding MART1 or gp100 for cancer therapy. J Immunol 156:700–710.
786. Sun WH, Burkholder JK, Sun J, et al. (1995) In vivo cytokine gene transfer by gene gun reduces tumor growth in mice. Proc Natl Acad Sci USA 92:2889–2893.

787. Lehmann F, Marchand M, Hainaut P, et al. (1995) Differences in the antigens recognized by cytolytic T cells on two successive metastases of a melanoma patient are consistent with immune selection. Eur J Immunol 25:340–347.

788. Strominger J. (1995) Peptide vaccination against cancer? Nat Med 1:1140.

789. Boon T. (1995) Tumor antigens and perspectives for cancer immunotherapy. Immunologist 3:262–263.

790. Mor F, Cohen IR. (1995) Vaccines to prevent and treat autoimmune diseases. Int Arch Allergy Immunol 108:345–349.

791. Janeway CA Jr, Travers P. (1994) Immunobiology. Current Biology, London, pp. 9–11.

792. Ada GL. (1994) Immune response. In: Webster RG, Granoff A, eds. Encyclopedia of virology, vol 2. Academic Press, New York, pp. 696–703.

793. Gala S, Fulcher DA. (1996) Managing HIV. 3.4. How HIV leads to autoimmune disorders. Med J Aust 164:224–226.

794. Feinberg M. (1995) Host virus relationships in pathogenic and nonpathogenic HIV and SIV infections. Seventh Annual Conference, Australasian Society for HIV Medicine (Abstract), p. 195.

795. Holoshitz J, Naparstek Y, Ben-nun A, Cohen IR. (1983) Lines of T cells induce or vaccinate against autoimmune arthritis. Science 219:56–58.

796. Maron R, Zerubavel R, Friedman A, Cohen IR. (1983) T lymphocyte lines specific for thyroglobulin produce or vaccinate against autoimmune thyroiditis in mice. J Immunol 131:2316–2322.

797. Linington C, Izumo S, Suzuki M, et al. (1984) A permanent rat T cell line that mediates experimental allergic neuritis in the Lewis rat in vivo. J Immunol 1984:1946–1950.

798. Caspi RR, Roberge FG, McAllister CG, et al. (1986) T cell lines mediating experimental autoimmune uveoretinitis (EAU) in the rat. J Immunol 136:928–933.

799. Kakimoto K, Katsuki M, Hirofuji T, et al. (1988) Isolation of T cell line capable of protecting mice against collagen-induced arthritis. J Immunol 140:78–83.

800. Eliass D, Markvits D, Reshef T, et al. (1990) Induction and therapy of autoimmune diabetes in the non-obese diabetic (NOD/Lt) mouse by a 65 kd heat shock protein. Proc Natl Acad Sci USA 87:1576–1580.

801. Fricke H, Mendlovic S, Blanc M, et al. (1991) Idiotype-specific T-cell lines inducing experimental systemic lupus erythematosus in mice. J Immunol 73:421–427.

802. Cohen IR, Weiner HL. (1988) T-cell vaccination. Immunol Today 9:332–335.

803. Liblau RS, Singer SM, McDevitt HO. (1995) Th1 and Th2 CD4+ T cells in the pathogenesis of organ specific autoimmune diseases. Immunol Today 16:34–38.

804. Renno T, Krakowski M, Piccirillo C, et al. (1995) TNF alpha expression by resident microglia and infiltrating leukocytes in the central nervous system of mice with experimental allergic encephalomyelitis. Regulation by Th1 cytokines. J Immunol 154:944–953.

805. Katz JD, Benoist C, Mathis D. (1995) T helper cell subsets in insulin-dependent diabetes. Science 268:1185–1188.

806. Vandenbark AA, Hashim G, Offner H. (1989) Immunization with a synthetic T cell receptor V-region peptide protects against experimental autoimmune encephalomyelitis. Nature 341:541–544.

807. Howell MD, Winters ST, Olee T, et al. (1989) Vaccination against experimental allergic encephalomyelitis with T cell receptor peptides. Science 246:668–670.

808. Weiner HL, Friedman A, Miller A, et al. (1994) Oral tolerance: immunological mechanisms and treatment of animal and human organ-specific autoimmune diseases by oral administration of autoantigens. Annu Rev Immunol 12:809–837.

809. Friedman A, Weiner HL. (1994) Induction of anergy or active suppression following oral tolerance is determined by antigen dosage. Proc Natl Acad Sci USA 91:6688–6692.

810. Miller A, Zhang ZJ, Sobel RA, et al. (1993) Suppression of experimental autoimmune encephalomyelitis by oral administration of myelin basic protein. VI. Suppression of adoptively transferred disease and differential effects of oral versus intravenous tolerization. J Neuroimmunol 46:73–82.

811. Clayton JP, Gammon GM, Ando DG, et al. (1989) Peptide-specific prevention of experimental allergic encephalomyelitis. Neonatal tolerance induced to the dominant T cell determinant of myelin basic protein. J Exp Med 169:1681–1691.

812. Wraith DC. (1995) Induction of antigen-specific unresponsiveness with synthetic peptides: specific immunotherapy for treatment of allergic and autoimmune conditions. Int Arch Allergy Immunol 108:355–359.

813. Dresser DW. (1962) Specific inhibition of antibody production. Protein overloading paralysis. Immunology 5:161–168.

814. Weigle WO. (1973) Immunological unresponsiveness. Adv Immunol 17:61–122.
815. Scherer MT, Chan BMC, Ria F, et al. (1989) Control of cellular and humoral immune responses by peptide containing T cell epitopes. Cold Spring Harb Symp Quant Biol 54:497–504.
816. Gammon G, Sercarz E. (1989) How some T cells escape tolerance. Nature 342:183–185.
817. Zamvil SS, Mitchell DJ, Moore AC, et al. (1986) T cell epitope of the autoantigen myelin basic protein that induces encephalomyelitis. Nature 24:268.
818. Zamvil S, Nelson P, Trotter J, et al. (1985) T-cell clones specific for myelin basic protein induce chronic relapsing paralysis and demyelination. Nature 317:355–358.
819. Wraith DC, Smilek DE, Mitchell DJ, et al. (1989) Antigen recognition in autoimmune encephalomyelitis and the potential for peptide-mediated immunotherapy. Cell 59:247–255.
820. Gautam AM, Pearson DJ, Smilek DE, et al. (1992) A polyalanine peptide with only five native myelin basic protein residues induces autoimmune encephalomyelitis. J Exp Med 176:605–609.
821. Wraith DC, Bruun B, Fairchild PJ. (1992) Cross-reactive antigen recognition by an encephalitogenic T cell receptor. J Immunol 149:3765.
822. Mason K, Denny DW Jr, McConnell HM. (1995) Myelin basic peptide complexes with class II MHC molecules I-A^u and I-A^k form and dissociate rapidly at neutral pH. J Immunol 154:5216–5227.
823. Fairchild PJ, Wildgoose R, Atherton E, et al. (1993) An autoantigenic T cell epitope forms unstable complexes with class II MHC: a novel route for escape from tolerance induction. Int Immunol 5:1151–1158.
824. Fairchild PJ, Wraith DC. (1992) Peptide-MHC interaction in autoimmunity. Curr Opin Immunol 4:748–753.
825. Liu GY, Fairchild PJ, Smith RM, et al. (1995) Low avidity recognition of self antigen by T cells permits escape from central tolerance. Immunity 3:407–415.
826. Liu GW, Wraith DC. (1995) Affinity for class II MHC determines the extent to which soluble peptide tolerize autoreactive T cells in naive and primed adult mice—implications for autoimmunity. Int Immunol 7:1255–1263.
827. Brocke S, Gijbels K, Allegrretta M, et al. (1996) Treatment of experimental encephalomyelitis with a peptide analogue of myelin basic protein. Nature 379:343–346.
828. Samson MF, Smilek DE. (1996) Reversal of acute experimental autoimmune encephalomyelitis and prevention of relapses by treatment with myelin basic protein analogue modified to form long-lived peptide-MHC complexes. J Immunol 155:2737–2746.
829. Kearney ER, Pape KA, Loh DY, Jenkins MK. (1994) Visualization of peptide-specific T cell immunity and peripheral tolerance induction in vivo. Immunity 1:327–339.
830. Wiener HL, Mackin GA, Matsui M, et al. (1993) Double blind pilot trial of oral immunization with myelin antigens in multiple sclerosis. Science 259:1321–1324.
831. Dirnhofer S, Berger P. (1995) Vaccination for birth control. Int Arch Allergy Immunol 108:350–354.
832. Talwar GP, Raghupathy R, eds. (1995) Birth control vaccines. Medical intelligence unit. RG Landes, Austin, TX.
833. Hill JA. (1991) Implications of cytokines in male and female sterility. In: Chaouat G, Mowbray J, eds. Cellular and molecular biology of the materno-fetal relationship. John Libbey Eurotext, pp. 123–129.
834. Best CL, Hill J. (1995) Natural infertility due to immunological factors. In: Talwar GP, Raghupathy R, eds. Birth control vaccines. Medical intelligence unit. RG Landes, Austin, TX, pp. 5–28.
835. Talwar GP, Sharma NC, Dubey SK, et al. (1976) Isoimmunization against human chorionic gonadotropin with conjugates of processed β-subunit of the hormone and tetanus toxoid. Proc Natl Acad Sci USA 73:218–222.
836. Dirnhofer S, Wick G, Berger P. (1994) The suitability of human chorionic gonadotropin (hCG) based birth-control vaccines. Immunol Today 15:469–474.
837. Deshmukh US, Talwar GP. (1995) The hCG birth control vaccine. In: Talwar GP, Raghupathy R, eds. Birth control vaccines. Medical intelligence unit. RG Landes, Austin, TX, pp. 75–88.
838. Rose NR, Lynne Burek C, Smith JP. (1988) Safety evaluation of HCG vaccine in primates: autoantibody production. In: Talwar GP, ed. Contraception research for today and the nineties. Springer, New York, pp. 231–239.
839. Moudgal NR, Suresh R. (1995) Follicle stimulating hormone (FSH) and FSH-derived vaccines. In: Talwar GP, Raghupathy R, eds. Birth control vaccines. Medical intelligence unit. RG Landes, Austin, TX, pp. 89–102.
840. Silverman AJ, Crey LC, Zimmerman EA. (1979) A comparative study of the luteinizing hormone releasing hormone (LHRH) neuronal networks in mammals. Biol Reprod 29:98–110.

841. Pal R, Talwar GW. (1995) The LHRH vaccine. In: Talwar GP, Raghupathy R, eds. Birth control vaccines. Medical intelligence unit. RG Landes, Austin, TX, pp. 63–74.
842. Khodr G, Siler-Khodr TM. (1978) The effect of luteinizing releasing factor on human chorionic gonadotropin secretion. Fertil Steril 30:301–304.
843. Tsong Y, Shaposhnik Z, Thau R. (1993) Mechanisms of action and safety of BhCG-tetanus toxoid vaccine. (Abstract) 75th Annual Meeting of the Endocrinology Society, Las Vegas, p. 282.
844. Talwar GP, Singh O, Pal R, et al. (1994) A vaccine that prevents pregnancy in women. Proc Natl Acad Sci USA 91:8532–8536.
845. Jones WR, Judd SJ, Ing RMY, et al. (1988) Phase I clinical trial of a World Health Organization birth control vaccine. Lancet 1:1295–1298.
846. Dirnhofer S, Klieber R, de Leeuw R. (1993) Functional and immunological relevance of the COOH-terminal extension of human chorionic gonadotropin β: Implications for the WHO birth control vaccine. FASEB J 7:1381–1385.
847. Naz RK. (1995) Sperm antigen-based birth control vaccines. In: Talwar GP, Raghupathy R, eds. Birth control vaccines. Medical intelligence unit. RG Landes, Austin, TX, pp. 29–40.
848. Goldberg E. (1986) Sperm specific lactate dehydrogenase and development of a contraceptive vaccine. In: Clark DA, Croy BA, eds. Reproductive immunology. Elsevier Press, New York, pp. 137–142.
849. Primakoff P, Lanthrop W, Woolman L, et al. (1988) Fully effective contraception in male and female guinea pigs immunized with the sperm protein PH-20. Nature 335:543–546.
850. Lin Y, Kimmel LH, Myles DG, et al. (1993) Molecular cloning of the human and monkey sperm surface protein PH-20. Proc Natl Acad Sci USA 90:10071–10075.
851. Herr JC, Flickinger CJ, Homyk M, et al. (1990) Biochemical and morphological characterization of intra-acrosomal antigen SP-10 from human sperm. Biol Reprod 42:181–189.
852. Liu MS, Abersold R, Fann CH, et al. (1992) Molecular and developmental studies of a sperm acrosome antigen recognised by HS-63 monoclonal antibody. Biol Reprod 46:937–948.
853. O'Rand MG, Porter JP. (1982) Purification of rabbit sperm autoantigens by preparative SDS gel electrophoresis: amino acid and carbohydrate content of RSA-1. Biol Reprod 27:713–721.
854. Naz RK, Alexander NJ, Isahakia M, et al. (1984) Monoclonal antibody to a human sperm membrane glycoprotein that inhibits fertilization. Science 225:342–344.
855. Hall J, Engel D, Naz RK. (1994) Significance of antibodies against FA-1 human sperm antigen in immune infertility. Arch Androl 32:25–30.
856. Naz RK, Morte C, Garcia-Framis V, et al. (1993) Characterisation of a sperm-specific monoclonal antibody and isolation of 95-kilodalton fertilization antigen-2 from human sperm. Biol Reprod 49:1236–1244.
857. Naz RK. (1992) Effects of antisperm antibodies on early cleavage of fertilized ova. Biol Reprod 46:130–139.
858. Mahi-Brown CA, Tung KSK. (1995) Vaccines against egg antigens and pathogenesis of ovarian autoimmune disease. In: Talwar GP, Raghupathy R, eds. Birth control vaccines. Medical intelligence unit. RG Landes, Austin, TX, pp. 41–61.
859. Wassarman PM. (1988) Zona pellucida glycoproteins. Annu Rev Biochem 57:415–442.
860. O'Hern PA, Bambra CS, Isahakia M, Goldberg E. (1995) Reversible contraception in female baboons immunized with a synthetic epitope of sperm-specific lactate dehydrogenase. Biol Reprod 52:331–339.
861. Miller SE, Chamow SM, Baur AW, et al. (1989) Vaccination with a synthetic zona pellucida peptide produces long-term contraception in female mice. Science 246:935–938.
862. Rhim SH, Millar SE, Robey F, et al. (1992) Autoimmune disease of the ovary induced by a ZP3 peptide from the mouse zona pellucida. J Clin Invest 89:28–35.
863. Quayle AJ, Anderson DJ. (1995) Induction of mucosal immunity in the genital tract and prospects for oral vaccines. In: Talwar GP, Raghupathy R, eds. Birth control vaccines. Medical intelligence unit. RG Landes, Austin, TX, pp. 149–165.
864. Ogra PL, Yamanaka T, Losonsky GA. (1981) Local immunologic defenses in the genital tract. Prog Clin Biol Res 70:381–394.
865. Kutteh WH, Mestecky J. (1994) Secretory immunity in the female reproductive tract. Am J Reprod Immunol 31:40–46.
866. Edwards JNT, Morris HB. (1985) Langerhans' cells and lymphoid subsets in the female genital tract. Br J Obstet Gynaecol 92:947–982.
867. Haneberg B, Kendall D, Amerongen HM, et al. (1995) Induction of specific IgA in small intestine, colon-rectum, and vagina measured with a new method for collection of secretions from local mucosal surfaces. Infect Immun 62:15–23.

868. Lehner T, Bergmeier LA, Panagiotidi C, et al. (1992) Induction of mucosal and systemic immunity to a recombinant simian immunodeficiency viral protein. Science 258:1365–1369.
869. Lehner T, Brookes R, Panagiotidi C, et al. (1993) T- and B-cell functions and epitope expression in non-human primates immunized with simian immunodeficiency virus antigen by the rectal route. Proc Natl Acad Sci USA 90:8638–8642.
870. World Health Organization. (1992) Fertility regulating vaccines. Report of a meeting between women's health advocates and scientists to review the current status of the development of fertility regulating vaccines. WHO/HRP/WHO/93.1 World Health Organization, Geneva, pp. 7–8.
871. Concepcion M, Mundigo A, Reeler AV. (1992) Social aspects related to the introduction of a birth control vaccine. In: Ada GL, Griffin PD, eds. Vaccination for fertility regulation. Cambridge University Press, Cambridge, pp. 233–247.
872. Holden C. (1992) Birth control for animals. Science 256:1390.
873. Tyndale-Biscoe CH. (1994) Virus-vectored immunocontraception of feral mammals. Reprod Fertil Dev 6:281–287.
874. Cooperative Research Centre for Biological Control of Vertebrate Pest Populations. (1995) Annual report. Commonwealth Scientific and Industrial Research Organization. Canberra, Australia.
875. Fenner F, Ratcliffe FN. (1965) Myxomatosis. Cambridge University Press, Cambridge, UK, p. 379.

Index

Numbers followed by an *f* indicate a figure; *t* following a page number indicates tabular material.

DNA vaccination, against protein
    antigens, 165–167, 171
DNA viruses, antigenic variation of,
    108–109
Domain replacement technology, 35
DTH. *See* Delayed-type hypersensitivity
    (DTH)
DTP. *See* Diphtheria-tetanus-pertussis
    (DTP) vaccine

E
EAE, 182, 184
EBV, 105, 175
Edmonston-Zagreb strain, 29
Edna McConnell Clark Foundation,
    38
Efficacy
    assessment of products, 11
    of vaccines, 30–34
Ehrlich, Paul, 6, 8
Emerging infectious diseases, 42,
    43t
Endogenous antigen pathway, 60
Eosinophils, 49, 95
EPI. *See* Expanded Programme of
    Immunization (WHO/EPI)
Epithelial immunity, 76–77
Epitopes, 55, 56f
Epitopes and determinants, 115
Epstein-Barr virus (EBV), 105, 175
"Escape from tolerance" concept,
    185
Escape mechanisms, 113–114
Exogenous antigen pathway, 59
Expanded Programme of Immunization
    (WHO/EPI)
    formation of, 9–10
    and global immunization, 39
    immunization programs of, 36–37
    infant immunization schedule, 37t
Experimental autoimmune
    encephalomyelitis (EAE), 182,
    184
Experimental chronic-relapsing
    autoimmune conditions, 186
Extracellular infectious agents, immune
    responses to, 96t

F
FCA, 123, 126
FDCs, 57, 71–73
Female reproductive tract, 197–198
Fertility control. *See* Animal fertility
    control; Human fertility control
Fetus, immune system of, 85–86
Fever, 47–48
FIA, 123, 126
Follicle-stimulating hormone (FSH),
    190–191
Follicular dendritic cells (FDCs), 57,
    71–73
Foxes, rabies vaccine for, 154
Freund's complete adjuvant (FCA), 123,
    126
Freund's incomplete adjuvant, 123, 126
FSH, 190–191

G
GALT, 79–80
Gene coding, isolation of, 145
Gene guns, 165
Genetic reassortment, 107
Genetic vaccination, 164–167
Global Programme on Vaccines and
    Immunization, 39, 171
Global Program on AIDS, 38
GM-CSF, 166, 179–180
GnRH, 190–191
Gonadotropin-releasing hormone (GnRH),
    190–191
Granulocyte-macrophage colony-
    stimulating factor (GM-CSF),
    166, 179–180
Gut-associated lymphoid tissues (GALT),
    79–80

H
Haemophilus influenzae type B infections,
    33f
Haptens, 6
HCG, 189–193
Heat shock proteins (HSPs), 134
Helper T cells, response to infections, 90
Hepatitis A vaccines, 19, 21